An Introduction to Neonatal Nursing Care

An Introduction to Neonatal Nursing Care

Second Edition

Edited by

Doreen Crawford PGCE, BSc (Hons)
SRN, RSCN, ENBs 405, 870, 998
Senior Lecturer

and

Wendy Hickson BA (Hons)
RSCN, RGN, ENBs 405, 998
Senior Clinical Nurse

T

First published in 1994 by:
Chapman & Hall

Reprinted in 2000 by:
Stanley Thornes Publishers Ltd

Second edition published in 2002 by:
Nelson Thornes Ltd
Delta Place
27 Bath Road
CHELTENHAM
GL53 7TH
United Kingdom

02 03 04 05 06 / 10 9 8 7 6 5 4 3 2 1

A catalogue record for this book is available from the British Library

ISBN 0 7487 6469 0

Illustrations by Margaret Sparshott
Page make-up by Acorn Bookwork

Printed and bound in Spain by GraphyCems

H|th Sci
RJ
253
.I57
2002

CONTENTS

LIST OF CONTRIBUTORS   vii
PREFACE   x
ACKNOWLEDGEMENTS   xi

PART ONE: *NEONATAL NURSING CARE*

1   NEONATAL CARE TODAY   *Kerry Bloodworth and*
    Doreen Crawford   3

2   ETHICAL ISSUES IN NEONATAL NURSING   *Kevin J. Power*   13

3   RIGHTS, WELFARE AND PROTECTION IN NEONATAL
    PRACTICE   *Fay Valentine*   31

4   PLAY FOR THE NEONATAL INFANT   *Tina Clegg*   58

PART TWO: *CLINICAL CONDITIONS*

5   RESUSCITATION AND PROBLEMS OF INFANTS BORN TOO
    SMALL OR TOO SOON   *Bernadette Byme and Wendy Hickson*   71

6   NURSING CARE OF AN INFANT WITH JAUNDICE
    Doreen Crawford   104

7   NURSING CARE OF AN INFANT WITH A DISORDER OF
    THE RESPIRATORY SYSTEM   *Doreen Crawford and Jill Fairhurst*   117

8   NURSING CARE OF AN INFANT WITH A GASTRO-INTESTINAL
    CONDITION   *Wendy Hickson*   148

9   NURSING CARE OF AN INFANT WITH A DISORDER OF THE
    CARDIOVASCULAR SYSTEM   *Doreen Crawford and Jill Fairhurst*   171

10 CARE OF INFANTS WITH RENAL DISORDERS   *Eileen Brennan*   204

11 NURSING CARE OF AN INFANT WITH A NEUROLOGICAL
    DISORDER   *Doreen Crawford*   226

Part Three: *Treatment and Care Strategies*

12   Nursing care of the infant in pain and discomfort
  Margaret Sparshott   245

13   Transport of infants   *Alison Gibbs and Andrew Leslie*   266

14   Neonatal infection   *Ann and Daniel Dooley*   285

15   Neonatal nutrition   *Sarah Illingworth*   300

16   Neonatal pharmacology   *Helen Chadwick*   314

17   Home discharge   *Doreen Crawford and Liz Sampson*   329

Appendix i: Using the edinburgh post-natal
             depression scale   346
Appendix ii: Methods of assessment of gestational age   348
Appendix iii: Normal values   352
Appendix iv: Abbreviations and glossary of key terms   353
Index   357

LIST OF CONTRIBUTORS

Kerry Bloodworth, MA, RGN, RSCN, ENBS 405, 904, Cert Ed
Kerry is currently Regional Leadership Facilitator in Nottingham. She has extensive experience of neonatal intensive care and in the past has been involved in implementing re-engineering and the Shared Governance initiative. Kerry's main interests include keeping her neonatal clinical skills up to date and aspects of teambuilding.

Eileen Brennan, RGN
Eileen is Senior Sister from the renal ward at Great Ormond Street Hospital, which remains one of the world leaders in the care of infants in renal failure.

Bernadette Byrne, PGCE, RGN, ENBs 998, 405
Senior Nurse Educator on the NNU at the Liverpool Royal Infirmary, one of the busiest NNUs in the country, Bernadette has responsibility for staff training and development needs in the ITU/HDU areas. She is well known in the Neonatal Nurses Association and has made frequent contributions to the neonatal literature.

Helen Chadwick, BSc (Hons), Dip. Clin. Pharm., Cert. Pharm. Practice
Helen is an experienced clinical pharmacist, who has presented at several symposia and conferences on pharmaceutical topics. Helen has a special interest in teaching. In the past, she has been responsible for the teaching of doctors and nurses and the training of junior pharmacists.

Tina Clegg, PGCE (Post Compulsory Education), HPS, NNEB, DPQS
Tina teaches on the hospital play specialist course and is a play coordinator on the children's units of the University Hospitals of Leicester. Tina has contributed to a number of symposia on play and the neonate and is well known in the field of nursery nursing.

Doreen Crawford, PGCE BSc (Hons), RSCN, SRN, ENBs 405, 870, 998
Doreen was editor of the text *Neonatal Nursing*, from which this book is derived. She is a senior lecturer at De Montfort University, where she is responsible for the High Dependency modules. Her research interests have included teaching resuscitation skills to parents and SIDs. Doreen holds informal contracts with the Leicester General Hospital NNU and the Children's Hospital to retain clinical skills and hopes to embark on doctorial studies in the near future. She has published many works in a variety of journals.

Ann Dooley, RGN, RSCN, ENB 405
Ann is a practising nurse on the NNU and Children's Hospital in Leicester University Hospitals NHS Trust.

Dan Dooley, MSc, PGCE, BSc (Hons)
Dan has a Masters degree in microbiology. He has been a biomedical scientist for the past 11 years and is now teaching.

Jill Fairhurst, BA (Hons), SRN, RM, ENBs A19, 405, 870, 997
Jill has a unique role in the University Hospitals of Leicester NHS Trust. She uses her skills as an Advanced Neonatal Nurse Practitioner to support the nursing and medical staff in the clinical area and is involved in teaching the ENB 405 at De Montfort University. Her research interests include the use of saturation monitoring and aspects of ventilation. Jill is reviewing the extended role in the NICU.

Alison Gibbs, RGN, ENB A19
Alison is an Advanced Neonatal Nurse Practitioner and coordinator of the Nottingham Neonatal Transport Service.

Wendy Hickson, BA (Hons), RSCN, RGN, ENBs 405, 998
Wendy is a part-time postgraduate lecturer at De Montfort University with responsibility for the ENB 405 course and is a Senior Nurse on the NNU at Leicester General Hospital. Her research interests include family-centred care, particularly focusing on the role of the father in the NICU.

Sarah Illingworth, BSc (Hons), State Registered Dietician
Sarah is Senior Children's Dietician for the University Hospitals of Leicester with a specialist interest in nutrition of the newborn infant and oncology.

Andrew Leslie, RGN, ENB A19
Andrew is an Advanced Neonatal Nurse Practitioner and has specialised in the field of transport. He has lectured and written extensively on his specialty.

Kevin J. Power, MA, BA, RGN, RSCN
As a Senior Lecturer at De Montfort University, Kevin's Masters degree is in Ethics and he is well known in the children's nursing field. He chairs the University ethics committee and reviews and writes for *Paediatric Nurse*.

Liz Sampson, RGN, RM ENBs 405, 998
Liz is currently a member of the Neonatal Outreach Team within the University Hospitals of Leicester. Her role includes clinical work within the NICU. Liz is Chairman of the Shared Governance Committee and her research interests include infant massage and breast-feeding the pre-term infant.

Margaret Sparshott, SRN
A recognised authority on neonatal pain, Margaret has advised government bodies on the extent of foetal and neonatal pain in an effort to guide current policy. Margaret is well known and respected in the field of neonatal nursing

and has produced a number of publications. Much of the chapter is derived from the author's own original research.

Fay Valentine, PGCE, RSCN, RGN
Senior Lecturer at De Montfort University, Fay was until recently the Senior Nurse responsible for Birmingham City Children's Services. She contributes to the RCN Child Protection Policy Board. She is well known in the children's nursing field and is frequently published in her specialties.

Preface

The first edition of this book was the UK's first neonatal nursing text. Like that book, the second edition is also written mainly by experienced neonatal nurses, with some chapters, such as those on play, microbiology and pharmacy, having been written by the appropriate specialists. This edition is intended primarily as an introduction for nurses who look after sick infants. It is not intended to be an exhaustive reference of all that can go wrong with an infant but to address some of the current issues and concepts of neonatal care today.

Terms

The term 'infant' has been used in this book to refer to both male and female infants. Equally, the terms 'nurse' and 'doctor' are intended to refer to both male and female practitioners. The term 'neonatal nurse' applies to any person who is professionally involved in the nursing care of a sick infant; that is to say, both male and female nurses, midwives or students.

The changing face of neonatology

As long ago as 1907, Pierre Budin, one of the founders of the art and science that we now call neonatology, wrote that 'the lives of the little ones have been saved but at the cost of the mother'. Today, nurses and doctors are partners, with the parents, in the care of the sick infant, but Budin's words remain as important now as they were then.

Neonatology keeps a relatively low profile these days. In the past, tiny and premature individuals were exhibited to the curious at fairs. Fortunately, much has changed over the years. It is not that society's fascination for the small does not still exist; it is not because we are reticent to show off the hi-tech environment in which we work – indeed, the neonatal unit is a tribute to modern technology; it is not because these infants are so vulnerable that a passing stranger is a fearsome infection risk. The reason for our low profile is because these infants, like any other sick human being, are entitled to privacy, peace and dignity in which either to recover or to die.

Doreen Crawford

ACKNOWLEDGEMENTS

The editors wish to express thanks and gratitude to family and friends who tolerated the stress and strain of the writing of this book and never gave up hope that it would be published. Thanks also to Neil Stevens and Dennis Crawford for their computer skills; to our colleagues and contributors; and especially to the infants and families with whom we have worked and who have taught us so much. Last but not least, thanks are due to our commissioning editor, Helen Broadfield, who has the natural ability to apply the big stick with such tact and grace that we never knew we were being chased.

In respect of Chapter 8, the editors would like to acknowledge the work of Maryke Morris, who was responsible for the original chapter in the first edition.

Doreen Crawford would like to thank Marie-Claire Turrell for the inspiration for and the draft of the original Chapter 9 in 1994, and her nursing colleagues at Glenfield General Hospital (part of the University Hospitals of Leicester) for their help and support. They are pushing back the frontiers of children's cardiac care on a daily basis.

In writing Chapter 16, Wendy and Doreen would like to acknowledge the work of Ian Costello, who was responsible for the original chapter in the first edition.

The Edinburgh Post-natal Depression Scale in Appendix 1 (page 346) is reproduced by kind permission of the Royal College of Psychiatrists and the method of assessing gestational age in Appendix 2 (page 348) by kind permission of Dubowitz, Dubowitz and Goldberg (1970).

In addition, the editors would like to thank the following for permission to use material in this book: The Controller of Her Majesty's Stationery Office for Table 3.3 on page 44 and Figure 3.1 on page 49; Nottingham Neonatal Service for Figure 13.1 on page 268, Figure 13.3 on page 279 and Figure 13.4 on page 280; and The Royal College of Paediatrics and Child Health for Table 3.1 on page 39.

PART ONE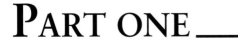

NEONATAL NURSING CARE

1 NEONATAL CARE TODAY

Kerry Bloodworth and Doreen Crawford

Aims of the chapter

This chapter considers some of the issues and challenges that present when organising the structure of care for neonates today. It provides a historical context of care, examines some of the changes that face neonatal nurses and suggests some fairly radical managerial perspectives that may enhance the provision of care.

INTRODUCTION

In the UK, the National Health Service is theoretically available to all, irrespective of economic status or social class. In fact, equal opportunity and equal quality of care are not equally available to all. The intense pressure on cots and poor staffing levels often result in no cots being available, and in cot closure. This can mean that infants have to be transferred many miles to the nearest available cot, with detrimental effects on the infant itself and on its family. Sadly, twin and higher-order births may be split between units. The geographic availability of specific therapy, such as nitric oscillation or extra corporeal membrane oxygenation (ECMO), makes the type of care an infant may receive a variable. National standards are yet to be set. The UK is a multicultural society and the way in which parents can relate to and communicate with staff will also have an impact on the overall quality of their care experience.

All organisations face difficulties when attempting to balance the various demands and expectations of society against the limits of staffing and budgeting. In neonatal care, a number of ethical and emotive issues further complicate the management of care. The highly technical neonatal speciality of today has evolved from the dual disciplines of medicine and nursing – specifically, the branches of midwifery and sick children's nursing (although the 'generic' nurse with general training has often also contributed to the staffing of the units). This care is not provided in isolation; neonatal nurses and doctors owe a significant amount to those who provide their support services. Quite simply, they could not function without the support of an extended team of porters, domestics, and laboratory, radiology and dietetic staff, as well as those who develop and maintain the equipment, although these people often remain in the background.

The neonatal unit (NNU) is a small part of a greater NHS, which operates as a vast public-sector organisation within a huge political and public context. This makes the functioning and management of the NNU, if not different, then much more complex than that of a department in a private-sector organisation. NNU nurse leaders need to combine skills of management, technical ability and professionalism with their greater responsibility towards the general public.

The method of financing to date means that NNU managers have had to compete for resources with different elements within the NHS system. This may change to a more devolved pattern of funding, which may put the front-line professionals more in charge; this would be a radical and largely welcome innovation.

INFLUENCES ON CARE

From a purely organisational perspective, public-sector organisations can appear very similar, if not identical, to private-sector organisations. However, their history makes them unique. Public-sector organisations have largely been sheltered from competition and even comparison mainly because of their monopoly position.

The NHS became very bureaucratic and this tendency towards bureaucratisation is still with the service today, reinforced by specific administrative rules and regulations. There have been repeated attempts to resolve this, and in the 1990s there was radical restructuring and the formation of an internal market. Trusts were established and a division between purchasers and providers was created. Key services were put out to tender. The existence of more than one hospital Trust in one city, offering the same or similar services, was considered to be good for patients; in the competitive market, the successful and more effective Trusts would succeed and the less successful would succumb to market forces.

The changes of the 1990s were unsettling for clinical staff and failed to resolve the load of bureaucracy; in some cases, they added to it. The facelessness of the bureaucracy has meant that there is a tendency for no one to accept responsibility. Today there is an increasing trend in cities with several units providing neonatal care for the units to merge, or at least to co-operate and streamline their services. It is important to reverse those competitive attitudes fostered by the previous reorganisation. There is some evidence that managers will have a difficult time in dealing with the uncertainties and fears of staff in response to further change (Maguire, 1998).

Methods of financing health care vary considerably but in all developed countries there is a mix between state funding, insurance and direct payments. A major concern of all governments, whatever their method of financing health care, is the control of costs. In the UK, the NHS Review leading to the publication of *Working for Patients* (DoH, 1989) studied the various systems for financing health care. It concluded that the present method, largely dependent on taxation, was probably better than any alternative. The UK system is apparently simpler than others and this is reflected in lower administrative costs. In the USA, administrative costs equal approximately 20% of the health care budget. This compares with 10% in France and only 5% in the UK. The NHS is often regarded as the best value for money of all health-care systems in the western world (Levitt *et al.*, 1999), although evidence relating to the effectiveness of reforms to health-care systems is scarce and studies have not used consistent frameworks for measurement (Evans *et al.*, 2001).

INFLUENCES ON THE MANAGEMENT OF CARE

The management of neonatal units in some hospitals is located within the directorates of obstetrics and gynaecology and in others within the provision of child health. Additionally, some neonates may need services that are located in other directorates. For example, they may require the services of the cardio-thoracic department, which has a more adult-based philosophy. This results in the fragmentation of the provision of neonatal care and no overall strategy to plan for and provide neonatal services.

Care planning for neonates has had to contend with continual change resulting from a macro-political viewpoint and from local political influence. (Indeed, the whole of the NHS has suffered from its status as a high-profile political football.) Senior management can have difficulty in implementing major policy changes and adjusting to funding modifications, particularly when being constantly audited, restructured and re-engineered. An examination of the smaller political agendas will reveal that the balance of power when planning care is not equal. Traditionally, the medical hierarchy has exerted more power and influence within the care settings (DoH, 2001). Arguably, the more senior that management becomes, the more detached they are from what is happening at the interface of care.

The hierarchical model of management is an outdated concept, since it alienates staff from the decision-making process. In the management of neonatal units, it is apparent to the nurse that the ideal structure would be viewed from the point of care outwards. This contrasts with the downward approach adopted in the traditional hierarchical manner.

For the working nurse who is so distant from the decision-making process, there is no direct link between the controlling 'core' and the point of service delivery. This may result in apathy towards management, and resistance to change and development. This form of managerial framework appears not to recognise or value clinical and professional skills or developing nursing practice. A better organisational model would have team-building and collective learning as the building blocks of the organisation. Such a model would be more likely to lead to quality care and to value the skills of the participants, engendering a feeling of individual and group responsibility.

AN ALTERNATIVE MANAGERIAL FRAMEWORK

The NHS needs to orientate towards a management perspective that focuses attention more acutely on the real issues that affect the experience and quality of care. The organisation of the management needs a flatter basis. One possible management strategy is the framework of shared governance.

Some frameworks are deliberately designed to facilitate the sharing of expertise, ideas and learning, and to unravel the ambiguities of organisational life. Using a framework of shared governance, the nursing contribution – currently an untapped potential in terms of patient care and advanced nursing practice – can be utilised. Shared governance promises, among other things, to improve staff retention rates, boost morale and raise clinical skills. All these factors would enhance the quality of patient care, and are highly topical and current issues in neonatal care today.

Shared governance is a form of participative management and has been credited with giving hands-on nurses and midwives a real voice in decision-making. In both the USA and the UK, a range of positive outcomes has been attributed to it, including the creation of an empowered nursing workforce, increased professional autonomy, improved job satisfaction, more effective nurse-led innovations in clinical practice, and improved overall quality of patient care (Bernreuter, 1993; Hess, 1998; Porter O'Grady, 1994; Geoghegan and Farrington, 1995).

There is much to learn from the repeated crisis in the NHS. Staff must move forward from a 'culture of blame' (DoH, 2001). It is critical to create an organisational climate in which professional and individual needs can flourish. This must begin with a focus on healthy interpersonal relationships, which must be anchored by trust, mutual respect, consistent, visible support, and open, honest communication. It must be accepted that nursing, like medicine, is not a perfect science and that even the best people can make mistakes (DoH, 2001). What is worse than making mistakes is not learning from them and not using the information to devolve a system that will minimise risk. The clinical situation on a neonatal unit often exposes staff to extraordinary events, including situations that require sensitivity and empathy. This is an area where ethical issues have to be faced on a daily basis (Crawford and Power, 2001).

High ethical standards are essential in situations of uncertainty, in which nurses are encouraged to find their own answers to practice-based problems. Values such as these should not be mere platitudes appearing in Trust nursing strategies; instead, they should be central to nursing philosophy and everyday practice. This may be difficult to achieve in the current hectic clinical environment, but the development of shared governance could allow it to happen.

DEVELOPMENT AND CHANGE IN PROFESSIONAL NURSING

The changes envisaged in the NHS are not unique to the nursing profession. All professionals are challenged by a rapidly changing knowledge base, new working practices and environments, increasing public expectations and risk of litigation. The possible impact on their practice of the latter may cause anxiety to neonatal nurses (Browne, 1999), who have witnessed an increasing tendency in their midwifery and medical colleagues to practise defensively. The very public suspension of senior doctors in Leicester, Birmingham and Bristol is certain to have caused unease. No doubt nurses will also have mixed feelings about the enquiries and reviews that have pilloried doctors' decisions to retain organs and perform surgery (Hunter, 2001).

A nurse's best defence against litigation is to practise within set protocols. These are increasingly being developed, based on best evidence and review by experts and peers. Unfortunately, in the care of neonates there are quite a few examples of care that are contentious and await good-quality definitive research. In some cases, such as suctioning and tube feeding, there is, indeed, contra-dictory evidence. Where neonatal practice is rapidly changing, the protocols have to be reviewed frequently in order for them to keep pace.

It is not comforting, but it is quite easy to envisage the neonatal nurse at the centre of a high-profile legal wrangle regarding practice. Nurses often lack the power and influence of their medical colleagues and many are not trained or kept informed about the legal implications of their practice. In addition, many worry about the level of support that they would enjoy within the current managerial model if they were required to answer for their practice in a court of law.

Making a Difference (DoH, 1999) states that ward sisters and charge nurses are the backbone of the NHS and that their leadership potential must be developed. In the neonatal unit there is a constantly shifting scene, combined with extraordinary technological advances. Nursing is no longer a routine, task-oriented role. Neonatal nurses are infant- and family-focused, and base their care on a holistic partnership. They are flexible, adaptable practitioners and in many cases welcome change and advances in technology, as a means to better care.

The pressure on cots is matched by the pressure on staff as the dependency of the occupants increases. Quite simply, sicker, smaller and more technology-dependent infants take more looking after and place a greater emotional and physical strain on staff. Neonatal units have a high staff turnover and a high sickness and burn-out rate. There is an urgent need to consider stress and career breaks in order to protect individuals who are suffering, and to retain their services. Such breaks would represent a significant departure from the 'tradi-tional' culture of nursing.

The changing workforce

There have been some interesting developments in neonatal care with the advent of Advanced Neonatal Nurse Practitioners (ANNP) and Nurse Consultants. The development of the role of the ANNP has the capacity to bring about real reform in neonatal care. One example is the Ashington innovation. This small maternity unit had about 2000 deliveries a year but had no on-site paediatric facilities. This made the provision of experienced medical cover difficult to justify. In order to keep the maternity services open when neonatal medical cover was withdrawn, in 1996, a team of ANNPs was established to take over the SHO role. Full evaluation of this project is yet to be completed but initial findings are favourable, reflecting high standards and quality of care (Hall and Wilkinson, 2001).

Watts (2001) reviewed ANNP-led transport teams and found the role compatible with the government's strategic intentions, although not specifically considered. She warned that there was a risk of ANNPs becoming doctors' assistants rather than being involved in advancing neonatal nursing practice. Bringing on a few individuals in a limited career framework may be ultimately detrimental to the profession as a whole, especially as the ANNP role lacks the status and authority accorded to senior doctors. For example, although nurse prescribing is now common, doctors and the government seem unwilling to extend this to many of the drugs required in an intensive-care setting. Nurses may not be given the authority to make a referral to a senior doctor from another specialty, or even request an X-ray. One argument asserts that there are insufficient numbers of nurses available to perform essential care, and that expanding the nursing role could cause skilled nurses to be diverted from nursing priorities. In addition, many nurses have no desire to function on a more medical basis, particularly with the increasing threat of litigation.

Workforce expectations are also changing. The declining numbers of young people entering nursing and the ageing profile of nurses already in service often drives these changes. Part-time, term-time and school-friendly contracts are increasingly made available in an effort to retain staff or enhance the prospects of skilled staff returning. This is a welcome development but care is a 24-hour requirement. Sufficient numbers of core staff are required to work round the flexible contracts so that no one is put under undue pressure. The number of informal and unqualified carers in the NHS is also increasing. The neonatal unit is seeing a return of the nursery nurse to supplement the care of the neonatal nurse. There are valid concerns that these skilled nursery personnel are not always sufficiently educated and equipped for this specialist role (Crawford, 2000). Males and the ethnic minorities are hugely under-represented and positive recruitment strategies are needed to encourage them to enter the profession.

Educational development of staff

One key concern of management is the development of nursing staff. As the risk of litigation increases, one defence strategy must be evidence-based practice. It would be ideal if management, education and research went hand in hand, but there is a paucity of sound, replicated, validated research in neonatal care and the practitioner is entitled to ask why. However, the imposition of national standards might constrain creativity, innovation and flair, and inadvertently hinder nursing progress. There is a growing tendency for teaching and learning in the workplace to be seen as a managerial function rather than the responsibility of educationalists (Knowles, 1990; Pedlar et al., 1991). This is seen by some as a positive step; perhaps the best research, teaching and training is provided by those who actually do the job, supported by and in partnership with educationalists.

As managers prepare to take a more active role in facilitating education, they need to consider the extent to which their organisation facilitates the learning of professional skills. This approach offers the opportunity to merge an individual's professional development with the performance review process, perhaps linked with the professional portfolio. This will ensure timely and relevant professional development.

Given the demands on a manager's time, there is some concern that education and training may be relegated to second priority, as practice will inevitably dominate. There is also a risk of poor practice being perpetuated, as students will learn from practitioners who have always (unquestioningly) performed a procedure in a particular way. These staff may be skilled and trained, but they may not have had the benefit of being educated in the techniques of research and reflective practice in an independent academic institution.

The establishment of NHS universities is an interesting development. Training staff together could lead to a greater sense of teamwork and shared identity, common purpose and goals. With control over the curriculum, the NHS could equip its practitioners for their future role better than the purely academic institutions. The Service is best placed to know what skills are required and how many staff need to be trained to meet demand. Costly repetition in the delivery of some subjects – core life sciences, communication skills, structure and function of the NHS – could be avoided by training students together.

The contrary argument states that such a curriculum would take a superficial view. The emphasis and depth of content would differ according to the profession and the number of suitable shared sessions might be limited. This makes the argument for streamlining education and cutting training costs less convincing. There is also a concern that the medical curriculum could dominate and the power imbalance between the professions would remain. This imbalance has been detrimental to patients in the past and ought to be addressed. Too much standardisation might be a retrograde step, affecting the purity of the teaching. Academic freedom is important for encouraging independent thinking, innovation and the undertaking of research that perhaps does not conform to the political standpoint of the day.

More planning of development from within might lead to less independent auditing and assessment; the service would be so good there would be no room for improvement. However, some believe that there is already too much political interference in and influence on the NHS. If the Service were to act as gatekeeper to the professions, and educator of the professionals and service providers, it would be even more vulnerable to political manipulation.

There is certainly a case for greater co-operation between the services and the educational providers. Widening participation and opportunity in education should not lead to a drop in educational standards. The education and training that students receive should equip them to perform well in the role for which they are being prepared.

The macro-political factors involved in education may seem a million miles away from the needs of the neonatal nurse at the cot-side. However, the future of the neonatal service rests with the staff of tomorrow and the education and preparation that they receive will influence what sort of practitioners they will become.

SHARED GOVERNANCE

Shared governance was first popularised in the 1980s (Porter O'Grady and Finnigan, 1984) and has been described as a system that relies on authority, responsibility and accountability. It is important to emphasise that shared governance was regarded as a method of better supporting the delivery of nursing care, rather than a 'new' method of care delivery. It grew out of the recognition that staff nurses were dissatisfied, not with nursing itself, but with the institutions in which they practised.

Shared governance is a collaborative management structure characterised by a balance of power between management and staff, and reciprocation through sharing of information. It is claimed that shared governance will achieve the following (Porter O'Grady, 1992):

- increased participation in decision-making;
- development of collaborative relationships, leading to the realisation of team goals;
- staff feeling valued, leading to greater commitment and higher morale;
- appropriate implementation and evaluation of ideas at ward level;
- improvement in the quality of nursing care.

Given that change is inevitable, the shared governance framework is an ideal tool for its implementation. It has the potential to include all nurses in the decision-making process, and can change the way nurses work and help them flourish. Surely, the rapidly changing and uncertain environment of the NHS is fertile ground for the shared governance concept.

The advocates of shared governance see the framework as a method for the recruitment and retention of staff, but it should not be seen as a quick fix for the problem. Until the blame culture expires and nurses shed their collective victim mentality (Malby, 1998), nursing may remain a relatively unattractive option to potential recruits in the wider society. The philosophy behind shared governance will produce assertive nurse leaders at all grades. These individuals will be unwilling to continue playing the 'doctor-nurse' game, and capable of using the media to change stereotypes and generate an informed understanding of the nursing contribution to health. This will create interest in the profession and eventually improve recruitment. Owing to the lack of research, only anecdotal evidence is available. In order to ensure lasting change, a slow evolutionary approach to implementing shared governance, requiring persistence and determination, is necessary.

CONCLUSION

According to the philosopher Ly Tin Weedle, chaos is found in greatest abundance wherever order is being sought. It always defeats order, because it is better organised (Pratchett, 1994). Ly Tin Weedle would have found many examples to support his philosophy in the management of neonatal care today.

A greater level of co-operation and teamwork can only be beneficial. If this higher level of co-operation and teamwork is to be achieved, all those involved in sustaining the NHS will need to recognise the worth of others, and build effective working relationships on the basis of trust through agreed ethical principles. Above all, the neonatal team should not lose sight of its reason for being – the care of the infant and its family.

REFERENCES

Bernreuter, M. (1993) The other side of shared governance, *Journal of Nursing Administration* **23**(10), 12–14

Browne, A. (1999) The increasing threat of litigation: neonatal nurses' perception of how litigation impinges on their practice, *Journal of Neonatal Nurses* **5**(3), 23–8

Crawford, D. (2000) The education of child-care professionals – a cause for concern, *Paediatric Nurse* **12**(6), 9–10

Crawford, D. and Power, K. (2001) Neonates on the edge of survival, *Paediatric Nurse* **13**(5), 16–20

Department of Health [DOH] (1989) *Working for Patients*, Department of Health, London

DoH (1999) *Making a Difference*, Department of Health, London

DoH (2001) *Learning from Bristol*, Department of Health, London

Evans, D., Tandon, A., Murray, L. and Lauer, J. (2001) Comparative efficiency of national health systems: cross-national econometric analysis, *BMJ* **323**(7308), 307–10

Geoghegan, J. and Farrington, A. (1995) Shared governance: developing a British model, *British Journal of Nursing* **4** (13) 734–5

Hall, D. and Wilkinson, A. (2001) Neonatal services provided by Advanced Neonatal Nurse Practitioners at Ashington: what have we learned in the first five years? Report by David Hall, Professor of Community Paediatrics, Sheffield, President of the Royal College of Paediatrics and Child Health; and Andrew Wilkinson, Professor of Paediatrics Oxford, President of the British Association of Perinatal Medicine, Northumberland Health Authority

Hess, R. (1998) Measuring shared governance, *Nursing Research* Jan/Feb **47**(1), 35–42

Hunter, M. (2001) Alder Hey Report condemns doctors, *BMJ* **322**, 255

Knowles, M. (1990) *The Adult Learner: A Neglected Species* (4th edition), Gulf, Houston, Texas

Levitt, R., Wall, A. and Appleby, J. (1999) Chapter 14. In: *The Reorganised National Health Service* (6th edition), Stanley Thornes, London

Maguire D. (1998) Tips to merge by, *Neonatal Network* **17**(7), 69–70

Malby, B. (1998) Clinical leadership, *Advanced Practice Nursing Quarterly* **3**(4), 40–3

Pedlar, M., Burgoyne, J. and Boydell, T. (1991) *The Learning Company*, McGraw-Hill, London

Porter O'Grady, T. (1992) *Implementing Shared Governance*, Mosby Yearbook, USA

Porter O'Grady, T. (1994) Whole systems shared governance: Creating the seamless organisation, *Nursing Economics* **12**(40), 51–2

Porter O'Grady, T. and Finnigan, S. (1984) *Shared Governance for Nursing: A Creative Approach to Accountability*, Aspen, Rockville MD

Pratchett, T. (1994) *Interesting Times, Victor Gollancz, London*, p. 4

Watts C. (2001) The role of the ANNP: Nurse-led neonatal transports, *Journal of Neonatal Nursing* 7(6), 196–200

2 ETHICAL ISSUES IN NEONATAL NURSING

Kevin J. Power

Aims of the chapter

This chapter aims to help the neonatal nurse clarify what a study of ethics may achieve and show how an ethical issue can be identified. It has been designed to stimulate the interest of the reader to consider some of the ethical issues that may arise when caring for infants on the NNU. Perhaps the most ambitious challenge of this chapter is to enable the reader to internalise ethics and see it not as an independent study but as a topic integral to everyday practice. The intention is not to provide easy answers to ethical questions that can be identified in neonatal nursing, because these can occur as a dilemma, with no single correct answer, but rather to offer the reader an opportunity to think critically about the questions and to develop reasoned arguments in support of or opposing a variety of standpoints. This chapter will not consider philosophical methods as a means of developing the skills of justifying any decision or action. For these the reader is guided to the excellent texts of Edwards (1996), Reed and Ground (1997), and Seedhouse (2000).

INTRODUCTION

Nurses, midwives and health visitors are accountable to the Code of Professional Conduct (United Kingdom Central Council, 1992a), so each individual has to justify any decisions made or positions adopted.

This chapter is set out in several sections:

1   The first section will justify the inclusion of this chapter in the book and clarify what a study of ethics might achieve.
2   The second section will establish how the nurse might identify an ethical dilemma and outline the decision-making frameworks that may assist in the analysis of these.
3   Third, some ethical issues in neonatal nursing will be examined; not in order to give answers to questions but rather to raise questions for analysis. It is important to consider some of the big questions (such as when to and when not to treat, and how to distribute finite health care resources). Some of the more everyday problems will also be considered (such as the balancing of professional obligations with the responsibilities of staff for themselves and their families).

4 The final section will consider the debate surrounding the nurse's role as advocate in neonatal practice.

The practical issues surrounding the rights of the child will be considered in Chapter 3.

Ethics is an enormous subject and some ethical issues are given little or no consideration here, not because they are unimportant, but because space is limited. Health-care ethics is an applied subject and cannot be viewed simply as an academic exercise. The reader will need to reflect on the content of this text and apply it to practice. The intention is to stimulate the reader to identify dilemmas that may result from practice; to look for and challenge assumptions that may exist in themselves or in others; then to formulate their own analyses of ethical situations and identify strategies for resolving these dilemmas.

WHY STUDY ETHICS?

One question needs to be considered from the outset: why should a neonatal nurse be required to (or even wish to) develop a knowledge of the ethics of health care? Surely the advance in evidence-based practice means that there is no need to debate the rights and wrongs of any action? Cannot the best available evidence guide all practice?

In fact, many other questions need to be answered in addition to what is the best treatment for any particular health problem. These questions include the following:

- What is in the best interests of the infant?
- What is in the best interests of the parents and family?
- What is in the best interests of society?
- Should an infant endure treatment with little prospect of survival?

The evidence may suggest a particular set of interventions, but questions remain as to whether those interventions should be implemented, and in whose interests are the interventions being carried out.

Neonatal nurses work with vulnerable people – parents and families who are often confused, uninformed and anxious, as well as neonates incapable of speaking for themselves. Neonatal care deals with extremes, at the beginning of extra-uterine life (often at the edge of viability) and at the end of life. As a result, neonatal nurses have to deal with moral dilemmas on a more regular basis than in everyday life.

The technological advances in neonatology have created new opportunities for treatment at those extremes (Rennie and Bokhari, 1999). Muraskas et al. (1999) have suggested that parents and infants are being 'held hostage by technology'. Their assertion is based on the fact that there are so many uncertainties regarding the success of high-tech treatments. It is very difficult to determine the point at which a treatment might be deemed futile, and stopped. Spence (1998) has noted that neonatal nurses find the situations in which infants have an uncertain prognosis most challenging. Hefferman and Heilig (1999) have noted in particular the 'moral distress' of experienced nurses when caring for infants undergoing an aggressive course of treatment. Rennie and Bokhari (1999) pointed out that a number of high-tech treatments were the subject of research and suggested that the additional ethics of research added to the burden of decision-making.

Neonatal nurses may need to support and assist parents and families to make difficult decisions associated with these uncertainties. These are all potential sources of inner conflict and stress. A study of ethics and reflection upon individual cases may help to facilitate personal coping skills and give a clear direction to the nurse's actions.

Finite resources

The resources available for the provision of neonatal care are finite. Neonatology must compete with other health services for a share of the total health budget, and decisions have to be made with regard to the distribution of these resources. Who should receive treatment and who should not? In addition, individual nurses are faced on a daily basis with decisions regarding priority. Which infant should they assess and care for first and which should they leave until later? On what do they base their decisions? It will not be possible to answer all of these questions on a simple clinical need basis, so neonatal nurses will need to use their understanding of ethics.

Accountability

Nurses are accountable for any decisions they make, both by virtue of the duty of care owed under the civil law (Dimond, 1996), and because of their professional obligation to a code of conduct (United Kingdom Central Council, 1992a). Nurses cannot simply claim a defence of following orders; they must be able to give good rational reasons for their actions, or indeed for any decision not to act in a particular case.

Neonatal nurses implement care and, according to Elizondo (1991), they might be required to implement care decisions with which they personally disagree. A knowledge of ethics is essential to enable neonatal nurses to develop a credible voice in the decision-making process. A sound understanding of the ethical implications of practice from a variety of standpoints will enable them to practise credibly.

What is ethics?

Rowson (1990) defines the term 'ethics' as 'thinking and reasoning about morality'. Beauchamp and Childress (1994) assert that 'ethics is designed to illuminate what we ought to do by asking us to consider and reconsider our ordinary actions, judgements and justifications'. For Rumbold (1999), ethics is 'concerned with the basis on which people, individually or collectively, decide that certain actions are right or wrong'.

Notions of what is right or wrong are bound up in morals, a term which is sometimes used synonymously with the term 'ethics'. However, 'morals' does not mean the same as 'ethics'. The word *moral* stems from the Latin word *moralis*, meaning 'custom' or 'manners'. This does not mean manners as in polite behaviour, but a more formal definition of what society believes to be right and proper behaviour in life. What is considered to be right and proper will necessarily depend on the values and beliefs held by the members of that society. Morality can change over time as individual and societal values and beliefs change. For example, the death penalty was once seen in the UK as an acceptable punishment for certain crimes, but this is no longer the case in all sections of society. One important example within the health service involves the acceptability or otherwise of retaining human tissue and organs without the explicit consent of the patient or, in the case of children, their parents. However, following the revelations from the Alder Hey Children's Hospital, and the recognition of the distress caused by this practice, procedures and policies are being reviewed (Hunter, 2001). If notions regarding what is right or wrong are dynamic, there is a need continually to examine these notions and to justify actions and beliefs. That is the subject of ethics. Because of this dynamism, there can be very few simple or fixed ideas regarding what is right or wrong, and neonatal nurses, in common with other professionals, must continually examine their own values and beliefs about what is right. They must also take into account the differing values of others, particularly in a multicultural society, when considering how to – indeed, *if* to – act.

Ethics is sometimes referred to as moral philosophy, while nursing is an applied science (or art) based on interpersonal interaction. Nursing ethics is concerned with the application of ethics complicated by human relationships. In applying these ideas to nursing practice, it very quickly becomes apparent that there are no precise answers to the question 'How should I act in this situation?'. Ethical dilemmas will arise whenever a nurse must make a judgement and be prepared to defend that judgement. Clearly, there are some dilemmas that are wholly clinical in nature: 'Is intervention A better than intervention B in this particular case?' There are others that are wholly ethical: 'Do all neonates have a right to life?' However, most decisions in health care have an element of both the ethical and the clinical. What is important is not to assume that the clinical decision outweighs any ethical considerations. Merely because something *can* be done – because a treatment exists or is possible – it does not follow that it always *should* be done.

So, what is an ethical dilemma and how is it recognised? Richardson and Webber (1995) offer a simple definition: 'a situation in which conflicting moral principles are present and they generate conflicting demands'. They give the example of the person who steals food to feed his starving family. In most societies, stealing is believed to be wrong but this may, in certain circumstances, conflict with the moral obligation to feed a family.

Edwards (1996) suggests that a moral issue can be identified whenever any action or proposed action may lead to some harm or benefit to others. It is clarified further by suggesting that if it is possible to examine a situation, and terms such as right, wrong, good, bad, duty, obligation, should, ought, harm are used – for example, 'Should the nurse have told the parents the truth?' – then it is probable that an ethical component exists. Applying ethics to nursing requires nurses to make choices and justify those choices to others.

ETHICAL DECISION-MAKING

Making and being accountable for ethical decisions is fraught with difficulty throughout nursing. It is hard to make decisions that balance the many demands of care. In the NNU, nurses provide care for the parents and other family members in an emotionally charged atmosphere. An infant's life is often at stake, making these decisions even more problematic. McHaffie and Fowlie (1996) demonstrated, with their research, many of the difficulties in making life and death decisions. Neonatal nurses should avoid seeking rapid and simple answers to the problems and dilemmas presented in clinical practice. As Rostain and Bhutani (1989) asserted, ethical dilemmas are

> ... truly difficult to resolve. They are highly likely to elicit doubt, anxiety and discomfort in the decision-makers. This is a healthy sign. It is important to experience a certain amount of uncertainty and uneasiness when facing these decisions. To fail to do so might well be a sign of moral indifference or of self-protection. Decision-makers need to be sure they have given careful consideration to all sides of the dilemma, have left "no stone unturned", and have struggled with the agonising feeling that tough choices elicit.

In any dilemma nurses seek to answer the question, 'What is the right thing to do?', but this should not lead to the belief that there is only *one* right thing to do. Nurses should seek to answer instead the question, 'How can I justify a decision to act, or refrain from acting, in any particular case?' This means being able to identify the issues at stake, weigh them against each other, and reach a conclusion that can be defended against any objections. Others may claim that the decision was mistaken, naïve or just wrong, but Curtin (1982) has asserted the following:

> In all decision-making one is a finite being with limited capabilities.... . A person could be wrong ... but must act with integrity ... according to the knowledge he possesses in keeping with his obligations ... in the search for a satisfactory outcome. (p. 59)

Nurses should not be afraid to ask difficult questions. They should not be intimidated into thinking that there are others who are better placed to make ethical decisions. Medical and paramedical staff do not undergo any more ethical training than nurses. The opinion of the nurse is just as valid as that of anyone else. In addition, the moral obligation to ask challenging questions is equal to the obligation to make rational, well-informed decisions. Neonatal nurses must also recognise that if they decide not to speak up or become involved in an ethical debate regarding an infant's care and treatment, this in itself is an ethical decision for which they must be able to give an account.

The following theories may guide nurses who are thinking about ethical dilemmas:

- Kant's (1964) duty-based ethics;
- Mill's (1910) consequentialist theory;
- Aristotelian (1980) virtue ethics (Ross *et al.*, 1980).

These theories may help to guide a general approach to ethical analysis however, they rarely provide any practical help in everyday ethical decision-making (Edwards, 1996). Moral philosophers have formulated ethical principles to provide something with which to apply these theoretical perspectives (Thiroux, 1977; Beauchamp and Childress, 1994), but again these are too abstract for everyday use. Several authors have formulated ethical decision-making tools or frameworks to help guide thinking about an ethical dilemma (Curtin, 1982; Pelligrino, 1987; Husted and Husted, 1991; Greipp, 1992; Seedhouse, 1998). Some, such as Curtin's, are linear in nature and guide the nurse through the process of decision-making. Other frameworks, such as Seedhouse's Ethical Grid (1998), are more flexible in their application but are perhaps less helpful to the inexperienced ethical thinker. Seedhouse (Seedhouse and Lovett, 1992) also offers an algorithmic version of his model as an alternative that gives a more linear approach to problem-solving.

There are critics of these models (McHaffie and Fowlie, 1996), who rightly point out that they are too cumbersome for everyday clinical use, and may even encourage simplistic and mechanistic thinking. However, used with integrity and care, they can provide a useful guide to decision-making. The models are merely guides, and not to be followed slavishly, but their use can help to ensure that no moral 'stone is left unturned'. Nurses should not neglect to consider the impact of their personal values on ethical decision-making. They should reflect on and develop an understanding of what they themselves believe regarding right and wrong. This will affect the weight applied to certain considerations in any dilemma.

Most of the ethical decision-making guides call for some deliberation regarding ethical principles, which have been outlined by moral philosophers. Examples of these principles are considered below.

The principles approach

There are two versions of ethical principles in common usage. Perhaps the best known is that described by Beauchamp and Childress (1994): respect for autonomy, beneficence, non-maleficence and justice. Less well known are those set out by Jacques Thiroux (1977), which incorporate the former, as well as prompting thinking about additional issues:

- the principle of the value of life;
- the principle of goodness or rightness;

- the principle of justice or fairness;
- the principle of veracity (truth-telling or honesty);
- the principle of autonomy or individual freedom.

Despite criticism of the principles approach to ethical thinking (Clouser and Gert, 1994; Wulff, 1994; Edwards, 1996), it does provide a useful starting point for reflection and identification of where every individual stands in relation to a number of ethical problems. The principles are not there to tell a nurse what to do, but rather to encourage nurses to think, 'What is my position on this principle and how do I justify it?'.

The principle of the value of life
This is based on the premise that life must be valued but death must be accepted. It does not demand that life be preserved at any cost. If there is strong justification for not preserving a life, there may be occasions when an infant may be allowed to die or a foetus have its life taken away. Quality of life must also be considered wherever it is in question.

The principle of goodness or rightness
This principle asks nurses to consider what is good and right. It demands that nurses cause no harm – also termed 'non-maleficence' (Beauchamp and Childress, 1994) – and that they actively prevent harm, also termed 'beneficence' (Beauchamp and Childress, 1994). Of course it is impossible to cause no harm in a neonatal unit because distress and pain are natural consequences of the invasive procedures that are necessary to ensure the well-being of the infant. In any ethical dilemma the nurse must weigh up the good, or the benefits, of an action against the bad, or harm, of that action, and ensure that the balance is always on the side of least harm for most benefit.

The principle of justice or fairness
This asks that nurses consider what is fair and just. 'Justice' here has two meanings. The first relates to ensuring that an individual's moral rights are upheld. The second relates to the fair division of resources among all those who might have a legitimate claim on those resources. This second meaning will be discussed further below.

The principle of truth-telling or veracity
This prompts nurses to consider whether it is always right to tell the truth or whether there is any justification for not telling the truth. They should also consider within this principle whether total honesty is required or whether certain information may be held back from families.

The principle of autonomy or individual freedom
This is based on the right to self-determination. It is obvious that the neonate cannot have any autonomy, except in the future, providing it survives to develop

into childhood and adulthood. However, the family, particularly the parents, may have claims to determine what is best for their child. Nurses need to consider how to weigh the parents' rights in determining the neonate's future against the neonate's own rights. Clearly, if the parents, for example, request that supportive treatment is withheld, the neonate may be denied the opportunity to develop its own autonomy. On the other hand, the parents may demand treatment that is not beneficial to the infant by virtue of its futility or because it would prolong suffering. This would impinge on individual freedom, as it may not have been the choice of the neonate.

All of this ethical theory may seem to be the preserve of the moral philosopher until it is applied to practice. The following section examines some of the ethical issues that face neonatal nurses in practice.

ETHICAL ISSUES

Withholding and withdrawing treatment

Questions relating to the withholding or withdrawal of treatment represent an enduring problem for the neonatal nurse. This is particularly the case with the advances in sophisticated technological support for the immature neonate. Guidelines to aid such decisions have been formulated (Royal College of Paediatrics and Child Health, 1997), but Doyal and Larcher (2000) note some problems in applying them. In some respects they are too general and non-specific to assist in particular cases. Alternatively, some clinicians feel they are too restrictive and apply unnecessary constraints on clinical practice. In order to illustrate some of the ethical problems that neonatal nurses may face, the following two principles stated within these guidelines will be examined:

1   the axiom that there is no morally significant difference between withholding and withdrawing treatment;
2   the principle of how to serve the best interests of the child.

There may be no morally significant difference between withholding treatment and withdrawing treatment, assuming the same objective of preventing harm and relieving suffering. Clearly, the objective of either cannot lawfully be the demise of the infant. But there certainly may be a difference in the mind of the individual, particularly perhaps the neonatal nurse. *Withdrawing* treatment might be viewed as more acceptable because at least the neonate has been given a chance. Either the treatment has not been successful or the burden of treatment has become so great as to outweigh any slight chance that the infant may survive; or, in the event of survival, the prospect for the quality of life is so poor as to lead to life being intolerable. Ruark and Ruffin (1988, cited in Pace, 1996) suggest that it is more difficult to stop treatment once it has been initiated, especially if the death of the infant is the direct result of the cessation of treatment (Pace, 1996).

Decisions regarding the *withholding* of treatment are made on the same premise but may cause greater anxiety for the neonatal nurse. There is a chance that a mistake has been made, and that an infant who would have benefited from treatment has been denied it. This is likely to be made all the more acute because the decision to commence treatment, or not, is likely to be undertaken in very different circumstances from those in which withdrawal is considered. The majority of decisions to withhold treatment take place at the point of delivery of the infant, when the time available for deliberation regarding the relative merits of treatment is extremely limited. Decisions to withdraw treatment are more frequently made in a calm and relatively unrushed atmosphere because the infant is already being supported and any delay in the decision is unlikely to have irredeemable consequences.

The potential consequence of this analysis is that there will be a temptation always to initiate treatment and then to decide whether or not to continue. The problem with this is that it is not beneficent to the infant to initiate treatment where the benefits of that treatment are outweighed by the harms, in terms of prolongation of suffering, of that treatment.

The question regarding whether a treatment is futile and should be discontinued can be determined using a scoring system (Goh and Mok, 2001). (The scoring system identified relates to paediatric intensive care but could be adapted to a NNU situation.) There is an enduring difficulty in relation to decisions regarding whether or not to withhold treatment – predicting the outcome of any action is fraught with risk. Clinically experienced practitioners, basing their predictions on evidence, can and usually do make ethically sound decisions (Goh and Mok, 2001). The central question that needs to be addressed in these situations (assuming treatment is possible) is, 'Will initiation, or continuation, of this treatment promote the well-being of the infant (beneficence) and minimise harm (non-maleficence)?'

Best interests

The above question is usually answered with reference to what is in the infant's 'best interests'. What is meant by this term?

It is a well-worn maxim in paediatrics that any decisions taken with regard to health care should consider what is in the child's best interests. Examples include The Children Act (DoH, 1989), The UN Convention on the Rights of the Child (1989) and the Royal College of Paediatrics and Child Health guidelines for withholding or withdrawing treatment (Royal College of Paediatrics and Child Health, 1997). The UKCC Code of Professional Conduct (United Kingdom Central Council, 1992a) also demands that nurses act 'in the interests of their patients'.

It is rarely, if ever, made explicit what might be construed as the child's best interests. Rose (1995) considered a concept analysis of best interests and identified a number of themes associated with the notion. Principle among these is the intention to do long-term good. The implication is that sometimes it may be necessary to cause or allow harm in the short term, such as burdensome treatment for the neonate, in order to bring about long-term good, such as survival.

It might be assumed that it is always in the child's interests to live. However, there are some situations in which it is arguably in the child's interests *not* to continue to live with severe pain and suffering. It is possible to maintain life, or at least a certain level of physiological functioning, in infants with intensive therapy. But few could argue that this would be in the best interests of the child if, in the long term, the potential to live without such support is extremely limited or non-existent.

Dworkin (1993, cited in Ellis, 1996) identifies two forms of interest that may have a significant impact on moral judgements. The first relates to the notion of suffering and the second relates to those things that make life worthwhile. Clearly, there are judgements to be made with regard to how much pain is worth enduring to achieve the pleasure that a person expects from continued life. It is relatively easy to judge that it is worth putting an infant through the suffering of some surgical treatments in order to promote long-term comfort and well-being. One example might be the treatment of an eminently correctable disorder such as an inguinal hernia repair. It is perhaps equally simple to allow the continuation of some discomfort, providing the infant will survive to lead a life that will be enjoyed and valued.

The use of the concept of best interests may lead to differences in practice. Doyal and Larcher (2000) cite evidence that children receive more burdensome treatment than adults because it is felt to be 'in their best interests'. In the majority of instances, adults have the capacity to decide what is in their own best interests and to decline or accept treatments on that basis. Adults can also assert their own best interests even where their view conflicts with the opinion of medical practice. An infant cannot do either. The scales may therefore weigh more heavily on the treatment side of the argument for sick neonates. This may be even more likely in a society where litigation is becoming more prevalent (McHale, 1998).

Kennedy (1988) is sceptical regarding the usefulness of the notion of best interests with regard to children. It is asserted that in order to have interests a person must have an awareness of, or be conscious of, the existence of interests. Harris (1985), using the analysis of the philosopher Locke, characterises self-awareness as the ability to envisage and wish to experience a future. Current understanding of human development suggests that the neonate is not self-aware and so cannot be conscious of the existence of interests. The consequence of this logic is that no infant can have an interest in and, by extension, moral claim to life-saving or life-preserving treatment (Kennedy, 1988). However, this notion discounts the argument that contends that the infant has the potential to develop the capacity for self-awareness. This is the justification for striving to preserve the life of a neonate.

Kuhse and Singer (1985) suggest that, while the neonate cannot have interests, it may be pertinent to ask whether it is 'always in the interests of the person the child *may become* [author's emphasis] to do everything possible to keep the child alive' (p. 140). This leads on to the question of the quality of life. Unless a person can develop the capacity for interests it is difficult to imagine any quality of life as a human being. There are certainly those who believe that life under some circumstances is worse than death. This is evidenced by the fact that some people choose to establish a living will, which details the circumstances under which they would not wish treatment to be initiated. This does not entail a claim to allow euthanasia but rather the withdrawing or withholding of burdensome or futile treatment. Death may occur but this would be an anticipated result. The problem here is that notions of an intolerable life are necessarily subjective.

The central problem with regard to quality of life issues is that a prediction of the outcome is usually required. This is fraught with difficulty; even with the best prognostic indicators, the final outcome of any treatment is all but unknowable. Seedhouse (1998) reminds those taking ethical decisions to take into account any disputed facts. In neonatal practice this would include the validity of any evidence to support prognostic indicators, and also a questioning of the basis on which those indicators were founded.

If gestational age is a factor in determining the likely success of intensive treatment, the accuracy of any estimates of gestational age must not be taken for granted. This might be the case particularly if a mother was aware that it was a crucial factor in determining the appropriateness of continued treatment. The temptation to give false information regarding the date of conception could be overwhelming. Absolute faith in the accuracy of methods of estimating gestational age is misplaced (Lantos *et al.*, 1994). Utilising gestational age as a basis for prognostic judgements also assumes that the mother has received antenatal care. If no such care has been received, for whatever reason, then there is much greater chance of inaccuracy with regard to gestational age estimation (Wariyar, Tin and Hey, 1997), and an estimation of the likely success of intensive care has greater uncertainty.

It is usually recommended that, where there is uncertainty regarding prognosis, the presumption should be to initiate treatment (Lantos *et al.*, 1994; Royal College of Paediatrics and Child Health, 1997) and to consider withdrawal at a later date when the position has become clearer. This is not a justification for initiating treatment in all cases. The argument that there is always uncertainty with regard to prognosis and that treatment must always be initiated, leads to a significant risk of some infants being subjected to over-burdensome treatment and possibly even abuse.

The neonatal team may have a duty to preserve life where possible, but there can be no absolute duty to preserve life at all costs, especially if the burden of treatment outweighs any potential beneficial outcome. Acting in this way would result in a tremendous burden on society. Guidelines such as those produced by the Royal College of Paediatrics and Child Health (1997) can provide some assistance but they are not a substitute for sound moral reasoning in each individual case.

There are some (fortunately rare) instances in which the life of one neonate or foetus has to be weighed against that of another. This might occur, for example, in the case of a multiple pregnancy, when a selective abortion is judged to be necessary. The question may not be which foetus to abort, as some foetuses will be easier to access for the procedure than others. The question is whether any of them should be sacrificed in order to save the life of the others? Is it better to sacrifice one life in order to preserve another? Society tends to view as heroes people who sacrifice their own life in order to save others, but a foetus in a multiple pregnancy does not have the luxury of choosing to sacrifice its life.

Consider this example: the captain of a sinking ship can save some passengers by closing a bulkhead leading to the flooded part of the ship. The action would condemn those behind the bulkhead to death but, if there is a duty to preserve life where possible, it can be justified. The suggestion is not that one life has more worth than another, but that it is better to prevent everyone from dying, even if it means some may have to lose their life. In the case of the multiple pregnancy, if there is a good chance of preserving the life of one or more of the foetuses, then it is better to end the life of another or others than to allow all to die. Similar issues had to be addressed in the case of conjoined twins Jodie and Mary (Brykczynska, 2000).

The point is that one life is not worth more than any other – this may suggest that one of the lives is worth nothing. Each human life should at least be given equal weighting in terms of its intrinsic value.

Justice

The questions discussed above may lead to a consideration of the concept of justice. 'Justice' here has two meanings. The first relates to the upholding of an individual's moral rights to freedom from harm (non-maleficence), promotion of well-being (beneficence) and self-determination (autonomy) (*see* page 19). The second meaning is that of distributive justice or the allocation of resources, or perhaps (pejoratively speaking) rationing. The concept of distribution of resources in a fair manner can be divided into micro and macro levels. At the macro level the distribution of health-care resources for neonates must be balanced against other areas. At the micro level nurses must decide on priorities for care and which infant and family to care for first or most. An analysis of the relevant ethical duties and rights, utilising a guiding framework, can assist in answering these questions.

At the macro level, McFarlane (1999) suggests that the cost of providing intensive care for a very premature neonate may be in the region of £20 000, although this will depend on a number of individual factors. The costs per year for providing respite facilities for a severely disabled child are around £160 000 (McFarlane, 1999). On this basis, in a financially regulated health service, there may be serious questions about whether it is rational to provide intensive care to very sick neonates who, depending on survival, may require large financial input for the rest of their lives.

Rawls (1971, cited in Edwards, 1996) and Nozick (1980) offered two, dichot-omous views of distributive justice. According to Nozick (1980), justice has to take into account a person's relevant 'holdings'. This means that if someone has worked hard to develop a career and has been careful to save money, they are entitled to have a larger slice of the cake than others who have not done so. Using the same approach, it could be argued that those who refrain from behaviour detrimental to health – smoking, overeating, and so on – have more entitlement to health care than those who do not. This would place neonatal services at a disadvantage when competing with adult services, where clients may claim that they deserve more, having paid taxes all their life. Clearly, neonates can have no such 'holdings' of their own, although parents may claim that their holdings transfer automatically to their offspring.

Rawls (1971) contended that justice should be based on the notion of fairness and that all resources should be distributed to ensure the greatest liberty for all. Not everyone is entitled to the same, but any inequality in the allocation of resources is justifiable as long as those who are most in need benefit from it. Under this formulation, it is acceptable to pay doctors more if their skills are used for the benefit of those who are ill and in need. It is also acceptable for adult services to be allocated more resources than neonatal services, if that means that more adults are able to return to a productive life, and to contribute to the tax income that the state needs in order to maintain all services. This is just one interpretation. It could also be argued that increasing taxation for those in employment, in order to provide more financial resources to neonatal services, would be a better solution. It is clear that resources for neonatal service need to be balanced against the overall benefit for society.

Another approach to determining the allocation of scarce resources uses an economist's formula – Quality Adjusted Life Years, or QALYs (Lockwood, 1988; Williams, 1996). Setting priorities by the use of QALYs, or priority forums in Oxford (McFarlane, 1999) and the Oregon experiment (Dixon and Welch, 1991), is fraught with difficulties. Some believe that they represent a scientific and evidence-based tool for deciding who gets treatment and who does not, but there is a significant subjective element in the measurement of QALYs. The use of priority-setting systems in neonatal care is inherently flawed; they are applied by healthy adults who have not experienced the quality of life of the severely disabled infant (Williams, 1995). Given that there are serious reservations as to the validity of a measurement scale it could be argued that they provide no answer to the question of the allocation of finite health-care resources.

So what has the macro allocation of resources to do with neonatal nurses? The issue is dealt with at a policy level, and individual nurses may feel that there is little that they can do. However, all nurses are obligated by the UKCC Code of Professional Conduct (United Kingdon Central Council, 1992a) to 'promote and safeguard the interests and well-being of patients and clients'. It could, therefore, be argued that each individual nurse has an obligation to voice an effective opinion with regard to the allocation of health-care resources. Taking the argument to its extreme, a neonatal nurse who feels that resources are scarce might be obligated under the code to lobby parliament for a greater allocation of resources. Nurses would then need to understand the principles on which policy decisions are made.

Advocacy

The obligations of the nurse in relation to the code of conduct raise the question of his or her role as advocate for the neonate and its family. The work is based on the premise of preventing harm and promoting good, and one way of ensuring this may be for nurses to adopt the role of advocate. The concept of advocacy has been a topic of debate in nursing for a number of years. The UKCC (1989, 1992a,b, 1996) views it as integral to the role of the nurse, while others have suggested that a number of insurmountable problems may prevent nurses ever becoming effective advocates (Allmark and Klarzinksi, 1992; Sutor, 1993; Willard, 1996; Woodrow, 1997).

Problems with nurse advocacy in neonatal practice

Seedhouse (2000) takes issue with nursing theorists for defining advocacy rather imprecisely or attempting to make the word mean far too much. A brief review of the literature can reveal descriptions of as many as 20 different types of advocacy. This can only lead to confusion and is generally unhelpful. The normal meaning of advocacy is to speak on behalf of some other person as that person perceives his or her interests (Seedhouse, 2000). A number of factors may influence a nurse's decision to act as advocate:

- the nurse needs to have reasoned competently on the basis of adequate information;
- there may be a conflict with the interests of others;
- the nurse should be in agreement with the decision, or, if not, should effectively support that position.

Even if a neonatal nurse has undertaken the kind of detailed analysis that Seedhouse (2000) deems essential, there remains the question of exactly who is being represented. Neonatal nursing is founded on the principles of family-centred care, and this creates a potential conflict of interests between the neonate, the mother, the two parents and the family. Clearly, also, within the normal meaning of advocacy (see above), neonates cannot know their own interests, let alone express them to the nurse. There is naturally a need for something like advocacy on the behalf of the neonate but there are serious questions regarding whether nurses can or should fulfil such a role.

It is doubtful whether every single neonatal nurse could develop all of the skills and qualities required by an advocate (Copp, 1986; Sellin, 1995; Mallik, 1997). Allmark and Klarzinski (1992) suggest that nurses have insufficient autonomy to carry out the role effectively. Nurses are subordinate in a managerial sense and may risk conflict with management, and could even be accused of working outside contractual bounds. If nurses are not willing to risk dismissal, they must seriously question their ability to act effectively as advocates. Nurses may also have to develop a very thick skin to deal with situations in which they wish to uphold an infant's rights, when in conflict with the views of colleagues, medical staff and the family. There are further problems when advocacy for one neonate may entail working against the best interests of other neonates who are making competing demands on resources.

The Government recognises the problems that may be faced by health-care professionals in advocating for their patients, and have included proposals to create patient advocates as part of the NHS Plan (DoH, 2000).

None of the above means that neonatal nurses cannot act in the interests of the infants in their care (Charles-Edwards, 2001), merely that they should think carefully before claiming the role of advocate. A neonatal nurse who is able to recognise and analyse an ethical question is more likely to be equipped to uphold the principles of the Code of Professional Conduct (United Kingdom Central Council, 1992a), to be able to minimise the harm and ensure the well-being of infants and families in their care.

Ethical dilemmas at a personal level

In all of the above, the emphasis has been on ensuring that decisions that are taken in practice are in the best interests of the child and the family. However, it is worth remembering that neonatal nurses also have moral rights and an obligation to their own family. At times, they may need to weigh their moral obligations to neonates and their families against those of other nurses. For example, if a member of staff telephones to say they will be late, those going off duty have to ask themselves which is greater: their duty to remain at work to provide cover or their duty to themselves to return home to their own family, and to ensure that they are properly rested for their next shift?

CONCLUSION

There are no simple answers to questions of ethics but ethics is not simply a matter of personal opinion. It is an applied science, demanding careful consideration of many rights and principles that may conflict with each other. The principles of ethics, as outlined here, provide individual nurses with an opportunity to consider where they stand in relation to various dilemmas and to justify actions taken in response. Difficult decisions cannot be avoided. Indeed, it may be unethical to attempt to avoid them. Neonatal nurses should confront difficult decisions where there are questions relating to balancing the need to promote well-being, minimise harm, promote autonomy and ensure just treatment for infants and their families. It is essential in all of this to avoid assuming that health-care practitioners know what is in the infant's best interests, especially if this is based on the assumption that continued life is always in the best interests.

Neonatal nurses also need to be aware of the issues relating to the allocation of finite health-care resources, both at the day-to-day micro level (where the nurse is one of those resources), and at the macro level, where neonatal services compete with other services for a slice of the overall budget.

Neonatal nurses should think carefully about whether or not to act as an advocate for an infant. This is not to say that nurses have no role in upholding infants' moral rights and ensuring justice but rather that they should question the role within the given definition of advocacy. Neonatal nurses care for many infants; it would seem to run counter to common sense to suggest that nurses could readily advocate for just one of those infants especially if the interests of that infant conflict with those of another.

This chapter has attempted to provoke thought regarding the application of ethics in neonatal nursing. The nature of the neonatal nurse's work in dealing with the vulnerable at the limits of life necessarily means that ethical questions will be raised on a daily basis. If nurses are to be truly accountable, a good understanding of ethics is essential, to enable sound reasoning for action or inaction in a variety of clinical circumstances. The ethics of health care is sometimes viewed simply as an academic subject, remote from real clinical nursing, but this is far from the truth.

REFERENCES

Allmark P. and Klarzinski R. (1992) The case against nurse advocacy, *British Journal of Nursing* 2(1), 33–6

Beauchamp, T. and Childress, J. (1994) *Principles of Biomedical Ethics* (4th edition) Oxford University Press, Oxford

Brykczynska, G. (2000) Not quite the judgement of Solomon, *Paediatric Nursing* 12(9), 7–8

Charles-Edwards, I. (2001) Children's nursing and advocacy: are we in a muddle?, *Paediatric Nursing* 13(2), 12–16

Clouser, K. and Gert, B. (1994) Morality vs principalism. In: Gillon, R. (ed.) *Principles of Health Care Ethics*, John Wiley & Sons, Chichester

Copp, L. (1986) The nurse as advocate for vulnerable patients, *Journal of Advanced Nursing* 11, 255–63

Curtin, L. (1982) No rush to judgement. In: Curtin, L. and Flaherty, M. (eds) *Nursing Ethics: Theories and Pragmatics*, Prentice-Hall International, Englewood Cliffs, NJ

Department of Health (1989) *The Children Act*, HMSO, London

Department of Health (2000) *The NHS Plan*, The Stationery Office, London

Dimond, B. (1996) *Legal Aspects of Child Health Care*, Mosby, London

Dixon, J. and Welch, H. (1991) Priority setting: lesson from Oregon, *The Lancet* 337, 891–4

Doyal, L. and Larcher, V. (2000) Drafting guidelines for the withholding or withdrawing of life-saving treatment in critically ill children and neonates, *Archives of Disease in Childhood, Fetal and Neonatal Edition* 83, F60–F63

Edwards, S. (1996) *Nursing Ethics: a principle-based approach*, Macmillan, London

Elizondo, A. (1991) Nurse participation in ethical decision-making in the neonatal intensive care unit, *Neonatal Network* 10(2), 55–9

Ellis, P. (1996) Exploring the concept of acting 'in the patient's best interests', *British Journal of Nursing* 5(17), 1072–74

Goh, A. and Mok, Q. (2001) Identifying futility in a paediatric critical care setting: a prospective observational study, *Archives of Disease in Childhood* 84, 265–8

Greipp, M. (1992) Greipp's model of ethical decision-making, *Journal of Advanced Nursing* 17 734–8

Harris, J. (1985) *The Value of Life: An Introduction to Medical Ethics*, Routledge, London

Hefferman, P. and Heilig, S. (1999) Giving 'moral distress' a voice: ethical concerns among neonatal intensive care unit personnel, *Cambridge Quarterly of Healthcare Ethics* **8**, 173–8

Hunter, M. (2001) Alder Hey Report condemns doctors, management and coroner, *British Medical Journal* **322**, 255

Husted, G. and Husted, J. (1991) *Ethical Decision-Making in Nursing*, Mosby, St Louis

Kant, I. (1964) The Doctrine of Virtue, Part II of *The Metaphysic of Morals* (Gregor, M. transl.), Harper and Row, New York

Kennedy, I. (1988) *Treat Me Right: Essays in Medical Law and Ethics*, Clarendon Press, Oxford

Kuhse, H. and Singer, P. (1985) *Should the Baby Live? The Problem of Handicapped Infants*, Oxford University Press, Oxford

Lantos, J., Tyson, J., Allen, A., *et al.* (1994) Withholding and withdrawing life-sustaining treatment in neonatal intensive care: issues for the 1990s, *Archives of Disease in Childhood, Fetal and Neonatal Edition* **71**(3), 218–23

Lockwood, M. (1988) Quality of life and resource allocation. In: Bell, J. and Mendus, S. (eds) *Philosophy and Medical Welfare*, Cambridge University Press, Cambridge

Mallik, M. (1997) Advocacy in nursing – a review of the literature, *Journal of Advanced Nursing* **25**, 130–8

McFarlane, A. (1999) Rationing in child health services: a personal view, *Archives of Disease in Childhood* **81**(1), 1–2

McHaffie, H. and Fowlie, P. (1996) *Life, Death and Decisions: Doctors and Nurses Reflect on Neonatal Practice*, Hochland and Hochland Ltd, Cheshire

McHale, J. (1998) Introduction: The nurse and the legal environment. In: McHale, J., Tingle, J. and Peysner, J. (eds.) *Law and Nursing*, Butterworth Heinemann, Oxford

Mill, J.S. (1910) *Utilitarianism, Liberty and Representative Government*, JM Dent, London

Muraskas, J. *et al.* (1999) Neonatal viability in the 1990s. Held hostage by technology? *Cambridge Quarterly of Healthcare Ethics* **8**(2), 160–72

Nozick, R. (1980) Distributive justice. In: Sterba, J. (ed.) *Justice: Alternative Political Perspectives*, Wadsworth Publishing, Belmont, California, IL

Pace, N. (1996) Withholding and withdrawing medical treatment. In: Pace, N. and McLean, S. (eds) *Ethics and the Law in Intensive Care*, Oxford University Press, Oxford

Pelligrino, E. (1987) The anatomy of clinical ethical judgements in perinatology and neonatology: a substantive and procedural framework, *Seminars in Perinatology* **11**, 202–9

Rawls, J. (1971) *A Theory of Justice*, Oxford University Press

Reed, J. and Ground, I. (1997) *Philosophy of Nursing*, Arnold, London

Rennie, J. and Bokhari, S. (1999) Recent advances in neonatology, *Archives of Disease in Childhood, Fetal and Neonatal Edition* **81**(1), 1–4

Richardson, J. and Webber, I. (1995) *Ethical Issues in Child Health Care*, Mosby, London

Rose, P. (1995) Best interests: a concept analysis and its implications for ethical decision making in nursing, *Nursing Ethics* **2**(2), 149–60

Ross, W.D., Akrill, J.D. and Urmson, J.O. (transl.) (1980) *The Nicomachean Ethics*, Oxford University Press, Oxford

Rostain, A. and Bhutani, V. (1989) Ethical dilemmas of neonatal-perinatal surgery, *Clinics in Perinatology* **16**(1), 275–302

Rowson, R. (1990) *An Introduction to Ethics*, Scutari Press, Harrow

Royal College of Paediatrics and Child Health (1997) *Withholding or Withdrawing Life-Saving Treatment in Childen: A Framework for Practice*, RCPCH, London

Rumbold, G. (1999) *Ethics in Nursing Practice* (3rd edition), Ballière Tindall, London

Seedhouse, D. (1998) *Ethics – the Heart of Health Care* (2nd edition), John Wiley and Sons, Chichester

Seedhouse, D. (2000) *Practical Nursing Philosophy: The Universal Ethical Code*, John Wiley and Sons, Chichester

Seedhouse, D. and Lovett, L. (1992) *Practical Medical Ethics*, John Wiley and Sons, Chichester

Sellin, S. (1995) Out on a limb: a qualitative study of patient advocacy in institutional nursing, *Nursing Ethics* 2(1), 19–29

Spence, K. (1998) Ethical issues for neonatal nurses, *Nursing Ethics* 5(3), 206–17

Sutor, J. (1993) Can nurses be effective advocates?, *Nursing Standard* 17(7), 30–2

Thiroux, J. (1977) *Ethics: Theory and Practice*, Glencoe Press, Encino, CA

United Kingdom Central Council (1989) *Exercising Accountability*, UKCC, London

United Kingdom Central Council (1992a) *Code of Professional Conduct for Nurses, Midwives and Health Visitors* (3rd edition), UKCC, London

United Kingdom Central Council (1992b) *The Scope of Professional Practice*, UKCC, London

United Kingdom Central Council (1996) *Guidelines for Professional Practice*, UKCC, London

United Nations (1989) *UN Convention on the Rights of the Child* (20, xi, 1989 TS 44; Cm 1976), UNGA, Geneva

Wariyar, U., Tin, W. and Hey, E. (1997) Gestational assessment assessed, *Archives of Disease in Childhood, Fetal and Neonatal Edition* 77(3), 216–20

Willard, C. (1996) The nurse's role as patient advocate: obligation or imposition, *Journal of Advanced Nursing* 24, 60–6

Williams, A. (1996) QALYs and ethics: a health economist's perspective, *Social Science in Medicine* 43(12), 1795–1804

Williams, L. (1995) Is the money well spent? Use of resources in neonatal intensive care, *Child Health* 3(2), 68–72

Woodrow, P. (1997) Nurse advocacy: is it in the patient's best interests?, *British Journal of Nursing* 6(4), 225–9

Wulff, H. (1994) Against the four principles: a Nordic view. In: Gillon, R. (ed.) *Principles of Health Care Ethics*, John Wiley and Sons, Chichester

3 RIGHTS, WELFARE AND PROTECTION IN NEONATAL PRACTICE

Fay Valentine

Aims of the chapter

This chapter presents a critical discussion of the application of rights, welfare and protection within the neonatal intensive care setting. There are a number of complexities and contentions that can arise for the neonatal nurse in trying to maintain these rights to address key welfare and protection issues. The main theme of the chapter is the transferability of knowledge on rights, welfare and protection to the clinical setting through the following key areas:

1 Neonatal rights – a neonate's rights within health care include the right to effective pain management and certain rights within clinical research studies.
2 Parental rights – an overview of the principles as applied to neonatal practice includes a discussion on family-centred care, visiting, parental participation in decision-making and consent.
3 Neonatal welfare and protection issues in practice – certain welfare risks and child protection issues need to be considered by neonatal nurses within practice to ensure the safety and continued development of the neonate post discharge. Areas of need and risk are discussed from both the parental and neonatal perspective.
4 Child protection – an outline of the national framework and current strategies within child protection. Areas include the management of child protection concerns and the need for multi-agency working.

These are wide-ranging subjects and it is not the intention of this chapter to provide an in-depth theoretical discussion. Rather, the aim is to raise awareness among neonatal practitioners of some of the issues that they need to consider within their practice. They have a responsibility to ensure that rights, welfare and protection issues are addressed within the neonatal unit, and guidance is provided here.

INTRODUCTION

The importance of rights within the field of health care has been the subject of many debates over recent years. It has been recognised in various charters (DoH, 1996) and patient choice and consumer involvement have been highlighted within the NHS Plan. A number of high-profile public cases – including the Bristol, Royal Staffordshire and Alder Hey inquiries – have contributed to the debate regarding the rights of infants, children and their families within health care. With the enactment of The Human Rights Act (1998), there may be an increased focus on individual rights, which could have long-term implications upon health-care services.

Child protection legislation and the United Nations (UN) Convention on the Rights of the Child (United Nations, 1989) encompass the age range up to 18 years. With the increase in teenage pregnancies, neonatal nurses may also need to consider the application of rights, welfare child protection issues in relation not only to the neonate but also to the adolescent mother.

Neonatal nurses work in close collaboration not only with the neonate but also with its family. They are therefore in a good position to recognise sources of stress within a family that may have a negative impact upon a child's health, development and well-being. This could relate to either the neonate or to a child sibling.

NEONATAL RIGHTS

'Rights' can be defined as claims or entitlements that deserve respect (McHale *et al.*, 2001). Distinctions are made between legal and moral rights and between negative and positive rights. Negative rights are those that require other people not to take certain actions, for example, the right not to be smacked. Moral rights are universal in that they apply to all and are based upon principles that are intrinsically 'good'. As such, moral rights are constant, unlike legal rights, which can be subject to change. Legal rights are based upon what is right according to law and therefore may apply only to certain groups of people.

The area of children's rights remains one of contention despite the fact that the UN Convention on the Rights of the Child (United Nations, 1989) is the most widely ratified international human rights instrument (Alderson, 2000). The convention focuses attention on the psychological and emotional well-being of children and was ratified by the UK Government in 1991. Veerman (1992, p. 184) describes the convention as 'an important and easily understood advocacy tool that promotes children's welfare as an issue of justice rather than one of charity'. In relation to its application to health care, Noyes (2000) states that it represents a shift from a highly 'paternalistic' and medically orientated view of children to a rights-based approach.

The convention sets out 54 statements (called articles), which outline the rights that all children and young people should have up to the age of 18 years. It integrates civil and political rights, as well as social, economic and cultural rights. The convention has specific articles relating to health care, and health-care providers are also guided by the other principles set out in the convention, including the best interests of the child, freedom of expression or opinion and non-discrimination.

According to Alderson (2000), the convention describes three categories of rights:

1   provision rights;
2   protection rights; and
3   participation rights.

In October 2000, as a result of the Human Rights Act 1998, rights contained in the European Convention on Human Rights became part of UK legislation. Although the European Convention makes no direct reference to children and young people, many of the clauses are applicable to these groups. The long-term impact of this legislation on the health service and the rights of minors is open to debate and is something that health professionals will need to take into account (British Medical Association, 2001).

In the following review, articles from the UN Convention are in italics. Cross-references to the Human Rights Act 1998 are included.

Provision rights

These articles relate to the essential (not luxury) standards, resources and goods that children should have by right.

Standards

Article 3: *'All services and facilities responsible for the care of children shall conform to the standards established by competent authorities, particularly in the areas of safety, health, suitability of their staff as well as competent supervision.'*

Neonates, however premature, are seen by UK law as children and therefore are recognised as human beings attributed with rights and status. Within the UK several documents have laid down the desired health-care standards for children's services (DoH, 1991b). For all neonatal and children's health professionals non-compliance with these standards should be a concern and deficiencies should be highlighted through clinical audits and clinical governance frameworks, as advocated by the Royal College of Nursing (2001).

One area of contention regarding these standards concerns the most appropriate professional to nurse sick neonates. The English National Board and UKCC have stated that neonatal nursing specialist practitioner courses should be based upon an initial registration of Part 8 or 15 of the Professional Register (United Kingdon Central Council, 1997). National standards set by the Department of Health clearly state that qualified children's nurses are the most appropriately trained staff to care for children within hospital (DoH, 1991b). There have been many debates regarding the justification of this recommendation from the UKCC.

As stated by Long (1998), the ENB 405 provided very specialist knowledge and skills in neonatal nursing but it did not provide the opportunity to develop a wider and deeper knowledge of children's nursing in general. Such knowledge has many useful applications when nursing critically ill neonates and their families. Useful topics covered include child protection, children's rights, adolescent heath risks and care, and wider welfare issues within a family unit.

The prime responsibility and duty of a children's nurse is to the child. The philosophy of care is in partnership with the family. A children's nurse can draw upon a breadth and depth of knowledge and experiences to provide the support and facilitation that families, including siblings and a neonate, require to ensure a successful outcome for both the infant and family. However, the pre-registration children's course would benefit from a strengthening of the neonatal component (Long, 1998).

Transitional care is another area of neonatal practice where concerns have been raised regarding the appropriateness of staff caring for neonates. Is a nursery nurse qualification sufficient to provide the high-quality care, education and health advice that is required for the preparation of both the neonate and family for discharge?

Article 24: *'All children have a right to the enjoyment of the highest attainable standard of health and to facilities for treatment, rehabilitation of health especially to diminish infant and child mortality.'*

Article 6 (2): *'State Parties recognise that every child has the inherent right to life and … shall ensure to the maximum extent possible the survival and development of the child.'*

Technological advances and improved skills have led to the survival of very small infants with multiple complex health needs. It may need to be considered whether striving for an individual's rights in one area of practice does not breach an individual's rights in other areas. *See* Chapter 2 for more on the moral and ethical considerations of the right to life and 'passive neonatal euthanasia' (withholding and withdrawing treatment), which can be legally argued as child abuse or even manslaughter.

Article 25: *'Any child cared for by a competent authority for the purpose of care, protection or treatment has the right to periodic review of the treatment provided to them and all other circumstances relevant to their placement.'*

This article considers a placement being a health-care organisation. Neonatal nurses need to ensure that, once a neonate has been a patient on the unit for a period of three months, social services are informed.

Publicising rights
Article 42: *'State Parties shall undertake to make the principles and provisions of the Convention widely known, by appropriate and active means, to adults and children alike.'*

It could be argued that the rights of the neonate and their families should be made more visible. Posters and leaflets could be used in order to raise awareness within families and among health professionals.

Protection rights

These rights relate to the protection of children from neglect, abuse, discrimination and exploitation.

Abuse

Article 19 (3): *'All appropriate legislation, administration, social and educational measures are taken to protect the child from all forms of physical or mental violence, injury or abuse, neglect or negligent treatment, maltreatment or exploitation.'*

Article 3 of the Human Rights Act 1998 Prohibition of Torture: *'No one shall be subject to torture or to inhuman or degrading treatment or punishment.'*

In the UK, children are the only population group that can legally be hit. The current UK law has been criticised by the European Court, but the Department of Health (2000b) consultation document on parental smacking concluded that it would be unacceptable to outlaw all physical punishment of a child by a parent. If it is not acceptable for adults to be hit, why is it acceptable for infants or children? As Roberts (2000) states, everyone can agree that beating a child is worse than 'mild physical rebuke'. It does not follow, however, that 'mild physical' abuse should be legally permissible. There is a clear difference between a husband beating a wife unconscious and 'mildly rebuking' her, but the law prohibits both.

Research suggests that infants are a particularly vulnerable group in society, with over 90% of infants in the UK being smacked (Newson and Newson, 1989; Willow and Hyder, 1998; Leach, 1999). Preventing physical punishment and raising parental awareness of its potential effects on an infant (such as the associated risks of shaking) is an area where neonatal nurses can work towards upholding a neonate's rights.

To comply with Article 19, there also needs to be protection for neonates from staff who may potentially cause them harm. Neonatal staff need to consider whether their recruitment practices, staff induction and supervision programmes are in accordance with national guidelines. These include the Report on the Allitt Inquiry (DoH, 1994), *Children's Safeguard Review: Choosing with Care* (National Health Service Executive, 1998), *The Government's Response to the Children's Safeguard Review* (Secretary of State for Health, 1998) and The Protection of Children Act (DoH, 1999).

A number of identifiable key indicators point to an infant being at risk of abuse – physical, emotional or neglect – from parents/carers. The neonatal nurse is well placed to identify risk factors and thereby co-ordinate appropriate service and educational support prior to discharge in order to prevent potential long-term abuse.

Discrimination
Article 20 (14): *'Where infants are cared for due regard shall be paid to the desirability of continuity in a child's upbringing and to the child's ethnic, religious, cultural and linguistic background.'*

Within neonatal practice consideration needs to be given to the cultural sensitivity of toys, clothing, music and reading material. The environment should also generally reflect the cultural diversity represented by the local population.

Participation rights

Right to name, identity and family
Article 7: *'The child shall be registered immediately after birth and shall have the right from birth to a name. The child has the right to acquire a nationality and, as far as possible, the right to know and be cared for by his or her parents.'*

Neonatal nurses are able to communicate with parents and advise them of the need to register their infant and the process to accomplish this. The right to a name involves other people respecting the child's name and not altering it in any way, such as shortening it or using a nickname against parent's wishes. Respect includes spelling and pronouncing the name properly (Alderson, 2000).

Right to have a voice
Article 12 (10): *'State Parties shall assure to the child who is capable of forming his or her own views the right to express those views freely in all matters affecting the child, the views of the child being given due weight in accordance with the age and maturity of the child.'*

This article obliges health professionals to seek the opinion and participation of young people in all situations that affect them. Alderson (2000) suggests that infants express their views by sounds of contentment or distress. Neonatal nurses may also need to consider this article in respect of adolescent mothers and give them time and the opportunity to express their concerns and views. These will need to be respected in the same way as the views of any other mother. Whenever possible, their wishes should be adhered to.

Implications for practice
Charles-Edwards (2001) comments that it is difficult to act as an infant's advocate because of the infant's unrealised capacity to understand and communicate. Neonatal nurses, however, are ideally placed to act in an infant's best interests, to ensure that their needs are met and that they are safeguarded from harm. This is essential, as the infant's inability to verbalise its own rights mean that these are more likely to be ignored or forgotten than those of adults. For more on advocacy, *see* Charles-Edwards (2001) and Chapter 2 (pages 26–7).

Right to effective pain management

According to Fulton (1996), ensuring children's rights in practice includes paying rigorous attention to their pain control. Like all children and adults, the neonate has a right to be free from pain and not to undergo undue suffering. There is therefore an expectation that nurses will accurately assess the neonate's pain and manage it effectively. Treating pain in the neonate has been highlighted as essential, both for ethical reasons and because untreated pain can lead to neonatal complications (Carbajal et al., 1999). The ability to assess pain and monitor the effectiveness of analgesia is vital in the neonatal nurse (Royal College of Nursing, 1999).

A decade ago pain in the neonate was believed to be limited. This was due to a widely held belief that function above the level of the brain stem did not occur and myelinisation was incomplete. It is now accepted that neonates do feel pain. (Indeed, a foetus undoubtedly responds to pain; the current debate revolves around the extent to which it can feel it – Sparshott, 1998.) Recently, much effort has been expended in investigating the degree of pain experienced by neonates and the ways in which they express distress. There has also been an increased awareness of the need for post-operative pain relief in neonates (Charlton, 1999, 2000).

The RCN pain guidelines for children (Royal College of Nursing, 1999) recognise that neonates need particular attention in the identification and assessment of their pain. A neonate's resources for communication are limited and the correct interpretation of both physiological and behavioural responses is essential. These responses may be subtle, individualised and affected by ventilation, sedation and other medication that the neonate may be receiving.

At times, neonates may be in pain, or feeling it, but may be unable to respond. The less mature, critically ill, sedated or paralysed neonate is unable to display the same pain behaviour as the older or healthier infant. Johnson and colleagues (1999) have highlighted the fact that newborns that have undergone a recent painful event are less likely to demonstrate behavioural and physiological indicators of pain. They recommend that a systematic and detailed documentation of procedural timing, and the age and state of neonate, provides the potential for an increase in knowledge when assessing pain.

Physiological and behavioural markers of pain have been shown to be reliable. There are a number of pain assessment tools available, which combine these variables to establish the intensity of a neonate's pain. Twycross and colleagues (1998) suggests that these are the tools that are the most effective for the assessment of pain in the neonate.

Combined with pharmacological painkillers, there are a number of measures available to the neonatal nurse for the alleviation of pain (Brooks, 1999). These include the removal of environmental stress, the minimising of disturbances, and soothing strategies (see Chapter 12).

Implications for practice
Pain assessment in neonates will continue to be problematic due to:

- their inability to verbalise their pain experience; and
- factors that may dampen a neonate's response to pain, such as sedation and the use of muscle relaxants.

Because this aspect of care is problematic, it should not be left unchallenged. Nurses need to interpret other factors that may influence the neonate's pain response to enable the development of effective pain assessment tools.

Research and rights

Another important area is the application in practice of the neonate's rights when there is involvement in clinical research. Research is divided into two broad categories – therapeutic and non-therapeutic. Therapeutic research has a direct improvement on the research subject. Non-therapeutic research aims to enhance the knowledge base, in order to make improvements for future patients.

There has been recent debate as to whether parents are able to consent morally and ethically to non-therapeutic research where there is no direct benefit to their infant (British Medical Association, 2001). There has also been discussion about whether the terms 'therapeutic' and 'non-therapeutic' are outdated. Dropping them would enable one criteria to be developed for the assessment of research risks and benefits, to prevent parental confusion (Alderson, 1999). It would also enable the advancement of practice based on best evidence (Royal College of Paediatrics and Child Health, 1999).

Guidelines for undertaking research with children have recently been published by the Royal College of Paediatrics (1999) and Child Health Ethics Advisory Committee (Royal College of Paediatrics and Child Health, 2000). The former relates specifically to infants and the latter provides general guidance for research with children. There are two basic principles within these documents:

1   Research involving children is important to the benefit of all children; and
2   A research procedure not intended to benefit the child subject directly is not necessarily unethical or illegal.

The clinical research process with children, particularly a clinician's responsibility to act in the best interests of the neonate, has been discussed by Allmark *et al.* (2001). There has been concern about the methodology used for obtaining the consent of parents for neonatal research, especially under emergency situations (Robinson, 1998; Manning, 2000). This concern was a key theme in the Report on the Griffiths Inquiry (National Health Service Executive, 2000). The complexity of the process of obtaining parental consent was found to be particularly problematic during times of physical, psychological and emotional stress. The report also considered the need for greater openness with subjects and suggested that posters should be displayed in all hospital wards.

The Royal College of Paediatrics and Child Health (1999) provides specific guidance relating to parental involvement in clinical research. Their position statement outlines current best practice in informing and involving parents in the health care of their infants in a research-based clinical setting. The Royal College of Paediatrics and Child Health Ethics Advisory Committee (2000) published a checklist (*see* Table 3.1) outlining the issues that should be discussed by researchers and families.

Table 3.1   *Royal College of Paediatrics and Child Health guidelines (2000) for parental involvement in clinical research*

- Purpose of the research
- Whether the child stands to benefit directly and, if so, the difference between research and treatment
- Meaning of relevant terms (such as placebos)
- Nature of each procedure, how often or how long each may occur
- Potential benefits and harms (immediate and long-term)
- Name of the researcher whom they can contact with enquiries
- Name of the doctor directly responsible for the child
- How children can be withdrawn from the project

From Royal College of Paediatrics and Child Health Ethics Advisory Committee (2000) with permission

Implications for practice

The neonatal nurse may be involved in the research process as a researcher, research assistant or participant in the implementation of study protocols. The nurse may have to provide an explanation to parents or other family members, and have to instigate practice changes as a result of research outcomes.

Neonatal nurses need to be clear about national guidance and policy, as well as the local research study aims and objectives, the procedure for obtaining parental consent and the need to ensure parental understanding. Parents must be given the information they require in order to make a choice, utilising their power of proxy consent in the best interest of their infant.

PARENTAL RIGHTS

The emphasis on personal autonomy is today widely applied to all individuals, including the very young. The parent's role is often seen as serving the growth of the infant's autonomy. Traditionally and legally, parents are entitled to make decisions on behalf of their children. The Children Act 1989 (DoH, 1991a)

Table 3.2   *Parental responsibility*

Parental responsibility	Gaining parental responsibility
<ul><li>Both parents if married at time of conception, birth or soon after</li><li>Only mother if not married to the infant's father</li><li>Can be acquired by an unmarried father by court order or parental responsibility agreement with the mother</li><li>Retains following divorce</li></ul>	<ul><li>Child under a residence order</li><li>At the request of a parent</li><li>Appointed legal guardian following death of a parent</li><li>Adoption</li></ul>

Shared responsibility between local authority and parents when child subject of a care order states that parental responsibility consists of the parent's rights, duties, powers and legal responsibilities in respect of their child and his or her property. This includes the right to give consent to treatment.

Table 3.2 outlines who has parental responsibility.

Where parental responsibility is shared with a local authority, the local authority may determine the extent to which parents may exercise this responsibility. For example, there may be restrictions made on their ability to give consent to medical treatment.

Consent and decision-making

The law sets limits on parental authority and parents may not jeopardise the safety of their infant. When it comes to parental consent to medical treatment, there are a number of considerations:

- In the majority of cases, lawful consent to treatment is required from only one parent. If there is disagreement between the parents it is deemed good practice to address both parents' concerns relating to the treatment.
- In cases where there are differing views regarding treatment decisions between health professionals and parents, and it is unclear what is in the child's best interests, the courts may be asked to decide. For example, in the case of the conjoined twins Mary and Jodie (Watt, 2000), the parents refused treatment on behalf of their infants, but clinicians believed that it was essential for the survival of at least one twin. The case was settled in the courts.
- Parents cannot force involved health professionals to provide certain treatments if the involved health professionals do not believe it to be clinically appropriate. Parents may seek a second opinion.

Paediatricians and neonatologists often claim for themselves the role of the infant's advocate. The growing acceptance of the patients' best interest standard as a criterion for decision-making can leave little consideration for the interests of other family members, and may reduce parental autonomy (Yeo, 1998; Emery, 2000). McHaffie and colleagues (2001) found that parents wanted to be given the opportunity and responsibility for decisions on the limitation of treatment. Withholding information for fear of upsetting parents could be seen as demonstrating a paternalistic approach. There are a number of reasons for keeping the responsibility of making the final decision with the consultant as nurses tend not to be the ones to decide to withdraw care. This is discussed more fully in Chapter 2.

Smith (1999) recommends a model for decision-making in the NNU, adapted from models of rational decision-making by Carroll and Johnson (1990) and Bond and Kendall (1990). Utilising the principles of the nursing process, it incorporates seven key stages. At each stage, active participation and interaction and a supportive approach with the parents is expected to ensure effective communication between staff and parents. The ultimate aim is to give care, which is individualised to meet the needs of the parents, and to ensure that their parental rights to information are upheld. As Emery (2000) highlights, neonatal nurses caring for infants have a legal responsibility to ensure that parents are given adequate information in a sensitive manner and in a way that they can understand.

Implications for practice
Neonatal nurses are in a prime position to assess the standard of the consent process and to address any deficiencies. Neonatal nurses need to consider not only the amount of information that is given to family members, but also the quality and depth of that information. This will enable parents to make informed decisions regarding the care of their infant. Parents should be provided with all available information in an impartial manner, and with the underlying rationale to back up the for-and-against of each individual treatment option (McHaffie *et al.*, 2001).

Family-focused care
Partnership with parents is a routine principle and philosophy of care for children in hospital. A philosophy of family-focused care requires considerable parental involvement, autonomy and control, in order for parents to become true partners, and to make informed decisions about the care and treatment of their infant. Many studies have examined the key components of, and antecedents for, this philosophy from both a parental and nursing perspective. These include partnership, negotiation, empowerment and models of care in practice (Gill, 1993; Valentine, 1998).

Enhancing technology
There is a potential conflict between the advances in health-care technology and the ability to achieve a family-focused care philosophy (Gordin and Johnson, 1999). Technology may contribute to the alienation of parents and can become an obstacle to human interaction (Cooper, 1993).

The neonatal nurse needs to encompass technological expertise within a family-focused care framework. This will ensure that parents feel involved, and supported in learning to care for their infant, while knowing that their infant is receiving the best technological care. It is imperative that any parent who is intimidated by the complex equipment of the NNU is reassured, to enable them to participate in the care of their sick infant. Several studies, largely focused on mothers, have highlighted the relinquished role of the parent as the primary care-giver as a key source of stress in the NNU (Lau and Morse, 1998; Holditch-Davis and Miles, 2000). This perceived loss of the parental role can affect a mother's ability to advocate and make decisions for her infant.

Parents can spend a lot of time at the cot-side. They should not be made to feel like redundant onlookers. They should be supported, educated and actively involved in the care of their infant, with a view to developing a cohesive independent family unit.

Implications for practice
Within an NNU environment, infants have the right to be seen as more than an extension of a vital piece of medical equipment. The clinical management of an infant can appear to be overwhelming. This may take precedence over the rights of the infant to be recognised as a new individual family member who needs to bond with its parents. By focusing on the infant and family, the neonatal nurse may encourage holding and touching, and participation in care decisions. This can overcome some of the dehumanising aspects and sources of parental stress that may be a facet of highly technological care.

Visiting
Contention exists when balancing the needs of nurses with the needs of parents (Griffin, 1998a, 1998b; Cuttini *et al.*, 1999). It is important to remember the needs and the rights of the infant to be part of a family. Neonatal infants are not owned by nurses or doctors but are key individuals within their own family. According to Griffin (1998b), 'It is ironic that we refer to parents as "visitors" when it is we who are truly visitors in the infant's life.' The Human Rights Act 1998 (Articles 8 and 11) may have an impact upon visitation policies.

Griffin (1998a) has commented that even where there is an 'open visiting policy', and visiting is not restricted, in reality parents experience some restrictions. Parents may be asked to leave the cot-side during doctor's rounds or some procedures, while new admissions are being made, or during nursing handover, under the pretext of patient confidentiality. Of course, the request may be legitimate, for example during busy periods, when other parents and nurses are talking (when confidential information may be overheard), and in some emergency situations. There are also inconsistencies as to who may stay overnight.

Within children's nursing it is common practice to include both the parents and the child within ward rounds and nursing handover. They are seen as vital participants and these opportunities allow them to participate actively in decision-making, impart their own information, gather information and communicate their own views. Yeo (1998) believes that parents should be seen as partners in the care of their infants and must be kept informed and updated, and be given choices of treatment regimes. In this way, parental autonomy may be achieved.

Restrictions are sometimes placed on the number of visitors, other than nursing and medical staff, that an infant may receive, and on the relationship of those visitors to the infant. Parents, however, have rights to choose who should visit their infant and when. In today's society, there are many different models of the family unit. To ensure a truly family-focused philosophy, siblings should be encompassed within the visiting policies. Families should be able to determine if they wish their other children to visit the infant. A study by Smith (1998) highlighted restrictions placed upon sibling visitation, with one NNU not allowing siblings under the age of five to visit and another not allowing siblings under two. Unless the siblings are ill, which would be truly against the best interests of all the infants in the NNU, restrictions should not be placed upon sibling visits. Play areas and toys may help to focus sibling activities or behaviour on the ward.

Implications for practice
In order to support parents effectively, neonatal nurses must understand their experiences, anxieties and sources of stress. This will enable them to develop effective strategies and policies. Parents should be seen as key participants within the care of their infant and need to be allowed to be with their infant when they wish. With good communication and information-giving practices there are no reasonable grounds for restricting visitation.

NEONATAL WELFARE AND PROTECTION ISSUES IN PRACTICE

Views of child protection, both within the public and among professionals, have altered in recent years. Following the publication of *Messages from Research* (DoH, 1997b) and *Childhood Matters* (National Commission of Inquiry into the Prevention of Child Abuse, 1997), there has been a national debate termed 're-focusing'. There has been overwhelming support for a move towards a more preventative approach to the problem of child abuse. This needs to be achieved without placing vulnerable children at an increased risk of harm.

Sources of stress within families may have a negative impact upon a child's health, development and well-being. This may be direct, or because the stressors affect the capacity of a parent to respond to their child's needs (DoH, 1999). Sources of stress may include social exclusion, domestic violence, mental illness of a parent/carer, and drug or alcohol misuse (DoH, 1999). Polnay (2001) has suggested that teenage motherhood, single parenthood and prematurity increase the risk. A sick infant may itself act as an increased source of stress.

To protect children from potential abuse, professionals must identify a situation in which a particular family or a particular adult poses a risk to a child. Action must then be taken within a multi-agency framework to prevent the risk of abuse occurring.

Impact on parenting of parental mental health, alcohol and drug misuse and domestic violence

There are many ways in which parental mental health, alcohol and drug misuse and domestic violence can impact upon a parent's ability to look after their child (Cleaver *et al.*, 2000). These include the following:

- parenting skills;
- parents' perceptions;
- control of emotions;
- neglect of physical needs;
- attachment;
- separation.

Social factors, which may arise as a result of the above, may indirectly affect the outcomes for the neonate. Social consequences identified by Cleaver and colleagues (2000) include the impact of poor living standards, the loss of friends and family, and the disruption of family relationships.

Domestic violence

The Department of Health has defined domestic violence as physical, sexual or emotional abuse inflicted on a spouse or partner by the other partner (National Health Service Executive, 1997). Several studies have identified the fact that in approximately 50% of child protection referrals, or children's care proceedings at court, domestic violence was an issue (Farmer and Owen, 1995; NSPCC, 1997).

Indicators of domestic violence have been identified as having physical, emotional and behavioural characteristics. (*See* Table 3.3).

Table 3.3   *Indicators of domestic violence*

Physical indicators	Behavioural indicators	Emotional indicators
• Unexplained injuries • Inappropriate injuries • Injuries to chest, breast and abdomen • Injuries to face, neck or head • Frequent use of analgesia • Evidence of sexual abuse	• Evasive, frightened • Denial or minimisation of partner violence • Reluctance to disagree with or speak in front of partner • Partner remains close and answers all questions	• Feelings of isolation • Panic attacks/anxiety/depression • Suicidal attempts • Alcohol or drug abuse • Frequent use of tranquillisers

From National Health Service Executive (1997), with permission

Maternal/parental mental health

Brockington (1999) confirmed that there is an association between obstetric complications and child abuse. Maternal mental health problems could incorporate the following:

- post-natal blues;
- post-natal depression;
- puerperal psychosis;
- fictitious or fabricated illness by proxy (Munchausen syndrome by proxy);
- infanticide.

Post-natal depression (PND) has been linked to behavioural and psychological problems in the infants of these mothers (DoH, 1999). Post-natal depression occurs in approximately 15–20% of women with its peak onset at between two and four weeks post delivery (Scottish Executive Health Department, 1996). Through parent–nurse interactions, neonatal nurses are in a prime position for identifying post-natal depression in mothers. Warning signs include lack of energy and excessive anxiety about an infant's health. The mother may question her parenting abilities and appear to lack confidence in holding or feeding the infant. Physical symptoms include sleep disturbance and depression. The mother may also express suicidal thoughts or fears of harming the infant. For guidelines on detection and management of post-natal depression, *see* Appendix I and refer to the Edinburgh Post-natal Depression Scale (Scottish Executive Health Department, 1996).

Falkov (1996) has suggested that the majority of fatal child abuse cases occur within families where there is parental mental illness. Although not all parents with a mental health problem pose a danger to their infant, a risk assessment needs to be undertaken. Weir and Douglas (1999) identified the following risk factors to children of parents with a mental health problem:

- withdrawal from social contact;
- parental detachment;
- neglect and failure to thrive;
- inconsistent and manipulative parenting strategies;
- difficulty in managing difficult or distressed infants;
- potential threat of or violent act.

For a detailed analysis of the issues, dilemmas and practice implications of parental mental illness upon child welfare and protection, *see* Weir and Douglas (1999).

Alcohol and drug abuse

Drug or alcohol use by parents does not automatically indicate child neglect or abuse. However, a comprehensive assessment of the relationship between the infant and parental alcohol and drug use and child care is indicated. The potential risks associated with alcohol and drug misuse include:

- foetal alcohol syndrome causing central nervous system (CNS) damage (Abel, 1997);
- abortion and neonatal deaths (RCP, 1995);
- pre-term delivery and low birthweights (Martinez *et al.*, 1999);
- infants born addicted to drugs;
- transmission of HIV with intravenous drug use (Pratt, 1999);
- complications with withdrawal from drugs (Plant, 1997).

Cleaver *et al.* (2000) have suggested that physical abuse is commonly associated with excessive alcohol use by the father, while maternal drinking has been more frequently linked to neglect. A study undertaken by the NSPCC (1997) concluded that, in two out of three calls to their services reporting neglect, the parent was using drugs or alcohol.

Neonates exposed to alcohol and drugs in utero can suffer a wide range of short-term and long-term side-effects. It has been identified that there is an increased risk of abuse and neglect for infants who exhibit symptoms of drug and alcohol withdrawal. This is heightened if combined with the emotional instability of a mother who is still dependent (Ohio Research Institute, 1992). Neonatal nurses are in an ideal position to ascertain whether the mother is still using drugs and, if so, to offer assistance to the mother in order to address the problem. An awareness of community resources, referral mechanisms and an integrated approach to the family will produce a better outcome for the infant (Reinarz and Ecord, 1999).

If a neonate is being screened for exposure to drug abuse, it is essential that the social services department is notified, along with a member of the liaison health visiting team. This allows them the opportunity to develop a relationship with the family and gather background information even before the result is known. *See Drug-using Parents: Policy Guidelines for Inter-agency Working* (Standing Conference on Drug Abuse, 1997) for specific guidance relating to drug-using parents.

Low-birthweight infants
Intrinsic factors within a neonate may also make them more vulnerable to abuse by their parents/carers. Low-birthweight infants can be less responsive to parenting efforts than those who have reached full term (Miles and Holditch-Davis, 1995). This may provide a negative perception of the infant. Immature behavioural cues are more difficult to interpret – there may be less frequent smiling, increased irritability and an inability to regulate distress when compared with full-term infants (Sachs *et al.*, 1999).

Teenage mothers
A teenage parent in the NNU is in a transitional state of adolescence to adulthood and childhood to motherhood, and this can stimulate a crisis. Adolescent pregnancy causes an early transition to parenthood. Coupled with the biological and psychological transformation of adolescence, this can present enormous challenges to the adolescent parent, their families and society (Schulenberg *et al.*, 1999). Parenthood for teenagers can cause disruptions to peer relationships and to education, and can lead to conflicts with family members.

Teenage parenthood has received a great deal of attention in the USA and the UK, where rates are high. Research tends to focus on the inadequacies of teenagers to parent as effectively as older mothers (Richardson, 1999; Payne, 2001). However, the skills and abilities of adolescent parents may be overlooked. It is clear that, given appropriate support, adolescents can be effective mothers and fathers. It is imperative that practitioners concentrate upon strategies that facilitate parenting skills among young people, rather than emphasising their limitations.

Neonatal nurses can play an active role in bringing about a positive resolution to this new role by facilitating adjustment through support systems, and encouraging participation in decision-making and care-giving practices.

Implications for practice
Certain factors within the parents and the neonate can serve as 'key indicators'. These should alert neonatal nurses to the special needs of families that may place the neonate or other children within the family at risk of harm.

Neonatal nurses are able to use their skills and knowledge to identify vulnerable families and infants. They can plan interventions that will reduce or eliminate any risks, before and after discharge. Neonatal care needs to be focused on the best interest for the infant while at the same time supporting the family. Neonatal nurses also need to widen their sense of professional responsibility. It should be remembered that other children besides the infant in the NNU, for example the infant's siblings, could also be at risk from adult members.

CHILD PROTECTION

National structure

The most important legislation underpinning the protection of children is The Children Act 1989 (DoH, 1991a). Sections 17 and 47 relate to the welfare and safety of children. Section 17 outlines the general responsibilities that local authorities have to safeguard and promote the welfare of children in need. Section 47 pertains to the statutory duty that local authorities have in investigating where there are reasons to suspect a child may be suffering, or may be at risk of suffering significant harm. Local authorities are granted the power to request assistance from other professionals and agencies. All health professionals, including neonatal practitioners, are statutorily obligated to co-operate with social services and to share information regarding an infant in their care. This includes significant information relating to the parents, carers and other adults who may pose a risk to the infant or other children within the family.

Working Together to Safeguard Children (DoH, 1999) explains how agencies and professional groups should work together in a multi-agency framework to promote children's welfare and protect them from abuse and neglect. The guidance reflects the principles contained within the UN Convention on the Rights of the Child and is informed by the requirements in The Children Act 1989.

Working Together to Safeguard Children (DoH, 1999) is split into several key sections, outlined in Table 3.4.

Local structures

Each local authority has an Area Child Protection Committee (ACPC). These have key strategic responsibilities for safeguarding and protecting children within their local area. The local ACPC comprises representatives from the local authority, the lead child protection agency, social services department, police, health, education, probation and voluntary services.

One of several key responsibilities of the ACPC is the development of local child protection procedures, outlining the professional responsibilities of individuals and the actions required when concerns are raised regarding a child's welfare and safety.

Table 3.4   *Implications for neonatal nurses of Working Together to Safeguard Children*

Working Together to Safeguard Children	Key issues raised	Implications for neonatal practitioners
Working together to support children and families	• Emphasises the shared responsibility and need to work within a multi-agency framework to support families and safeguard children	• Need to recognise role in relation to the broader remit of child protection/welfare and the need to work co-operatively with other agencies
Lessons from research and experience	• Impact of abuse and neglect; concept of significant harm; sources of stress for children and families	• Need to acknowledge preventative as well as protective role in child protection, recognising issues within an adult parent/carer that can affect their ability to care for their infant, or can pose a risk for their infant
Roles and responsibilities	• Main role of each statutory agency and their responsibilities towards safeguarding children	• Need to be aware and appreciate roles and responsibilities of other agencies and the need for joint working
Area Child Protection Committees handling individual cases	• Outlines the role and responsibilities of the ACPC and its key membership • Sets out clear expectations about the ways in which agencies and professionals should act if they have concerns about a child's welfare or fear that the child is at risk of abuse	• Need to be aware of health authority representatives: named doctor and named nurse • Need to be aware of local child protection procedures, processes, responsibilities and key professionals available for advice and support
Child protection in specific circumstances	• Children living away from home; Protection of Children Act 1999 and allegations of abuse by a professional; abuse of disabled children; investigating organised or multiple abuse and abuse by children and young people; child prostitution and internet pornography	• Recruitment and selection practices; local procedures for special circumstances
Some key principles	• Working in partnership with children and families; race, ethnicity and culture; sharing information; record-keeping; support, supervision and professional guidance	• Standard of record-keeping; disclosure of information; multi-agency working
Case reviews	• Purpose of, reason for and management of a review	• Day-to-day good practice; record-keeping; implementing recommendations
Inter-agency training and development	• Determining audience, levels and outcomes of training and the systems for its delivery and evaluation	• Attend relevant inter-agency training

Table 3.5 *Neonatal practice examples of child protection roles and responsibilities*

Role (DoH, 1999)	Neonatal practice example
• Recognising children in need of support and/or safeguarding, and parents who may need extra help in bringing up their children	• Recognising risk factors within an adult carer: mental health, domestic violence, drug and alcohol misuse, families in crisis
• Contributing to enquiries about a child and family	• Participating in requests for assistance from social services and other child protection agencies
• Assessing the needs of children and the capacity of parents to meet their children's needs	• Discharge planning and parental education and co-ordination of continuing support and follow-up; recognising responsibilities to child visitors to the unit
• Planning and providing support to vulnerable children and families	• Domestic violence; discharge planning and co-ordination
• Participating in child protection conferences	• Providing views and evidence of parents' capacity to meet their infants' needs; documentation
• Planning support for children at risk of significant harm	• Discharge education and co-ordination of continuing care and support services post discharge
• Providing therapeutic help to abused children and parents under stress	• Initiation of support services and providing ongoing care that is participative in nature and non-judgemental
• Playing a part, through child protection plan, in safeguarding children from significant harm	• Neonates on the unit that are under an emergency protection order
• Contributing to case reviews	• Ensuring clear and accurate record-keeping to facilitate reviews

Working Together to Safeguard Children (DoH, 1999) clearly states the responsibility of the health providers within the field of child protection. It also highlights the importance of the role that health professionals have at all stages of work with children and their families. Table 3.5 explains these key roles, and gives examples of how they may relate to neonatal practice.

The *Framework for the Assessment of Children in Need and their Families* (DoH, 2000a) (*see* Figure 3.1, page 50) provides a systematic basis for collecting and analysing information. This is to support professional judgements of how to help children and their families in the best interest of the child. Although the framework is to be used by social services for the assessment of all children in need, it could be utilised by neonatal nurses to guide and inform their judgements about a neonate's welfare and safety.

Child Protection Register

The principal purpose of the Child Protection Register is to make agencies and professionals aware of those children who are judged to be at continuing risk of significant harm and in need of active safeguarding (DoH, 1999). The social services department on behalf of the ACPC maintains the Child Protection Register.

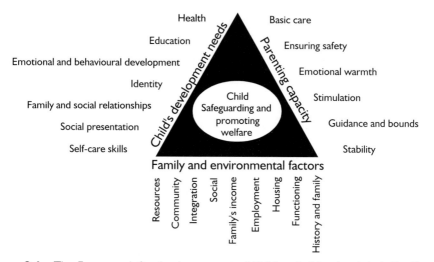

Figure 3.1 The Framework for the Assessment of Children in Need and their Families
From DOH (2000a), with permission

Any qualified health professional, police officer, social worker or designated education employee can seek access to the register. It is essential that health professionals and police can have access to the register outside office hours. Neonatal nurses need to be familiar with the procedure used to access the register, both within and outside office hours.

Procedures

Child protection procedures apply to all children under the age of 18 within the area that the local ACPC represents. Although there will be a local interpretation of the framework outlined in *Working Together to Safeguard Children* (DoH, 1999), procedures will be similar throughout the country. Individual Trust guidelines reflecting the local ACPC child protection procedures should identify referral procedures and specific details. This includes telephone numbers and whom to contact for advice.

In all acute health-care organisations there is a mandatory requirement to have identified the lead professionals for child protection, a named doctor and a named nurse/midwife (DoH, 1997a). These named professionals have clear roles and responsibilities for child protection. They are available to staff for support and advice regarding child protection or welfare concerns.

Neonatal practitioners should familiarise themselves with the local ACPC child protection procedures. They need to be aware of the services available at local level and know how to access them. Knowledge of when and how to make a child protection referral to the local authority social services department is required. Nurses need to be aware of who the key professional staff are, for communication, support and advice. In addition, they should know about their hospital's child protection and welfare documentation.

Key staff available within a local hospital will include some or all of the following:

- senior neonatal nursing and medical staff and senior staff who can be contacted out of hours;
- hospital-based social work team;
- children's liaison health visitor;
- named nurse/midwife/paediatrician with child protection responsibilities.

Emergency Protection Order

The courts may make an Emergency Protection Order (EPO) under Section 44 of The Children Act 1989. This may be issued if there is reasonable cause to believe that a child is likely to suffer significant harm if not removed from his or her present environment or not allowed to remain where he or she is safe.

If there are concerns that the infant's welfare will be at risk, a child protection conference will be undertaken before the infant is born. The outcome may state that when the infant is born, it will be placed under an EPO. An EPO places the child in protection for a maximum of eight days, with the possibility of an extension of a further seven days. A parent can appeal against this order after a period of 72 hours. If an infant is placed under an EPO, the neonatal practitioner needs to ensure effective communication and management of the child's welfare concerns. He or she should clarify the following issues with social services:

- any restrictions placed on parental visiting (for example, supervised access, or no access at all);
- any restrictions placed upon parental responsibility;
- any restrictions placed upon information to be shared with parents/carers;
- key observations that need to be recorded;
- key contacts in social services or the police if the infant is removed, or at risk of being removed.

Documentation

Accurate, clear documentation is required to facilitate multi-agency and disciplinary communication, and is useful for the preparation for child protection conferences and statements. The information contained in documentation may be vital for court appearances and Part 8 case reviews, when a case has involved a critical incident, perhaps leading to the death or near-death of a child. In such cases there is likely to be major public interest and the individual agencies will review all documentation and actions. A composite review is then produced by the Area Child Protection Committee.

Some key principles should be followed to ensure professional accountability is met:

- Concerns should be documented according to UKCC guidelines.
- Practitioners should be clear and accurate, and use body maps to document injuries or marks.

- Opinions or interpretations should be documented separately.
- In documenting professional communications, the name, designation, contact number and discussion details should be incorporated, along with the outcomes or decisions agreed, with the underpinning rationale.
- Records should be dated, timed and signed.
- A witness signature should be obtained if appropriate.
- Any referrals made in writing should be confirmed.

Communication with parents/carers

It is deemed good practice and a usual procedural requirement for parents to be notified when a referral is to be made to social services regarding a child welfare/protection issue. Within the hospital situation, a medical member of staff usually performs this act, as they normally instigate the referral process.

The Department of Health (1999) states the following:

While professionals should seek in general to discuss any concerns with the family and, where possible, seek their agreement to making referrals to social services, this should only be done where such discussion and agreement-seeking will not place a child at increased risk of significant harm.

This could be relevant in a case of suspected sexual abuse. If a 15-year-old teenage mother discloses to a nurse that the infant's father was also her uncle and that both he and her father took pornographic photographs of her, the nurse would not notify the teenager's parents that a referral was being made to social services, for fear of the following:

- the parent colluding with the perpetrator;
- pressure being placed on the teenage mother;
- evidence of abuse being obliterated.

CASE STUDY   SHAHID

Shahid is a 26-week gestation infant, who has been on the unit for 2 weeks. Over this time you have noticed that his father Kalhib has on three occasions smelt quite strongly of alcohol. Today you notice that Shahid's mother Sanitra has bruises on her face and arms. When you ask her what has happened, she breaks down in tears and informs you that Kalhib did it when he was drunk.

Response

- This is a welfare issue in view of the link between domestic violence and alcohol abuse with increased risk of child abuse and neglect.
- Kalhib poses a risk not only to Sanitra but also to Shahid and other children that he may care for.

Action

- Discuss with unit senior nurse and doctor.
- Check the Child Protection Register.
- Discuss concerns with liaison health visitor.
- Discuss with named nurse for child protection.
- Notify Sanitra of your concerns and tell her why you are referring to social services.
- Refer to social services.
- Record details of discussions.
- Follow up referral to ensure action has been taken.

CASE STUDY MARY

When Karen, the mother of 24-week gestation infant Mary, visits with her other daughter Josie you notice what you consider to be an adult slap mark on Josie's face. You discuss it with the paediatric registrar on the unit; the registrar's opinion is that, as Josie is not a patient, you should not interfere. However, you feel uncomfortable with this and wish to take further action.

Response

- For health professionals and for the hospital, there is a duty of care towards Josie as she is a minor.
- Nursing staff do not require the permission of medical staff to refer concerns regarding the welfare of an infant or child; it is routine good practice to do so.
- If there is a conflict of opinion and the nurse is still convinced the child is at risk or at potential risk, action must be taken.
- As there is a suspicion of non-accidental injury (NAI), and therefore a potential of further risk of harm, action is required and the nurse is accountable to take that action.

Action

To try to maintain good working relationships and communication the following actions should be taken:

- Discuss with senior member of staff.
- Check the Child Protection Register.
- Discuss with liaison health visitor.
- Discuss with named nurse/doctor for child protection.
- Notify Karen that you are referring to social services.

- Refer to social services.
- Record details of discussions.
- Follow up referral to ensure action has been taken.

IMPLICATIONS FOR NURSING PRACTICE

Effective child protection depends not only upon reliable and accepted systems of co-operation, but also on the skills, knowledge and judgement of all staff working with children. It is important that staff in direct contact with children receive training to raise their awareness of predisposing factors, signs and symptoms, and their knowledge of local child protection procedures (DoH, 1999).

Neonatal nurses need to be proactive in identifying the risks posed to infants by adults. They need to be aware of the indicators of abuse and become skilled in the detection of abuse. They need to maintain an up-to-date knowledge of local procedures and know to whom they can refer within their hospital. Above all they need to be prepared to refer to social services when they consider an infant or child to be at risk of harm.

REFERENCES

Abel, E.L. (1997) Maternal alcohol consumption and spontaneous abortion, *Alcohol and alcoholism* **32**(3), 211–19

Alderson, P. (1999) Did children change, or the guidelines?, *Bulletin of Medical Ethics* **150**, 38–40

Alderson, P. (2000) *Young Children's Rights: Exploring Beliefs, Principles and Practices*, Jessica Kingsley, London

Allmark, P., Mason, S., Gill, B.A. and Megone, C. (2001) Is it in a neonate's best interest to enter a randomised control trial? *Journal of Medical Ethics* **27**, 110–13

Bond, M. and Kendall, S. (1990) *Improving your Decision-making Workbook*, Distance Learning Centre, South Bank Polytechnic, London

British Medical Association (2001) *Consent, Rights and Choices in Health Care for Children and Young People*, BMJ Books, London

Brockington, I. (1999) *Motherhood and Mental Health*, Oxford University Press, Oxford

Brooks, M. (1999) Pain and the pre-term infant: mechanisms and management, *Journal of Neonatal Nursing* **5**(4), 27–33

Carbajal, R., Chauvet, X., Coulderac, S. and Olivier-Martin, M. (1999) Randomised trial of analgesic effects of sucrose, glucose and pacifiers in term neonates, *BMJ,* **319**, 1393–97

Carroll, J.S. and Johnson, E.J. (1990) *Decision Research: A Field Guide*, Sage, California, IL

Charles-Edwards, I. (2001) Children's nurses and advocacy: are we in a muddle? *Paediatric Nursing* **13**(2), 12–16

Charlton, A.J. (1999) Assessment of post-operative pain in neonates: a survey of nurses' practice, *Journal of Neonatal Nursing* **5**(5), 21–3

Charlton, A.J. (2000) Pain indicators in postoperative neonates: a study of nurses' preferences, *Journal of Neonatal Nursing* 6(2), 41–2

Cleaver, H., Unell, I. and Aldgate, J. (2000) *Children's Needs – Parenting Capacity: The Impact of Parental Mental Illness, Problem Alcohol and Drug Use, and Domestic Violence on Children's Development*, Department of Health, London

Cooper, M.A. (1993) The intersection of technology and care in the ICU, *Advances in Nursing Science* 15(3), 23–32

Cuttini, M., Rebagliato, M., Bortoli, P. *et al.* (1999) Parental visiting, communication and participation in ethical decisions: a comparison of neonatal unit policies in Europe, *Archives of Disease in Childhood* 81(2), 84–91

Department of Health [DoH] (1991a) *The Children Act 1989: An introductory guide for the NHS*, HMSO, London

DoH (1991b) *Welfare of Children and Young People in Hospital*, HMSO, London

DoH (1994) *The Allitt Inquiry*, HMSO, London

DoH (1996) *The Patient's Charter: Services for Children and Young People*, HMSO, London

DoH (1997a) *Child Protection: Guidance for Senior Nurses, Health Visitors, and Midwives and their Managers*, HMSO, London

DoH (1997b) *Messages from Research*, HMSO, London

DoH, Home Office, Department for Education and Employment (1999) *Working Together to Safeguard Children: A Guide to Inter-agency Working to Safeguard and Promote the Welfare of Children*, The Stationery Office, London

DoH (1999) *The Protection of Children Act*, Stationery Office, London

DoH (2000a) *Framework for the Assessment of Children in Need and their Families*, The Stationery Office, London

DoH (2000b) *Protecting Children, Supporting Parents: A Consultation Document on the Physical Punishment of Children*, The Stationery Office, London

Emery, M. (2000) Informed consent: keeping parents in the picture, *Journal of Neonatal Nursing* 6(3), 90–2

Falkov, A. (1996) *Working Together, Part 8 Reports: Fatal Child Abuse and Parental Psychiatric Disorders*, HMSO, London

Farmer, E. and Owen, A. (1995) *Child Protection Practice: Private Risks and Public Remedies*, HMSO, London

Fulton, Y. (1996) Children's rights and the role of the nurse, *Paediatric Nursing* 8(10), 29–31

Gill, K.M. (1993) Health professionals' attitudes toward parent participation in hospitalised children's care, *Children's Health Care* 22(4), 257–71

Gordin, P. and Johnson, B.H. (1999) Technology and family-centred perinatal care: conflict or synergy, *JOGGN* 28(4), 401–7

Griffin, T. (1998a) The visitation policy, *Neonatal Network* 17(2), 75–6

Griffin, T. (1998b) Visitation patterns: the parents who visit 'too much', *Neonatal Network*, 17(7), 66–8

Holditch-Davis, D. and Miles, M.S. (2000) Mothers' stories about their experiences in the neonatal intensive care unit, *Neonatal Network* 19(3), 13–22

The Human Rights Act 1998 (2000) The Stationery Office, London

Johnson, C.C., Stevens, B.J., Franck, L.S., Jack, A., Stemler, R. and Platt, R. (1999) Factors explaining a lack of response to heel stick in preterm newborns, *JOGGN*, Nov/Dec, 587–94

Lau, R. and Morse, C. (1998) Experiences of parents with premature infants hospitalised in neonatal intensive care units: a literature review, *Journal of Neonatal Nursing* 4(6), 23–9

Leach, P. (1999) *The Physical Punishment of Children: Some Input from Recent Research*, NSPCC, London

Long, T. (1998) Prerequisites for neonatal nursing and specialist practice: children should be nursed by qualified child health nurses, *Journal of Neonatal Nursing* 4(3), 17–20

Manning, D.J. (2000) Presumed consent in emergency neonatal research, *Journal of Medical Ethics* 26(4), 249–53

Martinez, A., Kastner, B. and Taeush, H.W. (1999) Hyperphagia in neonates withdrawing from methadone, *Archives of Disease in Childhood* 80(3), 178–82

McHaffie, H.E., Laing, I.A., Parker, M. and McMillan, J. (2001) Deciding for imperilled newborns: medical authority or parental autonomy, *Journal of Medical Ethics* 27, 104–9

McHale, J., Gallager, A. and Mason, I. (2001) The UK Human Rights Act 1998: implications for nurses, *Nursing Ethics* 8(3) 223–33

Miles, M.S. and Holditch-Davis, D. (1995) Compensatory parenting: how mothers describe parenting their 3-year-old, prematurely born children, *Journal of Paediatric Nursing* 10(4), 243–51

National Commission of Inquiry into the Prevention of Child Abuse (1997) *Childhood Matters*, The Stationery Office, London

National Health Service Executive (1997) *Domestic Violence*, Department of Health, HMSO, London

National Health Service Executive (1998) *Children's Safeguard Review: Choosing with Care*, HSC/212, HMSO, London

National Health Service Executive (2000) *West Midlands: Report of a Review of the Research Framework in Staffordshire Hospital NHS Trust (Griffiths Inquiry)*, NHSE, Birmingham

Newson, J. and Newson, E. (1989) *The Extent of Parental Physical Punishment in the UK*, APPROACH, London

Noyes, J. (2000) Are nurses respecting and upholding the human rights of children and young people in their care? *Paediatric Nursing* 12(2), 23–7

NSPCC (1997) Drunk in charge: substance abuse, *Community Care*, NSPCC, London

Ohio Research Institute on Child Abuse Prevention (1992) *Don't Shake the Baby*, League Against Child Abuse, Westerville, OH

Payne, D. (2001) Babies of teenage mothers 60% more likely to die, *BMJ*, 322–86

Plant, M. (1997) *Women and Alcohol: Contemporary and Historical Perspectives*, Free Association Books, London

Polnay, J. (2001) *Child Protection in Primary Care*, Radcliffe Medical Press, Oxon

Pratt, R. (1999) Perinatal HIV infection in 1999: effective preventative strategies, *Journal of Neonatal Nursing* 5(2), 37–41

RCP (1995) *Alcohol and the Young*, Royal Laversham Press, London

Royal College of Paediatrics and Child Health (1999) *Safeguarding Informed Parental Involvement in Clinical Research Involving Newborn Babies and Infants: A Position Statement*, RCPCH, London

Reinarz, S.E. and Ecord, J.S. (1999) Drug-of-abuse testing in the neonate, *Neonatal Network* 18(8), 55–60

Richardson, K.K. (1999) Adolescent pregnancy and substance use, *JOGGN* 28(6), 623–7

Roberts, M. (2000) Protecting children, supporting parents: government consultation on physical punishment, *Child Right*, 163, 3–5

Robinson, J. (1998) Was it informed? Was it consent? Lessons from the ECMO trial, *British Journal of Midwifery*, 6(3), 175

Royal College of Nursing (1999) *The Recognition and Assessment of Pain in Children*, RCN Publishing, London

Royal College of Nursing (2001) *Developing an Effective Clinical Governance Framework for Children in Acute Healthcare Services*, RCN Publishing, London

Royal College of Paediatrics and Child Health Ethics Advisory Committee (2000) Guidelines for the ethical conduct of medical research involving children, *Archives of Disease in Childhood* 82(2), 177–82

Sachs, B., Hall, L.A., Lutenbacher, M. and Rayens, M.K. (1999) Potential for abusive parenting by rural mothers with low birthweight children, *Image: Journal of Nursing Scholarship* 31(1), 21–5

Schulenberg, J., Maggs, J.L. and Hurrelmann, K. (1999) *Health Risks and Development Transitions During Adolescence*, Cambridge, UK

Scottish Executive Health Department (1996) *Report on Detection and Early Intervention in Post-natal Depression*, Clinical Resource and Audit Group (CRAG), Edinburgh

Secretary of State for Health (1998) *The Government's Response to the Children's Safeguard Review*, The Stationery Office, London

Smith, L. (1999) Family-centred decision-making: a model for parent participation, *Journal of Neonatal Nursing* 5(6), 31–3

Smith, M.B.E. (1998) A study of facilities for siblings on the neonatal unit: enhancing family care, *Journal of Neonatal Nursing* 4(5), 18–22

Sparshott, M. (1998) Pain and the foetus: the case for analgesia during invasive procedures, *Journal of Neonatal Nursing* 4(4), 21–3

Standing Conference on Drug Abuse (1997) *Drug-using Parents: Policy Guidelines for Inter-agency Working*, Local Government Drugs Forum, London

Twycross, A., Moriarty, A. and Betts, T. (1998) *Paediatric Pain Management*, Radcliffe Medical Press, Oxon

United Kingdom Central Council (1997) *Specialist Practitioner Qualification* [letter] Dpd/cp/letters/specprac, 10 September 1997, UKCC, London

United Nations (1989) *Convention on the Rights of the Child*, UNGA, Geneva

Valentine, F.A. (1998) Empowerment – family-centered care, *Paediatric Nursing* 10(1), 24–7

Veerman, P. (1992) *The Rights of the Child and the Changing Image of Childhood*, Martinus Nijhoff, Dordrecht

Watt, B. (2000) Justified murder? The separation of Jodie and Mary, *Child Right*, 171, 8–10

Weir, A. and Douglas, A. (1999) *Child Protection and Adult Mental Health: Conflict of Interest?* Butterworth Heinemann, Oxford

Willow, C. and Hyder, T. (1998) *It Hurts You Inside: Children Talking About Smacking*, National Children's Bureau/Save the Children, London

Yeo, H. (1998) Informed consent in the neonatal unit: the ethical and legal rights of parents, *Journal of Neonatal Nursing* 4(4), 17–20

4 Play for the Neonatal Infant

Tina Clegg

Aims of the chapter

This chapter introduces the neonatal nurse to the complex developmental needs of the infants in their care. It illustrates how the neonatal unit's environment is potentially damaging and how appropriate stimulation can be built into the neonate's day. As always, the parents and families should be regarded as partners in care. The way the infant is accepted into the family is crucial to the ongoing development of the individual and to the health of the entire family.

INTRODUCTION

Neonatal infants are complex in their needs. Advances in neonatology have resulted in increasing numbers of infants surviving their early traumas. They go on to spend a considerable amount of time in an NNU during their early formative period, before being discharged home. These early experiences are far from the normal ones that would be enjoyed by a new family member. The stimulation, touch, sounds and smells of a hospital, coupled with the medical and nursing interventions and the separation, are powerful influences on infants and on their families.

The developmental and play needs of infants are an essential element of neonatal care. Pre-term or sick infants have many disadvantages in the development process. If these disadvantages are exaggerated by a lack of stimulation, or by inappropriate stimulation, this can lead to further delay. Play that is assessed, organised and evaluated can be one of the ways in which the developmental care and the active participation of the families can be of benefit to all.

NEONATAL INFANT DEVELOPMENT

An understanding of the developmental milestones of infants, through the first six months of life, is essential in providing care. This needs to take into account developmentally sequenced progression. The infant's play needs should not be deferred. Deprivations in the developmental process can occur, depending on the experiences to which infants are exposed (Swanwick, 1990).

Development can be described as a process of continuous change; sometimes it is fast-paced and obvious and, at other times, it is slow and difficult to see. Developmental change is not haphazard but proceeds in an orderly fashion throughout life. All the infant's knowledge about the world comes through the senses of sight, hearing, taste, smell and touch. The sixth sense is proprioception, which tells the infant about the location of the mobile parts of the body, the legs and hands and their relationship to the rest of the body (Sylva and Lunt, 1990).

Developmental care in the neonatal unit is a philosophy that directs and forms the foundation for care provided for high-risk infants and their families. There are two main goals (Peters, 1999):

1 to decrease infant disruptions and handling by care-givers;
2 to modulate the infant's responses to the care they receive, in order to support each infant.

Early foetal and newborn experiences affect subsequent development in profound and long-lasting ways. Developmental care encompasses all care procedures as well as social and physical aspects in the NNU. An infant's physiological parameters and behavioural expressions in response to stimuli can be seen as a constant and reliable guide for care-givers (Peters, 1999). A plan of care can then be formulated and implemented to meet the needs of the individual infant. This will enhance each infant's opportunities without becoming a source of stress.

An infant's world is restricted to that which is provided by adults. There may be positive and negative experiences, and adults may have influence on the infant's environment in terms of temperature, light, noise, smell, taste, handling and positioning. All infants are individuals and will present a variety of challenges and opportunities to the health-care team looking after them.

The most vulnerable group of survivors is infants with extreme prematurity of less than 28 weeks gestation and extremely low birthweight (less than 1000 grams). They have a significant risk of developmental problems. Only a small number of these infants have major disabilities such as cerebral palsy but follow-up studies of school-age children suggest that more than half will have some sort of difficulty. Learning difficulties, perceptual and motor co-ordination problems, attention deficits and language delay are all examples of the diverse problems that are common among these infants (Warren, 1998).

WHAT IS PLAY?

Play, as a single concept, is exceptionally difficult to define but has come to be recognised as a normal and essential requirement for a child's well-being and development. It is the primary medium through which children learn and make sense of their environment (Organisation Mondiale pour L'Education Prescolaire, 1989). The works of Freud, Groos, Piaget and Erikson offer the reader an opportunity to study the philosophies of play in more depth.

Article 31 of the UN Convention on the Rights of the Child states that every child has the right to rest and leisure, to engage in play and recreational activities appropriate to the age of the child. The Children Act 1989 recognises that children's need for good-quality play opportunities changes as they grow up, but that they need such opportunities throughout childhood in order to reach and maintain their optimum development and well-being.

The neonatal infant needs play that provides suitable opportunities to strengthen the body, improve the mind, develop personality and acquire social competence. It is therefore as necessary for a child as food, warmth and protective care (Sheridan, 1997). Play and appropriate stimulation can compensate for the interruption of uterine life and promote the development that would normally occur in the uterus following the normal maturation sequence (Kroner, 1990).

The provision of play can cause anxiety and confusion in the health-care team and parents. The interaction between the infant's medical, nursing and developmental needs has to be balanced with the infant's responses and behavioural changes. These need to be documented by all carers so that a clear picture of toleration and behavioural changes is presented.

Developing play skills

Play stimulates a variety of skills that are physical, cognitive, social and personal (Goldstein, 1995).

- *Physical skills* include agility, balance, hand and eye co-ordination, physical co-ordination/dexterity, and strength.
- *Cognitive skills* relate to attention spans, creativity, imagination, intelligence, language, logical thinking, numeracy, memory, planning, problem-solving, and reading.
- *Social skills* include communication, co-operation and sharing.
- *Personal skills* involve adjustment, emotional development, popularity, and social development.

The quiet infant is too often labelled the 'good baby' and is at risk of under-stimulation (Verzemnieks, 1984).

Working with parents

The most common worry that mothers have about the future relates to their infant's development (Reid, 2000). Parents are very keen to support the developmental progression of their infant. One of the primary objectives of play specialists should be to encourage parents to be involved in their infant's play and to understand the value and consistency of the kind of care that only the parents can give (Reynolds, 1993). It is important to involve parents in all aspects of play, right from the early discussions of the need. The parents should be involved with the assessment of play needs, the planning and implementing of play activities, and the evaluating and recording of play, as well as monitoring the developmental progression. As partners in care they can have an active part in the delivery of play and help promote a normalising activity.

Play specialists can be involved in introducing siblings to the new infant. Using their skills, they can prepare the siblings for the alien and sometimes distressing world of the NNU as well as the events and procedures that the family will share. They can work with the older child to develop play opportunities that will eventually form part of the infant's play experiences. Hospital visits should be a positive experience for siblings.

PLAY PROGRAMMES

The outcome for low-birthweight infants could be improved by the provision of early developmental support through stimulation and play. Such a programme should be based on theory, be dynamic in nature and respect the infant's unique behavioural organisation, maternal child interaction and parenting needs (Wolke, 1991).

Play specialists use play programmes that are care plans for play and developmental sequencing. Like nursing care, many different models can used but these need to be based on the nursing notes and be accessible to the healthcare team.

PLAY AND DEVELOPMENT

Play and development sequences can be written under sub-headings or focuses:

- Sight
- Hearing
- Social interaction
- Oral stimulation
- Positioning
- Handling and touch
- Emotional care.

Sight

Sylva and Lunt (1990) cite the research by Frantz and describes how term infants just one week after birth showed a preference for more complex patterns when compared with simpler ones. Both patterns were shown at a distance of 10 inches. This research also suggested that infants preferred to look at real faces rather than face patterns.

To enhance the sight development of infants, using black and white pictures of simple and complex designs printed on cards and placed in the infant's field of vision can be helpful (Figure 4.1). They need to be used on a sessional basis

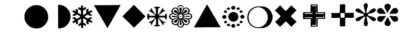

Figure 4.1   Pattern cards to stimulate the development of sight

allowing the infant to focus on and off these highly stimulating patterns. Parents and siblings could be involved in making these cards, which can be laminated if necessary to meet infection control policies.

Close face-to-face contact between the parents and infants (or photographs of their faces) can be used to aid visual stimulation. Attractive toys and mobiles can be used but these have to be in the field of vision and not at the end of the cot. They also need to be changed on a regular basis so that the infant does not get bored with the same view.

Example of a play and development plan designed to stimulate vision
The play therapist's aim would be to develop and encourage fixing and focusing. The designed activities would include:

- black and white pictures of simple and complex patterns in the infant's field of vision;
- close face-to-face contact with the infant, gaining eye contact, using different facial expressions and waiting for a response;
- photographs of the faces of family members.

An evaluation would take into account the way that the infant fixed and focused on the simple black and white pictures for a few seconds. Discussion with the parents would examine the extent to which the infant fixed on the parents' faces and held eye contact for several minutes. The evaluation would also include the extent to which they observed different facial expressions that mirrored their own.

As the parents are partners in care and have access to the care plans, the play programmes will need to be phrased sensitively and diplomatically. They are written after assessing the stage of the infant's development. Care must be taken that the programme is written in a positive format and based on what the infant has already achieved developmentally. 'Eyes open' is a positive statement but 'infant not fixing and focusing' is negative. The latter suggests another problem for parents whose infant already has so many.

Regular reviews and new developmental targets are essential, as progress will take place, even if this is slow or at times regressed due to the infant's medical condition. Evaluations of each play session need to be made so that a clear picture of the play input and developmental progress can be recorded. Parents should be encouraged to record their input into the evaluation, thereby gaining a sense of pride, and seeing the importance of their contribution to the infant's well-being.

On discharge, the parents will be confident about the developmental play required and their abilities to provide this. Parents' knowledge of child development and play will be enhanced along with good play skills and confidence.

Hearing

Hearing plays an important part in development. Infants need to develop the ability to hear and differentiate between sounds, to locate the direction of a sound, as well as to develop language and communication skills. When the perceptual abilities of newborn infants were tested by studying their reactions to sounds coming from various parts of the room, it was demonstrated that even a one-day-old infant attempted to look in the direction of the sound (Sylva and Lunt, 1990).

Infants in an NNU are exposed to a variety of external noises, including incubator fans, telephones, staff conversations and monitors (Purdy, 2000). Zahr and Balian (1995) found that covering incubators helped to reduce the exposure to outside noise but sources of 'white noise' will remain. These will cover up crucial auditory input and may lead to sensory deprivation.

Opportunities must be found for the infant to listen to, and concentrate on, specific sounds. Time must be given for the infant to respond to the bewildering array of sound stimuli, to find their direction and pitch, and to obtain reward for successful listening. Patterns for later speech development of speaking, listening and turn-taking are established and practised in these early exchanges.

Social interaction

Social interaction in the well infant takes place from the first contact with the parents and then with other significant carers. With sick infants, this social interaction is compromised due to the medical and nursing interventions and medical status of the infant. Social interaction is one of the important aims of the play specialist in supporting parents to play and bond with their infant. The reward of the first smile is a major developmental milestone for all parents. Infants in neonatal units need positive social interaction from all carers and not just delivery of care.

Oral stimulation

Oral stimulation is a challenge to all involved in neonatal care. Many pre-term infants have never developed the sucking response, and ventilated and naso-gastric-fed infants have not had the opportunity to practise sucking. Sucking is a complex set of actions, with taste, texture, smell and volume all being involved (along with breathing) in an area of the body where the infant has already experienced many unpleasant sensations. Oral stimulation is needed through play to introduce and encourage positive experiences. The cheeks and lips can be stroked and the infant's tongue can be gently pushed. The fingers or a dummy can be sucked. Taste, with a dummy, teat or spoon, can be gradually introduced with gentle encouragement and patience.

If breast-feeding is to be introduced, stroking of the lips, upper and lower gums with the nipple from the back to midline and stroking the infant's cheek with a finger may help the process along.

Positioning

Pre-term infants have poorly modulated muscle tone. Their movements tend to be disorganised and energy-consuming. They have difficulty working against gravity and tend to adapt to the shape of the surface on which they are placed. If nursed on a flat surface without support they may assume a flattened position. If allowed to persist, this may result in the characteristic postural pattern described as 'frog', which may interfere with development.

To encourage normal developmental patterns, the infant needs to be given opportunities to adopt flexed and tucked postures.

- Lying on the side is easiest for infants to adopt and stay in a flexed position. It helps them to succeed in self-calming strategies such as hand-to-hand, foot-to-foot and hand-to-mouth movements.
- The prone position may assist with breathing and the reduction of reflux. Infants are often more settled on their fronts than on their backs. They may move less, cry less and lose less heat.
- The supine position may be necessary for medical reasons. It is in this position that most heat and energy are lost and the infant finds it more difficult to control movements and to adopt a tucked position due to the effects of gravity (Warren, 1998).

There are many aids available to support the infant in a variety of positions and regular changes of position are required to maximise developmental opportunities.

Handling and touch

Handling and touching are vital for the infant's satisfactory development, although a balance must be struck so that handling is interspersed with periods of rest. Touch sensations are among the earliest to develop during gestation and ultimately provide stimulation, organisation, communication and emotional exchange (Montague, 1986). For term infants, touch is essential in the establishment of nurturing, protective attachment and relationships with the primary care-giver. This in turn establishes the foundation for learning, emotional regulation and social interaction (Brown, 2000). The five main factors of touch and handling are frequency, distribution, duration, type of handling (comfort or task) and the person initiating the handling.

In the NNU, the physiological stress responses are relentlessly re-activated with over-handling, painful procedures and changes in temperature. In most cases, there is little positive input given to counteract the negative stimuli that these sick infants receive. All infants need some form of positive touch during their day (Bond, 1999). Bond cites Adamson Macede's study on positive tactile touch and shows that, when compared to a control group, children in this study at the age of seven years scored higher in all measures of intelligence and achievement. It was felt that touch therapy helped to reduce the stress of the NNU and to promote healthy brain development.

The model of 'gentle human touch' with infants is the placing of hands to contain the infant at the head and lower back and buttocks or abdomen taking care only to provide support not intermittent stimulation. The results of this study indicated few detrimental effects and suggested that, in the short term, infants had less behavioural distress, more quiet sleep and less motor activity during procedures (Harrison, 1996).

Parental involvement in touch programmes can be beneficial. It may help to bring parents and infants closer, improve handling skills, self-esteem and positive thinking. It may also help to allay feelings of guilt and helplessness (Bond, 1999). Parents may instinctively want to stroke their infant but the infant may not be able to tolerate so much stimulation. Holding offers a more appropriate way of touching that is rewarding and enjoyable to both the infant and the parent.

Rest is an important feature of normal growth and development. Ensuring periods of undisturbed time is significant for high-risk infants. More than four hours without interaction is abnormal, while periods of less than one hour are insufficient to complete the sleep cycle (Fenwick et al., 1999).

Holding the infant for the first time has been described by mothers as a significant event (Reid, 2000). However, for many of these mothers, this event is delayed owing to the condition of their infant. Kangaroo care is the positioning of the near-naked infant between the mother's breasts (or on the father's chest) so that there is skin-to-skin contact between the two (Roberts et al., 2000). There are many positive benefits but the amount of time in quiet regular sleep increased and activity states significantly decreased with kangaroo care (Ludington et al., 1994). Conventional cuddling care can be used by other family members and the health-care team to provide comfort and contact with infants.

Infant massage is also being promoted in the NNU. It is a complex and intimate interaction, which staff or parents can perform. However, it needs to be taught, provided and monitored by suitably trained and confident people.

Emotional care

The aim is for consistency of care and as much parental contact as possible. A stable caring relationship is vital (Reynolds, 1993). Comfort, contact and bonding are vital processes in the development of the baby's emotional and social development. Tapes of family activities, the dog barking, other children playing and familiar music can all be played to the baby in the NNU.

Quiet time

It is important to reduce the environmental disturbances that can affect the infant whenever possible. Environmental modifications such as reducing noxious stimulation (light and sound) and the promotion of supported positioning and minimal handling are all key factors in stress reduction (Boxwell, 2000).

THE INFANT'S ENVIRONMENT

Hospitals are dangerous places to be, especially if you are small and sick! They are brightly lit and noisy, and full of high-tech equipment and dangerous organisms.

Light levels

Excessive light has been shown to be damaging to the infant's immature visual system. When light levels have been reduced in the nursery, the following changes have been noticed in infants (Warren, 1997):

- The face is more relaxed.
- Heart rate and breathing seem more stable.
- Oxygen saturation improves or oxygen requirement is reduced.
- More time is spent in deep sleep.
- Sleep is less active and more restful.
- They will wake spontaneously and open their eyes.
- They will open eyes with a relaxed face and focused expression.
- They are more able to persist with feeding.

Sound levels

Excessive noise levels may damage the immature structures of the ear leading to hearing loss. If steps are taken to reduce noise levels, the following changes may be noticed in infants:

- More time is spent in deep or restful sleep.
- They are less restless and show fewer big, tiring movement patterns.
- Respiratory rates, heart rates and oxygen levels are more stable.
- They are better able to concentrate on feeding.
- They are better able to stay in a relaxed, alert awake state.
- More energy is available for activities such as feeding and being sociable.

The sound that an incubator makes can mask the background noise of the unit. In addition, the sounds made by objects placed on top of the incubator will be magnified (Warren, 1998). It is important to reduce these negative effects on the infant. Positive steps by the care team to introduce quiet periods and not use the incubator surfaces as a worktop are beneficial to all in this environment.

OTHER CONSIDERATIONS

Effects of hospitalisation

Hospitalisation can be stressful and distressing, not only for the infant but also for parents and families. The parents' feelings of disempowerment, isolation and fear should not be under-estimated (Action for Sick Children, 1989). Siblings can be jealous and resentful of those who they perceive as taking what is right-fully theirs or who has things they themselves want (O'Hagen and Smith, 1993). Siblings are in a very vulnerable position when a pre-term or sick infant is cared for in an NNU following an unexpected or traumatic delivery. Little time or preparation will have been given to them and their needs. Many may not be able to visit or take an active part with the new family member but they will be aware of the distress around them.

Multicultural awareness

An awareness and understanding of cultural factors and backgrounds is important as they may have an influence and impact on parenting styles and attitude to play. Play resources must reflect the cultural diversity of the client group so that parents and siblings can fully participate with enjoyment and confidence in the play sessions.

Hospital play specialists

In 1991, the Department of Health recommended that there should be provision for play in all areas of the hospital where children are found, and that a play specialist should be employed. The training of hospital play specialists means that they are in a unique position to meet the play needs of infants and to work towards achieving the full potential of the infants in partnership with the health-care team and family.

It is essential that play specialists work as a part of the overall health-care team and liaises closely with staff members. There must be consultation on treatment plans, procedures and diagnostic implications so that a play programme can be designed to suit the individual infant (Action for Sick Children, 1989). Play specialists have the skills to observe an infant, monitor development, behavioural organisation and emotional state.

Play safety

The safety of the infant is paramount both in medical and play terms. Toys need to be cleaned and inspected on a daily basis in order to meet safety and infection control regulations. This process must be monitored regularly to ensure that high standards are maintained.

Play space in the incubator, cot, chair or floor needs to be provided so that monitoring equipment is not compromised or a hazard to anyone in the area. Close liaison with medical and nursing staff on play activities and times needs to be negotiated.

REFERENCES

Action for Sick Children (1989) *A Collection of Essays on Children's Health Care*, HMSO, London

Bond, C. (1999) Positive touch and massage for the neonate needing a means of reducing stress, *Journal of Neonatal Nursing* 5(5), 16–20

Boxwell, G. (2000) *Neonatal Intensive Care Nursing: Developmentally Focused Nursing Care*, Routledge, London

Brown J. (2000) Considerations for touch and massage in the neonatal intensive care unit, *Neonatal Network* 19(1), 61–3

Department of Health (1989) *The Children Act*, HMSO, London

Fenwick, J., Barclay, L. and Schmied, V. (1999) Activities and interactions in Level II nurseries: a report of an ethnographic study, *Journal of Perinatal and Neonatal Nursing* 3(1), 53–65

Goldstein, J. (1995) A question of play under five, *Contact*, June, 8–9

Harrison, L. (1996) The effects of gentle human touch on pre-term infants, *Neonatal Network* 15(2), 35–42

Kroner, A.F. (1990) Infant stimulation, *Clinics in Perinatology* 17(1), 173–84

Ludington, S. *et al.* (1994) Kangaroo care: research results and practical implications and guidelines, *Neonatal Network* 13(1), 19–27

Montague, A. (1986) *Touching: Human Significance of Skin* (3rd edition), Harper and Row, London

O'Hagen, M. and Smith, M.(1993) *Special Issues in Childcare*, Baillière Tindall, London

Organisation Mondiale Pour L'Education Prescolaire (World Organisation for Early Childhood Education, or OMEP) (1989) Cited in: *Hospital. A Deprived Environment for Children?* The case for hospital play. Play in Hospital

Peters, K.L. (1999) Infant handling in NICU: does developmental care make a difference?, *Journal of Perinatal and Neonatal Nursing* 13(3), 83–109

Purdy, I.B. (2000) Newborn auditory follow-up, *The Journal* 19(2), 25–33

Reid, T. (2000) Maternal identity in preterm birth, *Journal of Child Health Care* 4(1) 23–9

Reynolds, K. (1993) *Let's Play, No 1. Baby in Hospital*, National Association of Hospital Play Staff, NAHPS, London

Roberts, K.L., Paynter, C. and McEwan, B. (2000) A comparison of kangaroo mother care and conventional cuddling care, *Journal of Neonatal Nursing* 19(4), 31–5

Sheridan, M. (1997) *Spontaneous Play in Early Childhood from Birth to Six Years*, Routledge, London

Swanwick, M. (1990) Development and chronic illness, *Nursing* 4(16), 24–7

Sylva, K. and Lunt, I. (1990) *Child Development: A First Course*, Blackwell, Oxford

United Nations (1995) *UN Convention on the Rights of the Child*, HMSO, London

Verzemnieks, D. (1984) Developmental stimulation for infants and toddlers during the first year of life, *American Journal of Nursing* 8(4), 749–52

Warren, I. (1998) Supporting the development of infants on special care baby units: the NIDCAP programme, *Journal of Neonatal Nursing* 4(6), 18–22

Wolke, D. (1991) Annotation: supporting the development of low birthweight infants, *Journal of Child Psychology and Psychiatry* 32(5), 723–41

Zahr, L.K. and Balian, S. (1995) Responses of premature infants to routine nursing interactions and noise in the NICU, *Nursing Research* 44(3), 179–85

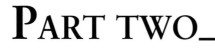

PART TWO

CLINICAL CONDITIONS

5 RESUSCITATION AND PROBLEMS OF INFANTS BORN TOO SMALL OR TOO SOON

Bernadette Byrne and Wendy Hickson

Aims of the chapter

This chapter is in two parts. The first will consider resuscitation and the second the problems of infants who are born too small or too soon. The chapter gives an overview of the procedure of resuscitation and equips the reader to participate in the process. The second part of the chapter provides working definitions of the terminology commonly heard in the neonatal unit, and identifies the differences between the classification of infants and the problems specific to them.

INTRODUCTION

The past few decades have brought many advances in neonatal care. Mortality and morbidity rates are progressively being reduced as a result of greater understanding of neonatal problems from birth, and concurrent advances in technology. Early detection of problems, accurate assessment and prompt intervention are essential. Once stabilised and transferred, infants will benefit from care that is appropriate to their specific needs.

RESUSCITATION

Following delivery and the clamping of the umbilical cord, the majority of infants take their first breath, cry and establish a steady heart rate of between 120/140 beats per minute within the first minute of extra-uterine life. There is a small proportion of infants, 1 in 50–100 (Roberton, 1999), who do not experience this sequence of events and for whom active resuscitation is imperative to ensure compatibility with life. The principle aims of resuscitation are to ensure a clear airway, support breathing and to support circulation (Drew et al., 2000).

Infants requiring resuscitation may be grouped as follows (Roberton, 1999):

- no respiratory output;
- cyanotic;
- bradycardic and with weak respirations;
- strong respirations but cyanosed; and
- muscle or CNS disorders.

Infants requiring resuscitation can be predicted in approximately 70% of cases (Roberton, 1999). As not all infants requiring resuscitation can be predicted, it is important for all staff to be competent at resuscitation techniques. Efficient, prompt action enhances the prognosis of the infant. When potential complications are suspected, it is important that a paediatrician is present at delivery.

The following factors predict infants that are likely to need support following delivery:

- mothers who have suffered major incident, such as massive haemorrhage or sudden eclamptic fits;
- mothers who suffer from a severe or chronic condition that has a known effect on the foetus;
- prolonged rupture of membranes;
- gestations of less than 35–36 weeks;
- malpresentations and cord prolapse;
- need for major obstetric interventions such as high forceps or caesarean section;
- severe intra-uterine growth retardation;
- display of foetal distress and/or compromise by delivery, and having inhaled meconium;
- a pre-natal diagnosis that suggests the infant will need expert care;
- twins and multiple births;
- rhesus incompatibility;
- drug-dependent mothers.

TRANSITION FROM INTRA- TO EXTRA-UTERINE EXISTENCE

The lungs are unnecessary to sustain existence until the moment of birth. Because of the high pulmonary vascular resistance, there is restriction to blood flow from the heart to the lungs. Only about 7% of the right ventricle output flows through the lungs in foetal life. The right-sided cardiac output is redirected through the foramen ovale and the ductus arteriosus. During the last moments of the second stage of labour, the umbilical cord is compressed and foetal circulation to the placenta is inhibited. This results in hypoxia sufficient to initiate gasping. For the majority of infants, this gasping coincides with birth; they take their first breath and all is well.

With the first few breaths, marked cardiovascular changes begin. The lung fluid is cleared and the alveoli expand and become capable of exchanging gas. With the exchange of gas, the O_2 tension rises and the CO_2 tension falls. The pulmonary arterioles dilate and pulmonary vascular resistance falls. This results in increased pulmonary blood flow. Decreased pulmonary pressure means that there is a reduction in blood flow through the ductus. Increased pulmonary blood flow raises the pressure in the left atria, which closes the foramen and reduces the flow between right and left sides of the heart (*see* Chapter 9).

Neonatal asphyxia

The pathophysiology of neonatal asphyxia is well documented; a brief overview is given here.

Neonatal asphyxia occurs when impaired gas exchange results in a rising foetal $PaCO_2$ and a decreasing PaO_2. This initiates gasping respiration. Unless this gasping results in satisfactory gas exchange and blood gas adjustment, the respiratory effort is temporarily suspended. This is known as *primary apnoea* and may last about 10 minutes. After this period, respiratory activity recommences, with rhythmic gasps of ever-increasing frequency and desperation. If gas exchange occurs at this point, spontaneous recovery is still possible. However, if satisfactory oxygenation exchange still does not take place, the respiratory activity will decrease, then, once again, cease. This is called *terminal apnoea* and animal studies suggest that respiration will not spontaneously recommence (Dawes and Jacobson, 1963). Roberton (1999) discusses animal studies where primary apnoea may occur for up to 10 minutes, when the last gasp is taken and apnoea occurs. The infant may survive 20 minutes of complete oxygen deprivation.

Although the term 'asphyxia' is used regularly, Stephenson and colleagues (2000) suggest that, due to poor definition, it should not be used. In their view, the term may cause distress to the parents and medical team and may override a variety of conditions.

The APGAR system

First developed in 1953, the APGAR scoring system (*see* Table 5.1) is used to assess the newborn infant. Five items are scored 0–2 at 1 minute, 5 minutes and, in some instances, 10 minutes of age (although the effectiveness of determining asphyxia at 1 minute of age is questioned – Roberton, 1996). Further questions as to the validity of the APGAR scoring system have been asked. These include the retrospective recalling of information and the application of the APGAR score and its accuracy when applied to an extremely premature or intubated infant (Marlow, 1992).

Table 5.1 APGAR scoring system

	Score		
Clinical feature	**0**	**1**	**2**
Heart rate	0	<100	>100
Respiration	Absent	Gasping or irregular	Regular or crying lustily
Muscle tone	Limp	Diminished or normal with no movements	Normal with active movements
Response to pharyngeal catheter	Nil	Grimace	Cough
Colour of trunk	White	Blue	Pink

Despite the reservations, the APGAR system is, however, used universally as a method of determining the need for active resuscitation in the newborn infant.

BASIC EMERGENCY RESUSCITATION OF THE NEWBORN

An essential element of any resuscitative procedure is to ensure that the infant is kept warm. Associated problems with cold stress include worsening hypoxia, hypoglycaemia, worsening respiratory distress syndrome, pulmonary haemorrhage and intracranial haemorrhage (Levene *et al.*, 1987). In addition, the production of surfactant slows down (Yeo, 1998). The asphyxiated infant cannot generate its own heat and will further cool down (Roberton, 1996). The pre-term and very low-birthweight infant is at greater risk of problems due to immaturity of organs, lack of brown fat and a smaller body mass. Even a healthy full-term infant may drop its body temperature to 35–35.5 degrees by 15–30 minutes of age if care is not taken in labour ward to prevent heat loss (Roberton, 1996).

Drying the infant following delivery, removing wet linen and placing the infant under a radiant heater are fundamental in the initial steps of resuscitation (Spiedel *et al.*, 1998; Boxwell, 2000; Drew *et al.*, 2000).

The following equipment is needed for resuscitation:

- flat surface;
- overhead radiant heater;
- dry towels;
- oxygen supply;
- wall or portable suction and suction catheters of various sizes;
- clock with second hand;
- stethoscope;
- gloves;
- resuscitation bag (low-inflating/self-inflating/valved T-piece; self-inflating is presently the most popular method);
- face masks (varying sizes);
- two laryngoscopes (check prior to procedure that they are working);
- ET tubes of varying size;
- introducer;
- hats of varying size;
- scissors/forceps/suture/adhesive tape;
- connector for ET tube;
- nasogastric tubes of varying size;
- cannulas/butterflies/syringes/needles;
- sterile pack for insertion of UAC/UVC;
- sterile bottles for blood cultures/specimens;
- emergency drugs/fluids;
- pen/paper (it is necessary to document at the time all drugs/fluids that are administered to the infant).

Method of resuscitation

When an infant requires resuscitation always ensure that there is help. Do not try and resuscitate an infant single-handed. If the infant does not improve after bag and mask ventilation and requires advanced life support there will need to be more than one extra person present, to ensure efficiency and safety. The administration of drugs and fluids must be drawn up and recorded, actions have to be documented and the parents need to be supported.

A – Airway

One common reason for failure to establish a good respiratory pattern at birth is the presence of copious secretions in the upper airway. Drew and colleagues (2000) recommend the use of electronic suction with a vacuum of no greater than minus 100mmHg to aspirate these secretions. The suction catheter should be a size 10FG for the term infant and a size 8FG for the pre-term infant. Gentle suction should be used, to ensure that there is no damage to the mucosa in the oropharynx. Initially the oropharynx should be aspirated and then, if needed, the nostrils. Often, once the secretions have been cleared by suctioning, no further intervention is needed and the infant can go with the mother to the post-natal area. These infants are usually vigorous and rate a high APGAR score in all other respects.

It is important for the nurse to realise that the majority of infants do not require suction of the upper airways. The lung fluid present in the infant's mouth can simply be wiped away with a clean piece of gauze. Suctioning may predispose the infant to problems of reflex bradycardia, apnoea and hypotension (Spiedel et al., 1998). As Roberton (1996) states, if the infant is fit and healthy, suctioning should not be carried out.

At delivery, evidence of meconium staining of the infant's fingernails, the cord and a general presence of meconium will alert the paediatrician to the likelihood of meconium aspiration. If the paediatrician identifies the presence of meconium at or below the vocal cords, he or she should, under direct vision with a laryngoscope, suction the pharynx and larynx (Spiedel et al., 1998, Drew et al., 2000). Alternatively, if meconium is present in the posterior pharynx or larynx, the infant should be intubated and suctioned via the endo-tracheal tube; the tube should be replaced as necessary (Kelnar et al., 1995; Spiedel et al., 1998).

B – Breathing

Infants who are making little respiratory effort, who are pale or blue, and inactive and floppy, need more vigorous attention. Ventilation may be by bag and mask or by intubation. The bag and mask method of ventilation should only be used for the infant who has made some attempt to breathe; it is extremely difficult to use in a non-breathing infant whose lungs are full of fluid (Roberton, 1996). Contra-indications for bag and mask ventilation include diaphragmatic hernia and meconium aspiration.

When the bag and mask are being used to ventilate the infant, for optimal airway opening the recommended position is the neutral position. This may be achieved by lying the infant flat, placing a small rolled-up towel under the shoulders and slightly extending the neck (Drew et al., 2000).

Delivery of air/oxygen is via an ambu bag or Laerdal system. The bag should have a large reservoir, to maintain an adequate pressure (Field et al., 1986). A round mask made of clear silicone is preferred as this allows for observation of secretions and a better seal over the infant's nose and mouth. The mask should fit comfortably over the mouth and nose, avoiding the eyes and not overriding the chin. An adequate seal needs to be maintained to ensure efficient ventilation.

To enable delivery of 100% oxygen flow should be set at 10 litres/minute. Rennie and Roberton (2002) recommend a supply of up to 5 litres/minute of O_2 or air, stating that the gas must be passed through a blow-off valve set at 30 cm H_2O. Initially, five sustained inflations should be delivered via a 500 ml bag with a maximum inflation pressure of 30 cm H_2O. The hand ventilation rate should be 30 breaths per minute (Spiedel et al., 1998; Drew et al., 2000). Compression of the soft tissue of the neck should be avoided. This may be achieved by holding the mask to the face with third, fourth and fifth fingers resting on the mandible (Niermayer and Clarke, 1998).

One study aiming to determine the effects of mask and bag ventilation on pre-term and term infants concluded that mask ventilation was efficient. However, certain factors, including adequacy of pressures and adequate ventilation of the alveoli (Palme-Kilander and Tunell, 1993), need to be carefully monitored. It has been suggested that face-mask resuscitation may lead to gastric distension. Applying pressures of less than 3.5 kPa has been shown to reduce the likelihood of gastric distension (Vyas et al., 1983). The majority of term infants respond quickly to bag and mask resuscitation (Roberton, 1996). It is imperative when ventilating an infant constantly to look out for chest movement, to establish that the lungs are being inflated.

Inadequate ventilation may result from an ill-fitting face mask, inadequate pressure, incorrect positioning of infant or secretions or obstruction in the upper airway.

If heart rate and colour have not improved and respirations have not commenced within one minute of bagging, then endotracheal intubation is required. An insertion of an oral airway is also necessary if the infant has bilateral choanal atresia or Pierre Robin syndrome.

Intubation is most often achieved using direct laryngoscopic vision although finger intubation has been described (Hancock and Peterson, 1992). Severely compromised or small premature infants do not usually require sedation for intu-bation. Intubation should be a calm procedure and there should only be 30 seconds between an unsuccessful intubation and the recommencing of bag and mask resuscitation. This should be continued for 30–60 seconds prior to re-intu-bation (Spiedel et al., 1998).

C – Circulation

Chest compressions are necessary to maintain circulation until resuscitative procedures are successful or stopped. Chest compressions should be commenced if after 15–30 seconds of ventilation the heart rate is below 60 beats per minute, or is 60–80 beats per minute and not increasing (Bloom and Cropley, 1994).

Compressions may be given by using the thumb technique or two-finger technique. The two-thumb technique is the preferred method of chest compression (Drew *et al.*, 2001). Because the chest wall is encircled by the hands, higher coronary artery perfusion pressures are produced and, being less tiring to perform, it can be sustained by the resuscitator for longer. Pressure should be applied by both thumbs to the lower third of the sternum; if the chest circumference is very small, the thumbs may have to overlap. The two-finger method can be used if there is only one resuscitator or in the case of a large infant, when the resuscitator's hands may be too small to encircle the chest wall.

The chest wall should be compressed to a depth of 1.5–2.5 cm at a rate of 120 compressions/minute (Spiedel *et al.*, 1998). Ventilation with 100% oxygen should be continued to ensure that the blood circulated as a result of the chest compressions is well oxygenated. The hand actions should be smooth and rhythmic and allow the chest to re-expand following each compression to allow circulatory return to the heart. Drew *et al.* (2000) suggest that a rate of 120 compressions/minute is difficult to achieve and virtually impossible to sustain and recommend 90 chest compressions and 30 ventilations per minute at a ratio of 3:1.

Drugs

Medication and intravenous fluids are administered to improve cardiac output and cardiac and cerebral perfusion. A member of staff should be responsible for documenting clearly and legibly all drugs administered, and the amount used.

Access may be via umbilical venous catheter, tracheal tube, intraosseous cannula, peripheral vein cannula or intramuscular injection (Drew *et al.*, 2000). Intravenous access is the most common, although in the collapsed infant this may be impossible. Umbilical venous access is usually preferred next. Although it is not commonly used, recent studies confirm that intraosseous access has great benefits in the early stage of resuscitation, including ease of access, higher rate of infusion (as there is no venous damage) and success of siting, and no apparent long-term adverse effects on bone growth (Ellemunter *et al.*, 1999; Fisher and Prosser, 2000). Although access may be limited in the very sick infant, access via the umbilical catheter should be avoided due to several factors, including the possibility of a blood clot being flushed into the infant, trauma of the umbilical artery and small amounts of drugs not reaching the circulation (Roberton, 1999).

The following drugs are used in advanced resuscitation:

- adrenaline;
- sodium bicarbonate;

- naloxone – should only be given if the mother has received opiates within 6 hours of delivery (Roberton, 1999);
- volume expanders – should only be given if the infant is hypovolemic or has an acute blood loss (Roberton, 1999; Drew *et al.*, 2000);
- glucose 10%.

For additional information on the use of these drugs and dosages, *see* Rennie and Roberton (2002), Drew *et al.* (2000), *British National Formulary* (British Medical Association, 2001) and *Medicines for Children* (1999).

In addition, local Trust and health authority drugs policies should be adhered to, as should the UKCC code of conduct relating to drug administration.

Resuscitation in the NNU

Discussion has centred on the infant who requires resuscitation following delivery. The fundamentals of care relate to the infant who requires resuscitation on NICU. Preparation is imperative, and knowledge of the skills needed to commence, participate or assist in resuscitation is essential. To educate staff caring for sick infants in the skills of resuscitation and keep those skills sharp most units have a rolling programme based on the Resuscitation Council UK (2000) recommendations. Most practitioners have now also taken the Neonatal Advanced Life Support (NALS) programme. All of the equipment needs to be instantly available and operational. Time is of the essence during the resuscitative procedure and searching for necessary items may be detrimental to the outcome of the infant.

The procedure needs to be undertaken in the optimal thermal environment. Windows and doors closed, radiant heater switched on, wet linen removed and where possible the infant should not be unnecessarily exposed. This further improves the infant's outcome.

When to stop resuscitation

There is no easy answer to the question of how long to continue resuscitation, and hospitals should develop their own policies regarding the commencement and abandonment of resuscitation. These are usually based on absence of cardiac output and respiratory effort when all reversible factors have been eliminated (Drew *et al.*, 2001). Successful recovery has taken place in primates after 20 minutes of complete oxygenation deprivation. Anecdotal evidence is all that is available for many cases of prolonged resuscitation of human infants.

The decision to abandon resuscitation should be taken by the most senior member of the team who is present at the time, after all reasonable methods have been tried. Often, the thought of having to give parents bad news keeps the team going far longer than is really justifiable. It is imperative that the parents are cared for at this extremely stressful time. Unfortunately, in an emergency event, the parents may be left on their own as all focus is directed towards keeping the infant alive. Whenever possible, a nurse should be available to care for the parents with regular updating of information. If resuscitation is not effective the parents should, if they wish, hold and spend time with their infant. A nurse or doctor should be available whenever the parents need support.

ETHICAL ISSUES IN RESUSCITATION

The debate as to whether an infant should have been resuscitated or not will be heard on a daily basis in hospitals all over the country. Decisions to resuscitate or not are fraught with legal and ethical dilemmas. The issues are not likely to be easily resolved by the use of protocols and policies based on weight or gestational age or extent of deformity. There are just too many variables and each case will need to be assessed on an individual basis. Shelton (2001) commented on the Dutch experience based on research indicating poor prognosis and outcome when resuscitation of infants of less than 25 weeks gestation took place. Whatever the situation, the decisions that are taken on behalf of the infant should be taken with the full participation of the parents.

For more on ethical issues in neonatal nursing, *see* Chapter 2.

CLASSIFICATION OF NEONATES IN THE NEWBORN PERIOD

Assessment of gestation and classification of birth weight is fundamental to any decision-making.

Definitions

There is no universal agreement on birthweight classification but the commonly accepted definitions are as follows (Chiswick, 1986):

- Normal birthweight (NBW)   2500 grams or more
- Low birthweight (LBW)   Below 2500 grams
- Very low birthweight (VLBW)   Below 1500 grams
- Extremely low birthweight (ELBW)   Below 1000 grams

Infants of low birth weight are further classified by maturity and how appropriate they appear for their gestational age. Infants who are term or pre-term and an appropriate size for gestational ages are termed 'appropriate for gestational age' (AGA). Infants who are term or pre-term and small for gestational age are termed 'small for gestational age' (SGA).

Gestational age is classified as follows:

- Pre-term   < 37 completed weeks (259 days)
- Term   37–42 completed weeks (259–293 days)
- Post-term   after 42 completed weeks (294-plus days)

RISK FACTORS FOR PRE-TERM AND SGA INFANTS

Table 5.2   Comparative factors affecting the pre-term and growth-restricted infants

Predisposing factor	Pre-term	SGA
Maternal		
Pregnancy-induced hypertension	+	+
Multiple gestation	+	+
Maternal smoking		+
Maternal substance abuse	+	+
Maternal disease, e.g. diabetes	+	
Placental		
Placenta previa	+	+
Placental infarction		+
Absent or reversed end diastolic flow	+	+
Infection, e.g. syphilis		+
Foetal		
Congenital infection TORCH		+
Chromosomal abnormality		+
Inborn errors of metabolism		+
Teratogenic		+

CONSEQUENCES OF PRE-TERM BIRTH

Birth weight and gestational age are both predictors of outcome for the newborn infant. When considering the mortality of extremely low-birthweight infants (500–800 grams), as little as 100 grams can make a significant difference to the likelihood of survival (Taeusch and Sniderman, 1998, p. 40).

Intra-uterine growth restriction (IUGR) and SGA

Intra-uterine growth restriction (IUGR) can adversely affect the foetus. The effects may also have long-term sequelae for the child. To appreciate the long-term sequelae of the small for gestational age (SGA) infant it is important to understand the concept of symmetrical and asymmetrical growth restriction.

Symmetrical growth restriction is associated with an early insult to the foetus. Growth restriction in the first 20 weeks of gestation will produce an undersized foetus with fewer cells but normal cell size. This insult globally resets the growth potential of most of the organs, limiting the overall organ and foetal size. Conditions that produce symmetrically small foetuses include chromosomal abnormalities, some syndromes and congenital infections. Neonates who are unaccountably symmetrically small should be investigated for congenital infection. The TORCH screen is the initial method. The acronym refers to toxoplasmosis, others (such as syphilis), rubella, cytomegalovirus and herpes simplex/hepatitis B.

Asymmetrical growth restriction reflects a reduction in oxygen and/or nutrient supply to the foetus occurring after completion of organ development. This reduction in oxygen and nutrient supply is usually the result of utero-placental insufficiency and maternal substance abuse or smoking. Vital organs such as the brain and heart are spared during asymmetrical growth restriction but there is loss of muscle and fat development.

Mortality is higher for SGA foetuses. The smaller the foetus, the higher the morbidity rate. Compared to normally grown infants the small term infant has a greater risk of foetal distress, acidosis, poor APGAR scores and increased risk of mortality (Charlton, 1998, p. 52). As much as 50% of this mortality can be attributed to anatomical development and chromosomal abnormalities of the foetus. A multi-centre researcher in the USA confirmed these findings (Vohr *et al.*, 2000).

The growth-restricted neonate is at risk of hypoglycaemia, hypocalcaemia, hypothermia and polycythaemia. The long-term consequences for the IUGR and pre-term infant is a neurological impairment. Studies have suggested that when compared with their appropriate weight/born at term counterparts they have lower IQ, a greater risk of developmental delay and cerebral palsy (Allen, 1998).

An important predictor for long-term sequelae is the head circumference of the infant at birth. When the foetus has been exposed to early growth restriction – for example, congenital infections – there may be poor head growth. The post-natal growth in head circumference may be a predictor of neurological outcome but should not be used in isolation.

GESTATIONAL ASSESSMENT

Gestational age assessment is based on the following:

- Date of last menstrual period – the accuracy is dependent on the woman having a regular menstrual cycle.
- Ultrasound scan based on bi-parietal diameter, femoral length, head circumference and/or abdominal circumference – ultrasound scans can be quite accurate provided they are performed early on in the pregnancy. As confidence builds in the interpretation of the scanning technique, the data provided is likely to become even more reliable.
- Date of first recorded foetal activity – this is first felt at around the 16th and 18th weeks of gestation although this may be later in the first pregnancy.
- Date of first recorded foetal heart sounds – these are detected between 10 and 12 weeks of gestation by ultrasound Doppler.

Characteristics of the newborn

Gestational age assessment may be obtained from a visual examination of the infant. External features of the newborn are valuable indicators.

Skin

The full-term infant has around 20 layers of stratum corneum, the tough, protective outer barrier layer. Pre-term infants have far fewer layers of stratum corneum. An infant of 30 weeks gestation will have around three to five layers and the infant of 24 weeks will have no stratum corneum. This is the reason why the pre-term infants appear extremely red. The blood vessels are visible, as the skin is transparent and gelatinous. The formation of the stratum corneum is accelerated during the first 10 to 14 days (Evans and Rutter, 1986). By 36 weeks the skin has lost its transparency and underlying blood vessels are no longer visible. As gestation progresses beyond the 38th week, the subcutaneous tissue begins to decrease, causing wrinkling and desquamation. The skin of a post-term infant is often dry and fissured as a result of vernix loss and depletion of subcutaneous tissue (Houska and Durand, 1998). Skin care for the pre-term infant will be considered later in this chapter (*see* pages 98–100).

Lanugo

The body of a 20–28-week infant is covered with fine downy hair called lanugo. By the 28th week this begins to disappear mainly from the face and the anterior trunk. A few patches may remain over the shoulders at term.

Sole creases

Creases first appear on the sole of the foot extending to the heel. These increase with gestational age. However, the SGA infant, with early loss of vernix, may have more sole creases due to drying. This indicator of gestational age is invalid after 12 hours of age due to the drying of the skin after birth.

Breast tissue and areola

By 34 weeks gestation, the areola is raised and by 36 weeks there is evidence of breast tissue.

Ears

Cartilage formation increases with gestational age. An infant of 36 weeks gestation will have well-formed cartilage and demonstrate robust recoil of the pinna when folded. The external ear of the extremely pre-term infant will be shapeless with little or no curving of the pinna edge.

Eyes

The eyelids are fused until 25 weeks gestation. Further assessment of the eyes is possible by examining the anterior vascular capsule of the lens. Assessment is based on the pattern and presence of the vessels of the vascular capsule (Hitter *et al.*, 1977; Lepley *et al.*, 1998).

Genitalia

In the female, the clitoris is prominent during the early gestation. During early gestation, owing to the absence of fat in the labia majora, the labia minora protrudes. By 40 weeks the labia majora completely covers the labia minora and the clitoris is hidden. In the male, at less than 28 weeks gestation, the testes are high in the abdominal cavity. By 37 weeks they can be felt high in the scrotum. The testes are fully descended by 40 weeks gestation.

Hair

Head hair is present by 20 weeks gestation, and eyebrows and lashes from around 23 weeks. The head hair of an infant of less than 34 weeks gestation is fine, woolly and sticks together. A term infant's hair lies flat and has a silky feel, with individual strands identifiable (Lepley *et al.*, 1998).

Posture

This is poor in extremely pre-term infants, as the skeletal muscle is under-developed resulting in hypotonia. At 30 weeks there is slight flexion of the feet and knees. By 34 weeks there is flexion of the hips and thighs and at 35 weeks this flexion has extended to the upper limbs. The term infant has full flexion of all limbs with immediate recoil.

For a comprehensive assessment tool, *see* either Dubowitz and colleagues (1970) or Ballard and colleagues (1991).

THERMOREGULATION IN THE SGA INFANT AND THE PRE-TERM INFANT

Using the above methods of assessment, the physical differences between mature low-birthweight infants and infants who are pre-term but appropriately sized can be described. Knowledge of the biology of neonates is essential for understanding their various problems and the nursing interventions required for maintaining homeostasis.

Thermal control

The neonate produces heat metabolically and lacks the ability to generate heat from shivering. The neonate has several ways of regulating and controlling body temperature.

Hypothalamus

The hypothalamus is able to detect changes in temperature and initiate an appropriate response to either lose or generate heat. However, the neonate's hypothalamus can be slow to respond to changes in body temperature. Sensation of cold by the skin triggers a much earlier response to cold stress although the two systems are integrated.

Skin

Sympathetic nerves present in the skin enable vasoconstriction to occur in response to sensation of cold. This vasoconstriction serves two purposes. First, it diverts the flow of warm blood away from the periphery to the central core reducing heat loss. Second, peripheral vasoconstriction places an insulating layer of fat between the core and the cold skin, again reducing heat loss.

Brown fat

Brown fat is the primary source of thermogenesis in the neonate. It is laid down during the third trimester of pregnancy. It is situated in the axilla, mediastinum and around the kidneys. It is highly vascularised and has a large supply of sympathetic nerves. During cold stress, there is an increased production of noradrenaline, which acts on brown fat causing lipolysis. The breakdown of brown fat into free fatty acids produces heat. As brown fat has a generous supply of blood vessels this heat is quickly transported around the body, raising its temperature.

Heat loss mechanisms

Convection
Convection occurs when ambient air temperature is less than the infant's body temperature. This mechanism is either passive or active. Passive convection involves connective heat loss from the skin to the still ambient air. Active convection occurs when the air around the infant is moving, for example, when there are breezes from open windows or doors.

Evaporation
Evaporation of water requires energy. All newborn infants have transcutaneous water loss (insensible water loss). The energy source used for the evaporation of this water is heat from the infant's skin. The more immature the skin, the greater the insensible water loss and the greater the potential for temperature loss.

Radiation
This can be described as the transfer of heat from the infant's body to cooler surrounding walls. The cooler the walls the greater the heat loss potential.

Conduction
This is the loss of heat from the skin to contact surfaces. For the term infant this loss is minimal because of bedding. However, for the exposed low-birthweight infant it may be a problem. Additionally, in small infants, the nappy may account for a large proportion of the skin surface; if that nappy is applied cold, the heat loss may be significant.

Implications of cold stress on the neonate

The infant's response to cold is to vasoconstrict the peripheral blood vessels (Figure 5.1). Vasoconstriction leads to anaerobic metabolism, which can lead to metabolic acidosis. This acidosis can result in pulmonary vessel constriction, leading to further hypoxia and metabolic acidosis.

A second consequence of cold stress is hypoglycaemia, the result of increased utilisation of glucose and the rapid depletion of glycogen stores. This situation is compounded by the hypoxia, which is associated with cold stress. This compromises the infant's ability to produce new glucose from gluconeogenesis.

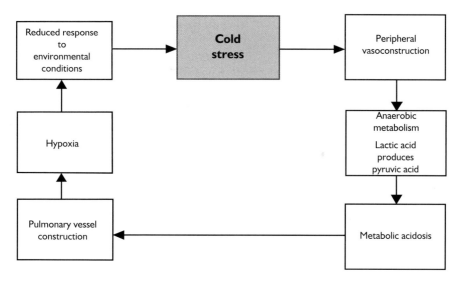

Figure 5.1   Implications of cold stress on the neonate

Nursing strategies to maintain the infant's temperature

Understanding of the concept of thermo-neutral environment is crucial to the care of the neonate. Essentially, it relates to the environmental temperature needed by the neonate to maintain normal body temperature using the least amount of oxygen and calories. Any strategy that aims to reduce heat loss in the neonate needs to include control of the environmental temperature and humidity.

Incubator temperature

Most sick neonates are nursed in an incubator for ease of access and observation, as well as for warmth. Choosing the optimal incubator temperature is vital. It is based not only on the infant's weight, but also on the ambient temperature. The calculation is complicated when double-walled incubators are used to reduce losses from radiation, but Table 5.3 gives a rough guide.

Table 5.3   Incubator temperature according to birthweight

Birthweight	Incubator temperature
1000 grams	35°C
1500 grams	34°C
2000 grams	33°C

Modified from Stephenson et al. (2000)

Nurses may employ a number of other strategies in order to reduce heat loss, and these are outlined in Table 5.4.

Table 5.4 Nursing strategies to reduce heat loss

Strategy	Effect
Pre-warm all bedding, nappies and clothing	Minimises conductive heat losses
Use correctly fitting clothes	Provides a more effective insulating layer
Keep handling to a minimum	Opening the portholes repeatedly will increase heat losses
Avoid stripping the infant naked	Reduces the surface area exposed
When weighing the infant, line the scales with a pre-warmed towel or blanket, or wrap the infant in the pre-warmed towel or blanket for the time on the scales (zero the scales with the blankets in place)	Reduces heat losses from convection, conduction, radiation and evaporation

Incubator humidity

Researchers are agreed that pre-term infants have an increased transdermal water loss (TDWL) when compared with their term counterparts. This may be as high as 80mls/kg per day. For an infant weighing 750 grams, TDWL may be as much as 60mls in 24 hours. This figure can be more than doubled when open warmers are used (Sedin, 1996). TDWL decreases rapidly following birth as the development of the stratum corneum is accelerated. However, nurses need to take measures to reduce TDWL losses. Reduction of TDWL is achieved through the use of incubator humidity. Raising incubator humidity to 80% can reduce TDWL by 75%.

TDWL will have decreased by 50% by day five and will be at term infant levels by approximately 2 weeks old (Sedin *et al.*, 1985). The extremely pre-term infant requires high humidity levels for the first five days, reduced to 'normal' environmental humidity levels by 2 weeks. As a general guide, the more immature the infant, the longer the epidermis takes to mature, and thus the longer incubator humidity is required.

FLUID AND ELECTROLYTE BALANCE

A term neonate is approximately 78% water. Of the total body water, 45% is extracellular (intravascular and interstitial) and 33% is intracellular. Following birth, the percentage of extracellular fluid increases and a diuresis occurs, accounting for the weight loss in the first 10 days of life.

The pre-term infant has a higher proportion of total body water and the percentage of extracellular fluid is greater. A post-natal weight loss in the pre-term infant can be attributed to an inadequate calorie intake. The theory is that the loss of weight from diuresis of extracellular fluid is offset by an increase in intracellular weight (Heimler *et al.*, 1993).

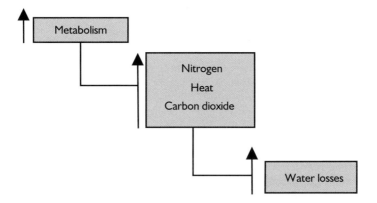

Figure 5.2 Water loss in relation to metabolic rate

Water loss is also dependent on the metabolic rate (Figure 5.2). The body uses carbohydrates, fats and protein to produce energy; the higher the metabolic rate, the higher the energy requirements. Waste from metabolism is excreted with water. The kidneys produce urine, which excretes nitrogen. The respiratory system excretes carbon dioxide with exhaled gas. As skin matures, glands within it produce sweat, which reduces heat loss. The higher the metabolic rate, the more water is lost.

As well as metabolic rate there are other factors to be considered when assessing fluid losses in the newborn:

- water loss from skin;
- phototherapy;
- tachypnoea;
- inadequate gas humidification;
- osmotic diuresis (hyperglycaemia).

Total body weight is not the only measure of hydration in the neonate. The neonate who is acutely ill and unstable may have increased vascular permeability, leading to reduced intravascular volume with interstitial oedema. Although the infant appears oedematous, it may have inadequate circulating volume.

In this situation, an assessment of the serum electrolytes is required.

Sodium

Sodium is the principal ion of extracellular fluid controlling the movement of water by osmosis, drawing fluid into the capillary. The kidneys are responsible for sodium balance. The glomeruli filters sodium and the tubules re-absorb sodium in exchange for potassium and hydrogen. The sodium balance is inter-linked to the potassium and the pH balance of the blood. If the serum sodium decreases (hyponatraemia), there is a drop in serum osmolarity, followed by the movement of water from the extracellular to the intracellular compartment.

Early hyponatraemia can be associated with other factors such as perinatal asphyxia and respiratory distress syndrome. When these situations arise, there is a degree of hypoxia, which affects the secretion of antidiuretic hormones. As the secretion of antidiuretic hormone increases more water is retained. The serum concentration of sodium is decreased relative to the water volume and there is a shift of water into the interstitial compartment.

This situation is compounded by the immaturity of kidney function, which leads to poor re-absorption of sodium by the tubules (Figue 5.3).

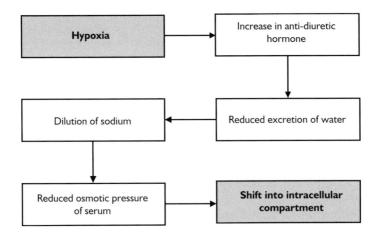

Figure 5.3 Hypoxia and its effects

Late-onset hyponatraemia is a consequence of inadequate supplementation. All low-birthweight infants require sodium supplementation to achieve a positive sodium balance. The smaller the infant, the greater the level of sodium supplementation required.

Potassium

Potassium is the principle cation of interstitial fluid and is responsible for regulating the flow of water in and out of cells. The kidney excretes potassium. Filtered potassium is re-absorbed in the proximal tubule and secreted by the distal tubule in exchange for sodium. Imbalance of potassium can be related to gastro-intestinal fluid loss, for example, excessive gastric aspirates and excessive ileostomy losses.

Nursing strategies to maintain an infant's fluid status

The purpose of any nursing strategy is the early identification of fluid imbalance. In order to achieve this, it is necessary to monitor and record the factors listed in Table 5.5.

Table 5.5 Factors to be monitored to achieve identification of fluid imbalance

• Blood pressure	• Low BP indicates reduced circulating volume
• Heart rate	• Increased HR indicates compensation for reduced circulating volume
• Capillary refill time > 2 secs	• Prolonged CRT suggests peripheral shut-down possible due to fluid imbalance
• Skin turgor	• Skin turgor is an indication of hydration
• Urine volume	• Urine output should be around 2 ml/kg
• Urine SG	• Normal urine SG is 1010
• Volume of gastric aspirates	• Pre-warning of potassium depletion
• Volume of ileostomy output	• Pre-warning of potassium depletion

METABOLIC COMPLICATIONS OF THE NEWBORN

There are many rare disorders of metabolism. Only the more relevant and common imbalances will be considered here.

Hypoglycaemia/ hyperglycaemia

One major challenge to the neonate is the regulation of levels of blood glucose. During foetal life, homeostasis is achieved through placental transfer of glucose and neonatal production of insulin. During the later stages of gestation, glycogen stores are laid down in the liver. Following delivery, the neonate is challenged to maintain normal levels of blood glucose. For effective management of these levels it is essential to have an understanding of neonatal glucose homeostasis. There is a physiological fall in blood sugars at around 4 hours post delivery. Plasma glucagon rises, triggering the endogenous production of glucose from the glycogen stores. Glucagon also activates lipolysis (breakdown of fats) and gluco-neogenesis (production of new glucose from muscles and protein).

With these mechanisms working, the neonatal blood glucose levels rise steadily during the first 24 hours following delivery.

The reasons why neonates become hypoglycaemic fall into two main categories: the increased utilisation of glucose and the decreased production of glucose or stores.

Increased utilisation of glucose

Infants of diabetic mothers

Glucose transfer across the placenta is necessary for foetal growth. However, if the level of glucose transfer is high, the foetus will develop islet cell hypertrophy, producing excessive amounts of insulin in response to high blood glucose levels. Following delivery and abrupt discontinuation of glucose transfer, the infant becomes hypoglycaemic almost immediately. The severity of neonatal hypoglycaemia is related to the level of maternal diabetic control during pregnancy.

As insulin is the main growth factor for the foetus during development the infant will be large for gestational age. A large body is called macrosomatic.

However, if the mother also has placental insufficiency, secondary to maternal diabetic vascular disease, the foetus may have a degree of growth restriction.

Cold stress and glucose

When an infant is exposed to cold stress, there is a corresponding increase in metabolic activity, in an attempt to increase body temperature. A consequence of this increased metabolic activity is increased utilisation of glucose stores. If steps are not taken to reverse the cold stress, hypoglycaemia will follow. This scenario is particularly relevant to the pre-term or growth-restricted infant or one who lacks the necessary glucose stores from which heat can be generated.

Birth asphyxia and glucose

During asphyxial episodes, blood is preferentially diverted to essential organs such as the brain, where there is also an increased need for energy (glucose). The brain is glucose-dependent, and has limited stores of glucose. The neonatal response is to increase the rate of glycogen breakdown in order to meet these increased needs and the net result is hypoglycaemia.

Polycythaemia

Erythrocytes are dependent on glucose for metabolism. If there is an abundance of erythrocytes, there is an increased need for glucose, resulting in hypoglycaemia. Additional causes of hypoglycaemia secondary to polycythaemia include increased production of insulin as a direct result of the polycythaemia, and decreased hepatic glucose production as a result of sluggish hepatic circulation.

Decreased production/inadequate stores of glucose

Typically, these two problems are associated with pre-term delivery and/or growth restriction.

The newborn infant maintains normal levels of blood glucose by glucogenesis, which is under the control of the hormone glucagon. Pre-term infants are disadvantaged on three counts. First, they lack the glycogen stores required to generate glucose. Second, they lack the muscle mass and protein levels to make gluconeogenesis feasible. Third, they lack the hepatic and hormonal maturity successfully to produce glucose from stores. The growth-restricted infant may have the hepatic and hormonal maturity but lack the glycogen stores and muscle mass from which glucose can be generated.

If the infant is born pre-term and growth-restricted, the incidence of hypoglycaemia may vary from 38% to 67% (Lubchenco and Bard, 1971).

Nursing management of abnormal glucose metabolism

It is important to identify the high-risk neonate because the neonatal brain is dependent on glucose for all metabolic activities. Other sources of energy such as fatty acids are bound to albumin and are too large to cross the blood brain barrier. Hypoglycaemia may therefore result in neurological injury to the neonate.

The following types of neonate may be at risk:

- pre-term infants;
- growth-restricted infants;
- infants with polycythaemia;
- infants of diabetic mothers;
- cold infants;
- infants with birth asphyxia;
- infants with poor APGAR scores.

To ensure early detection, blood glucose levels are initially monitored on an hourly basis. The time between observations is increased according to the infant's levels and the clinical findings. If the blood glucose does not respond to early and frequent feeding, an IV infusion of 10% dextrose may have to be commenced. This is sometimes commenced with a bolus of 10% dextrose followed by the infusion. Boluses of stronger solutions of dextrose are avoided where possible, to avoid rebound hypoglycaemia. When infusing high concentrations of dextrose, these should preferentially be given via a central line to reduce the potential risk of extravasation of hypertonic fluid into tissues. It should be noted that these lines are not without complications (DoH, 2001). Oral feeds are introduced as soon as the infant is stable. Initially, small oral feeds are given in addition to the dextrose, but as the infant improves the IV is weaned down and the oral feeding will be increased as tolerated.

Hyperglycaemia

Causes of hyperglycaemia include:

- stress;
- infusions of parenteral nutrition;
- sepsis;
- very low birthweight (<1000 grams).

Stress

During stress the secretion of the adrenal hormones, adrenaline and glucocorticoids is increased. This results in an increase in blood glucose levels. This is a physiological response to stress and once the stressor has been removed the blood glucose returns to normal. Such stressors include surgery or other stressful procedures (Pildes and Pyati, 1986).

Parenteral nutrition

Combined insulin resistance and a varying infusion of dextrose concentration can result in hyperglycaemia. This is more common in the infant who is receiving parenteral nutrition. The problem may be magnified if the infant is either very pre-term or of very low birthweight. In addition, infusions of lipids can also cause hyperglycaemia because the oxidation of fatty acids enhances gluconeogenesis (Pildes and Pyati, 1986).

Very low birthweight

There is no clear understanding why very low birthweight infants become hyper-glycaemic. Among the theories are the following:

- The insulin response is variable despite production of endogenous hepatic glucose.
- Insulin is resistant due to immature glycogenolysis enzyme systems (Pildes and Pyati, 1986).

Sepsis

Hyperglycaemia may be the first sign of sepsis in the neonate. The pathway for this is understood to be an inability to cope with the endotoxins resulting from bacterial infections. It is thought that endotoxins decrease glucose use (Cowett, 1985).

Nursing management of infants with hyperglycaemia

Following the identification of an at-risk infant, blood glucose is frequently monitored, and urine is required for analysis of glycosuria. This is not usually a problem, as these infants may be polyuric. Medical management will vary depending on the cause of the hyperglycaemia but IV access would be required and infusions of insulin may be given.

Hypocalcaemia/hypercalcaemia

Calcium metabolism

Calcium is central to many physiological functions:

- It is necessary for bone mineralisation.
- It maintains cell permeability.
- It plays a role in muscle contractions and nerve transmissions.
- It is vital for normal cardiac function.
- It also has a role to play in coagulation of the blood.

The regulation of serum calcium levels is under the control of parathyroid hormone and vitamin D. Parathyroid hormone regulates calcium levels by activating the mobilisation of calcium from bone and intestines and reducing the renal excretion of calcium. The precursor for this action is either low serum calcium or magnesium levels. The role of vitamin D is to act with the parathyroid hormone to increase absorption of calcium from the bones.

Calcitonin is the antagonist to this process, lowering the calcium levels by counteracting the effects of parathyroid hormone.

Hypocalcaemia

Pre-term birth is a risk factor for hypocalcaemia, especially if the delivery is before 34 weeks completed gestation as calcium is laid down in foetal bones after this time. Infants of diabetic mothers are also at risk because of a delay in parathyroid hormone production after birth. A third group of infants who are at risk of hypocalcaemia are those who have suffered birth stress or asphyxia. The pathway for this relates to a surge in calcitonin, which suppresses serum calcium levels. Tissue damage and glycogen breakdown associated with asphyxia cause a release of phosphorus into the circulation, which decreases calcium uptake, further compounding any hypocalcaemia.

Clinical presentation of hypocalcaemia

With mild hypocalcaemia the infant may have a subtle range of neuromuscular signs. It may be jittery and hyperactive, and exhibit a high-pitched cry. With more severe hypocalcaemia the infant may suffer from stridor, laryngospasm and fits. In severe hypocalcaemia the cardiac function may be affected, with a prolonged QT interval.

Low-birthweight infants and infants born before 34 weeks gestation have missed out on the period of most rapid accretion of calcium and phosphorous. If these infants are fed unfortified breast milk or standard formula milk, they will not be able to achieve an intra-uterine rate of accumulation. They will be at risk of bone demineralisation, fractures and rickets. Vitamin D is produced in the skin on exposure to ultraviolet irradiation (sunlight); the sick pre-term or low-birthweight infant may go many weeks without the benefit of exposure to sunlight. A vitamin D supplement can be given to pre-term or low-birthweight infants.

Vitamin supplementation is given to all infants below 1,500 grams birth-weight. Supplementation begins when enteral feeds are tolerated and continues until around 6 weeks post discharge. The recommended dose of vitamin D in the form of Calciferol is 600 international units daily.

Hypercalcaemia

More rare, hypercalcaemia is associated with neonatal hyperparathyroidism or maternal hypothyroidism with over-stimulation of the foetal parathyroid glands. It may be iatrogenic due to an over-infusion of calcium.

Clinical presentation of hypercalcaemia

The infant with hypercalcaemia may be hypotonic, irritable, feed poorly and have polyuria resulting in dehydration owing to the interference with the action of antidiuretic hormone (ADH).

Nursing management of hypercalcaemia

The methods are primarily supportive. Hypercalcaemia is corrected either by administration of Frusemide, to induce a diuresis, which will lower the calcium levels, or by the administration of glucocorticoids. Steroids decrease the intestinal absorption of calcium. An infusion of Calcitonin will inhibit the effects of the parathyroid hormone reducing calcium levels. Restricting the dietary intake of calcium is essential and increasing the phosphate intake may promote bone accretion of calcium, thus lowering serum calcium levels. For further information on the management of hypercalcaemia *see* Chapter 10.

FEEDING

All of the anatomical structures of the gastro-intestinal tract are well formed by the second trimester, although functional maturation of these structures occurs later. Maturation and growth of the gastro-intestinal tract is regulated by endogenous events such as release of hormones, and exposure to exogenous factors such as enteral feeding.

Amniotic fluid is swallowed throughout gestation providing about 3 grams of protein per day for foetal growth and development, as well as having a trophic effect upon the gut (Abbas and Tovey, 1960). Supporting evidence for this comes from studies of infants with complete atresia of the upper intestines. Infants born with duodenal atresia have some degree of hypotrophy below the atresia.

The pre-term infant lacks adequate hormone secretion. Physiologically, pre-term infants have decreased bile salts and pancreatic lipase, putting them at risk of fat malabsorption. They have reduced ability to absorb lactose as a result of decreased lactase and reduced enzyme levels lead to incomplete protein digestion. All these factors result in loss of protein and calories in the stool. Despite these limitations, early gut priming will stimulate the gut's functional maturation, whereas lack of enteral feeding can lead to intestinal mucosal atrophy.

Functional immaturity also relates to the organisation of gut motility. The pre-term infant lacks the muscle mass to enable forceful forward movement of gut contents and lacks co-ordination of gut activity. There is diminished oesophageal peristalsis and delayed gastric emptying time. Full distribution of the enteric nervous system is not present until the infant is close to term.

Gut motor activity is cyclical. The cycle consists of muscle stillness followed by irregular contractions interspersed by intense regular contractions, which migrate distally through the gut. Organisation of this cycle is present between 33 and 36 weeks of gestation. By term, fully organised gut motility is achieved.

Early versus late enteral feeding

The timing of the introduction of enteral feeding will be based on an assessment that includes not only cardio-respiratory stability but also on an antenatal history of placental blood flow and perinatal birth history. A maternal history that includes absent or reversed end diastolic flow will indicate caution when administering enteral feeds. Caution is also indicated if there is documented evidence of foetal hypoxia. Both these situations indicate potential for mesenteric ischaemia, increasing the potential for necrotising enterocolitis.

During periods of hypoxia and/or circulatory dysfunction there is circulatory shunting of blood selectively to perfuse vital organs at the expense of 'non-vital' organs such as the gut, resulting in ischaemic injury. Full enteral feeding may compound this. The neonatal gut has limited ability to regulate blood flow and oxygenation. During feeding there is increased need for oxygen and increased mucosal blood flow. If there is underlying respiratory disease, the infant may not be able to meet these increased needs. However, given the evidence for enteral feeding stimulating post-natal gut adaptation and maturation of functional ability, some enteral feed would be advised.

The early introduction of enteral feeding may result in a reduction in total parenteral feeding days. It is possible to extrapolate that reduced parenteral feeding days will equate to reduced cost, reduced risk of line sepsis, and the need for antibiotic therapy (Chapter 15).

Nursing management in feeding pre-term and growth-restricted infants

Both groups of infants are at risk of complications as a result of feeding. This needs to be balanced with the desirability of feeding. Stable pre-term and growth-restricted infants should have small volumes of milk administered via nasogastric tube. For example, 0.5 mls of colostrum or formula given, perhaps, 2-hourly. This milk should be commenced within 24 hours of age with parental knowledge and consent. The priming of the gut does not contribute to the nutritional needs of the infant. The purpose is to stimulate gut hormone activity in order to promote earlier tolerance of full enteral feeding. Initially, the volumes are not increased, to avoid gastric pooling and aspiration. The nasogastric tube is aspirated on a 4–6-hourly basis to check absorption.

Infants should be observed for:

- milky vomits;
- bile-stained vomits;
- bloody stool;
- abdominal distension;
- abdominal tenderness.

The first signs of necrotising enterocolitis (or NEC, a common and serious gut condition) may be systemic and subtle, such as:

- apnoea;
- bradycardia;
- decreased peripheral perfusion (temperature gap greater than 1.5 degrees);
- sluggish capillary refill time (greater than 2 seconds).

For further details of NEC, *see* Chapter 8.

Preferred milk

Ideally, breast milk should be given to the infant, as there are so many advantages. It contains bombesin, somatostatin and epidermal growth factor, all of which play an important role in the post-natal regulation and adaptation of the gut. In addition, breast milk contains protective factors that play a significant role in reducing the incidence of post-natal infections. Protective factors include:

- immunoglobulins;
- complement;
- lysosomes;
- lactoferrin;
- macrophages;
- lymphocytes.

Human milk protein is predominantly in the form of whey, which has the benefit of being easily digested, especially by the pre-term gut. Nutritional needs are considered in greater detail in Chapter 15.

Progression of feeding

With both pre-term and growth-restricted infants the feeding objective is to work towards fully independent feeding, either by breast or bottle, depending on parental wishes. Generally, the more mature growth-restricted infants are ravenous and keen to feed. In contrast, the pre-term infant has yet to learn what is involved. The manner in which feeding is established is influenced by local policy; a few general points are considered below.

- If an infant is demonstrating rooting and latching behaviour, it is giving out cues about a readiness to feed.
- The decision to offer breast or bottle feeds will depend on other factors such as cardio-respiratory stability.
- Offering breast or bottles is developmentally advantageous, will build patterns of appropriate feeding behaviour and will enhance bonding.
- If the infant is exhibiting feeding cues but is unable to take oral feeds, offering non-nutritive sucking opportunities may be beneficial. This can reduce the time taken to achieve full oral feeds. Behaviour may become more settled, enabling the infant to enjoy more prolonged sleep and may significantly shorten hospital stays. (For strategies used to settle infants *see* Chapter 12.)

RESPIRATORY CONSIDERATIONS OF THE PRE-TERM OR GROWTH-RESTRICTED INFANT

Following delivery the pre-term infant usually has a more compromised respiratory function than that of the growth-restricted. This is owing to interrupted development (*see* Chapter 7). Pre-term and growth-restricted infants can be exposed to complications during delivery, which can affect respiratory efficiency. Infants from either group can have co-existing pathology with implications for the respiratory function. In addition, infants of diabetic mothers who may seem large for gestational age can have respiratory difficulties similar to those of the premature.

During foetal life, the lungs are filled with fluid. The fluid volume in the lungs is around 20 mls/kg at term. This fluid is created from filtration of pulmonary capillary blood and secretions from alveolar cells. Foetal breathing movements account for around 600 mls of fluid shift per day. The role and function of foetal lung fluid is not well understood, however, evidence from clinical practice shows that, where there is prolonged reduction in amniotic fluid volume, there is pulmonary hypoplasia. Compression of the lung, for example as a result of diaphragmatic hernia, will also be detrimental to lung development.

Adaptation to air breathing

For the foetus to make a successful transition to air breathing, the lungs must be cleared of fluid. This process begins 2–3 days prior to delivery with a reduction in the volume of fluid being produced. Production ceases completely during labour in response to catecholamine release. Foetal breathing activity is interrupted and the stimulus for breathing activity to recommence is primarily the cooling following delivery. Stimulation by sound, light and touch are also important in increasing central arousal and exciting regular breathing activity. In addition, hypoxia also plays a role in stimulating the onset of breathing (Condorelli and Scrapelli, 1975).

With the first few breaths, residual foetal lung fluid is forced into the pulmonary lymphatic system and lung capillaries. This results in a fall in airway resistance and a rise in functional residual capacity. The compliance of the lungs increases over the first 24 hours following birth as lung fluid continues to be absorbed.

There are three overlapping post-natal developmental stages starting at birth and lasting for four days.

- Stage 1 – adaptation to extra-uterine life; spreading and thinning of endothelial cells; dilatation of the pulmonary arteries.
- Stage 2 – epithelial cells take up their final position and lay down connective tissue.
- Stage 3 – growth of the pulmonary vascularture.

Factors inhibiting lung maturation

Infants of diabetic mothers

The lungs of a foetus of a non-diabetic mother will be mature from a pulmonary perspective by 34 to 35 weeks gestation. The incidence of respiratory distress in the mature infants of diabetic mothers is higher.

There are several theories for this:

- Hyperinsulinaemia may block the cortisol effect in maturing lungs.
- It may delay the surfactant production.
- It may delay fluid clearance and restrict the thinning of the connective tissue in the lung (Kjos et al., 1993).
- Infants of diabetic mothers may be born by elective caesarean section before labour commences. This means that the surge in catecholamines, which may stimulate surfactant release, is missing (Marino and Rooney, 1981).

- Delivery by caesarean section can result in wet lungs. This is due to the absence of vaginal pressure on the chest, responsible for squeezing out the lung fluid.

This is true of any infant delivered by section. Generally speaking, the severity of the respiratory distress will be dependent on the gestational age at delivery. The more pre-term the infant, the more immature the lungs will be.

Perinatal asphyxia

During foetal asphyxia, lung perfusion falls, which can lead to epithelial damage to the air spaces within hours of birth. When the foetus recovers from the asphyxial insult, pulmonary hyper-perfusion occurs. There is a resultant leakage of plasma from the capillaries, which in turn inhibits the function of surfactant. Inadequate surfactant reduces lung compliance and increases atelectasis. This in turn reduces available surface areas for gas exchange, leading to worsening respiratory distress.

Foetal Rh disease

The association between respiratory distress and Rh disease is concerned with the chronic anaemia and pulmonary oedema that occurs in the iso-immunised foetus. This is complicated by the necessity for pre-term delivery. Improved obstetric care has reduced the incidence of severe Rh disease in recent times.

Factors accelerating lung maturity

The administration of antenatal steroids (glucocorticoids) have been shown to accelerate foetal lung maturity and thus reduce neonatal mortality and morbidity from respiratory distress syndrome (Gamsu *et al.*, 1989; Rosenberg *et al.*, 2001).

Growth-restricted infants who have been exposed to chronic stress in utero (maternal toxaemia, maternal hypertension, PROM and placental insufficiency) may have lung maturity in excess of their gestational age. An explanation for the accelerated lung development is the release of high levels of glucocorticoid as a response to the stress. The adrenal glands, which are found in growth-restricted infants, are large and active. Glucocorticoid steroids are secreted by the adrenal glands.

Management of the growth-restricted infant

Because of the factors that accelerate lung development, the growth-restricted infant is at less risk of developing respiratory disease than its appropriate-weight counterpart. The nurse's role is to assess and monitor developments, and facilitate early interventions to achieve and maintain respiratory stability irrespective of gestational age or birthweight.

CARE OF THE PRE-TERM INFANT'S SKIN

In the pre-term infant, the organ of the skin accounts for 13% of total body weight compared with approximately 3% in the older child. The skin of the foetus develops from a single-cell epidermal layer at 3 weeks gestation to fully formed skin and nails at 40 weeks gestation.

Composition of the skin

Skin is composed of three layers:

- epidermis;
- dermis;
- subcutaneous layer.

Epidermis

The horny outer layer of the skin is constructed of stratum corneum, which consists of closely packed dead cells. Exfoliated cells in utero form part of the vernix. New cells are produced at the base of the epidermis and take around 26 days to reach the stratum corneum. Contained at the lower levels of the epidermis are the keratin cells and the melanocytes.

Dermis

The dermis lies directly beneath the epidermis and is 2–4 mm thick at full-term birth. It is constructed of collagen, fibrous protein and elastin fibres. Nerves and blood capillaries are contained within the dermis.

Subcutaneous layer

Fatty connective tissue is the major component of the subcutaneous layer. It functions as a heat insulator, shock absorber and storage area for fat. Subcutaneous tissue is laid down in the final trimester.

Functions of the skin

- The skin acts as a barrier against infection.
- It protects internal organs.
- Skin contributes to thermal regulation.
- It plays a role in fluid balance.
- It provides sensory input.

Associated problems of the skin

The skin problems associated with pre-term birth can be divided into three distinct categories.

Dermal stability

Collagen is deposited in the dermis during the final trimester and prevents fluid accumulating in this layer. When birth occurs before collagen is laid down the infant will exhibit oedema and be at risk of dermal injury secondary to reduced blood flow to the oedematous areas.

Dermal-epidermal cohesion

In the mature skin, fibrils connect the dermis to the epidermis; in the pre-term infant, these connections are few and widely spaced. This puts the infant at risk of blister-type injuries from the removal of tape as well as friction and thermal injury.

Depth of the stratum corneum

The effectiveness of the barrier function of the stratum corneum is related to the depth of this layer. The stratum corneum is composed of keratinocytes coated in lipids. By 30 weeks gestation, this layer is only a few cells thick and below 24 weeks gestation there may be no development of stratum corneum.

Early research indicated that post-natal development of the stratum corneum was accelerated during the 2 weeks following delivery (Evans and Rutter, 1986). However, later research would suggest that in the extremely pre-term infant (less than 24 weeks gestation), the maturation process may take as long as 4 weeks (Sedin *et al.*, 1985).

The clinical implications for reduced thickness of the stratum corneum are related to the extent of transdermal water losses. Infants born at 23 to 24 weeks gestation may lose as much as 13% of total body weight as transdermal water loss in the first day of life in an ambient humidity of 50% (Lund *et al.*, 1999). Transdermal water losses are clinically significant when managing temperature control and fluids (*see* page 86).

Nursing management of the pre-term skin

Nursing management is aimed at preventing the multi-factorial problems of the skin (*see* Table 5.6). Care of the skin can pose more problems in the pre-term infant than in the growth-restricted infant.

Table 5.6   Nursing management of the pre-term skin

Problem	Nursing management
Dermal instability	• Regular change of position • Assess tightness of tapes continuously • Use flexible tapes for securing lines • Assess and review 'dependent' areas regularly • Monitor blood pressure from direct arterial source; if this is not available, release BP cuff after every measurement
Dermal-epidermal cohesion	• Minimal use of tape • Remove tape using a wet swab • Use water-activated electrodes • If facilities are available, monitor heart rate from arterial output not electrodes • Use lowest possible temperature for monitoring transcutaneous PaO_2 and $PaCO_2$ • Change probes 2–3-hourly (balance has to be made between the risk of blister injury and thermal injury)
Loss of temperature and fluid through a thin stratum corneum	• Use double-walled incubators • Use humidity up to 90% in the extremely pre-term infant for a minimum of 14 days

Neonatal skin care is a complex problem that may, on first inspection, appear to be of a lesser priority than cardiovascular or respiratory stability. However, maintenance of skin integrity is vital to the long-term well-being of the pre-term infant and must be considered to be as important as other aspects of neonatal management.

SAMPLE EXAMINATION QUESTIONS

Question 1
Identify some of the factors that may result in the birth of an infant who requires resuscitation. (*20 marks*)
During resuscitation, what are the nurse's priorities? (*80 marks*)

Question 2
What antenatal factors may contribute to an infant being born who is small for gestational age? (*100 marks*)

Question 3
How is heat lost to the environment? (*20 marks*)
What are the implications of cold stress to the infant? (*20 marks*)
What nursing strategies can be employed to maintain a small infant's body temperature? (*60 marks*)

Question 4
In what ways does the skin of a pre-term infant differ from that of a term infant? (*20 marks*)
What nursing steps can be taken to protect the skin of an infant in the NNU? (*70 marks*)

REFERENCES

Abbas, T.M. and Tovey, J.E. (1960) Proteins of the liquor amnii, *British Medical Journal* 1, 476–9

Allen, M. (1998) Outcome and follow-up of high risk infants. In: *Avery's Diseases of the Newborn*, (7th edition), WB Saunders, Philadephia, PA

Ballard, J., Khoury, J.C., Wedig, K., Wang, L. *et al.* (1991) New Ballard Score expanded to include extremely premature infants, *Journal of Pediatrics* 119, 417–23

Bloom, R. and Cropley, C. (1994) *Textbook of Neonatal Resuscitation*, American Heart Association/American Academy of Pediatrics

Boxwell, G. (2000) *Neonatal Intensive Care Nursing* (Chapter 3), Routledge, London

British Medical Association and Royal Pharmaceutical Society (2001) *British National Formulary*, BMA and RPS, London

Charlton, V. (1998) Fetal growth: nutritional issues (perinatal and long-term consequences). In: *Avery's Diseases of the Newborn*, (7th edition), WB Saunders, Philadelphia, PA

Chiswick, M. (1986) Commentary on current World Health Organisation definitions used in perinatal statistics, *Archives of Disease in Childhood* 61(7), 708–10

Condorelli, S. and Scrapelli, E.M. (1975) Somatic respiratory reflex and onset of regular breathing movements in lamb fetus in utero, *Pediatric Research* 9(12), 879–84

Cowett, R.M. (1985) Pathophysiology, diagnosis and management of glucose homeostasis in the neonate, *Curr Prob Pediatr* 15(3), 1–47

Dawes, G. and Jacobson, H. (1963) Treatment of asphyxia in newborn lambs and monkeys, *Journal of Physiology* 169, 167–84

Department of Health [DoH] (2001) *Review of the Deaths of Four Babies due to Cardiac Tamponade associated with the Presence of a Central Venous Catheter*, DoH, London

Drew, D., Jevon P. and Raby M. (2000) *Resuscitation of the Newborn: A Practical Approach*, Butterworth Heinemann, Oxford

Drew, D., Jevon, P. and Raby, M. (2001) Resuscitation of the newborn: a step-by-step guide, *Journal of Neonatal Nursing* 7(4) [supplement]

Dubowitz, L.M.S., Dubowitz, V. and Goldberg, C. (1970) Clinical assessment of gestational age in the newborn infant, *Journal of Paediatrics* 77(1), 1–10

Ellemunter, H., Simma, B., Trawoger, R. and Maurer, H. (1999) Intraosseous lines in pre-term and full-term neonates, *Archives of Disease in Childhood, Fetal and Neonatal Edition* 80(1), 74–5

Evans, N.J. and Rutter, N. (1986) Development of the epidermis in the newborn, *Biology of the Neonate* 49(2), 74–80

Field, D., Milner, A. and Hopkin, I. (1986) Efficiency of manual resuscitators at birth, *Archives of Disease in Childhood* 61(3), 300–2

Fisher, R. and Prosser, D. (2000) Intraosseous access in infant resuscitation, *Archives of Disease in Childhood* 83(1), 87

Gamsu, H.P., Mullinger, B.M. and Donnai, P. (1989) Antenatal administration of betamethasone to prevent respiratory distress syndrome in pre-term infants, *Journal of Obstetrics and Gynaecology* 96(4), 401

Hancock, P. and Peterson, G. (1992) Finger intubation of the trachea in newborns, *Paediatrics* 89(2), 325–7

Heimler, R., Doumas, B.T. *et al.* (1993) Relationship between nutrition and weight and fluid compartments in the pre-term infants during the first week of life, *Journal of Pediatrics* 122(1), 110–14

Hitter, H.M., Hirsch, N.J. and Rudolph, A.J. (1977) Assessment of gestational age by examination of the anterior vascular capsule of the lens, *Journal of Pediatrics* 91(3) 455–8

Houska, C. and Durand, D. (1998) Skin and skin care, Chapter 17. In: Merenstein, G. and Gardner, S. (eds) *Handbook of Neonatal Intensive Care*, Mosby, St Louis, IL

Kelnar, C., Harvey, D. and Simpson, C. (1995) Chapter 3. In: *The Sick Newborn Baby* (3rd edition), Ballière Tindall, London

Kjos, S.L., Henry, O.A. *et al.* (1993) Insulin requiring diabetes in pregnancy: a randomized trial of active induction of labor and expectant management, *American Journal of Obstetrics and Gynecology* 169(3), 611–15

Lepley, C., Gardner, S. and Lubchenco, L. (1998) Chapter 5. In: Merenstein, G. and Gardner, S. (eds.) *Handbook of Neonatal Intensive Care*, Mosby, St Louis, IL

Levene, M., Tudehope, D. and Thearle, J. (1987) Initial nursery care, Chapter 9, *Essentials of Neonatal Medicine*, Blackwell Scientific, Oxford

Lubchenco, L.O. and Bard, H. (1971) Incidence of hypoglycaemia in newborn infants classified by birthweight and gestational age, *Pediatrics* 47(5), 831–8

Lund, C., Kuller, J. and Lane, A. (1999) Neonatal skin care: the scientific basis for practice, *Journal of Obstetrics, Gynaecology and Neonatal Nursing* 28(3), 241–52

Marino, P.A. and Rooney, S.A. (1981) The effects of labor on surfactant secretion in newborn rabbit lung slices. Cited in *Avery's Diseases of the Newborn*, (7th edition), WB Saunders, Philadelphia, PA

Marlow, N. (1992) Do we need an Apgar score? *Archives of Disease in Childhood, Fetal and Neonatal Edition* **67**(7), 765–9

Royal College of Paediatrics and Child Health (1999) Medicines for Children, RCPCH, London

Niermayer, S. and Clarke, S. (1998) Delivery room care, Chapter 4. In: Merenstein, G. and Gardner, S. (eds.) *Handbook of Neonatal Intensive Care*, Mosby, St Louis, IL

Palme-Kilander, C. and Tunell, R. (1993) Pulmonary gas exchange during face mask ventilation immediately after birth, *Archives of Disease in Childhood* **68**(1), 11–16

Pildes, R. and Pyati, S.P. (1986) Hypoglycaemia and hyperglycaemia in tiny infants, *Clinics of Perinatology* **13**(2), 351–75

Rennie, J.M. and Roberton, N.R.C. (2002) *A Manual of Neonatal Intensive Care* (Resuscitation of the newborn, Chapter 6) (4th edition), Oxford University Press, Oxford

Resuscitation Council UK (2000) *Resuscitation at Birth: The Newborn Life Support Course Manual*, Resuscitation Council, London

Roberton, N.R.C. (1996) *A Manual of Normal Neonatal Care* (Resuscitation of the newborn, Chapter 4), (2nd edition), Arnold, London

Roberton, N.R.C. (1999) Resuscitation of the newborn, Chapter 16. In: Rennie, J. and Roberton, N.R.C. (eds) *Textbook of Neonatology*, (3rd edition), Churchill Livingstone, Edinburgh

Rosenberg, K.D., Desai, R.A., Na, Y., Kan, J. and Schwartz, L. (2001) The effect of surfactant on birthweight specific neonatal mortality rate in New York, *Annals of Epidemiology* **11**(5), 337–41

Sedin, G. (1996) Fluid management in the extremely low birthweight pre-term infant. In: Hansen, T.N. and McIntosh, N. (eds) *Current Topics in Neonatology*, WB Saunders, London

Sedin, G., Hammarland, K., Nilsson, G.E. *et al.* (1985) Measurement of transepidermal water loss in newborn infants, *Clinics in Perinatology* **12**(1), 79–99

Sheldon, T. (2001) Dutch doctors change policy on treating pre-term babies, *BMJ* **322**(7299), 1383

Spiedel, B., Fleming, P., Henderson, J., Leaf, A. *et al.* (1998) In the delivery room, Chapter 2. In: *A Neonatal Vade-Mecum*, (3rd edition), Arnold, London

Stephenson, T., Marlow, N., Watkin, S. and Grant, J. (2000) *Pocket Neonatology* (Early Care, Chapter 3), Churchill Livingstone, Edinburgh

Taeusch, H.W. and Sniderman, S. (1998) History and physical examination of the newborn. In: *Avery's Diseases of the Newborn*, (7th edition), WB Saunders, Philadelphia, PA

Vohr, B., Wright, L.L. and Dusick, A.M. (2000) Neurodevelopmental and functional outcomes of extremely low-birthweight infants in the National Institute of Child Health and Human Development, Neonatal Research Network, *Pediatrics* **105**(6), 1216–26

Vyas, H., Milner, A. and Hopkin, I. (1983) Face mask resuscitation:does it lead to gastric distension? *Archives of Disease in Childhood* **58**(5), 373–5

Yeo, H. (1998) *Nursing the Neonate* (Preterm labour and the birth of a small baby, Chapter 2), Blackwell Sciences, Oxford

6 Nursing care of an infant with jaundice

Doreen Crawford

Aims of the chapter

This chapter reviews the physiology of neonatal hyperbilirubinaemia (jaundice) and outlines the causes. It then focuses on the care of an infant with this condition.

Introduction

Jaundice can be described as a yellow discoloration of the skin and mucous membranes. From a biochemical perspective, it is a state of high bilirubin levels (in excess of 25 micromoles per litre, or μmol/l) in the circulation (hyperbilirubinaemia), and not usually evident until levels of 85–100 μmol/l are reached. Experienced neonatal nurses and midwives spot most cases of jaundice on visual inspection, although this method is subjective, and can be influenced by green or yellow clothing in the infant, or poor artificial lighting. Rose (2000) has outlined Kramer's rule, which involves a visual inspection of the areas of the body involved and blanching the skin to observe the colour of the tissues. However, caution is urged when applying this rule to the sick or the pre-term infant.

Locally, jaundice is expected to affect 80% of premature infants (the smaller and sicker the more likely the incidence) and probably as many as 50% of well term infants. It is not a disorder, but a symptom and there are many possible causes.

Frequently used terms

An awareness of the frequently used terms is crucial to an understanding of neonatal jaundice.

Physiological jaundice

This is part of the 'normal' process of adaptation from uterine life to self-sufficiency. It becomes apparent from the third day and has usually gone by a week. It is not part of a disease process and in normal infants who are feeding and are well hydrated there is unlikely to be any sequelae.

Pathological jaundice

This occurs as a result of hyperbilirubinaemia because of a disease process. For example, excess destruction of red blood cells (erythrocytes) which may have occurred because of blood incompatibility ABO or antibodies. More rarely, it may be because of a metabolic abnormality or may indicate serious liver malformation.

Conjugated bilirubin
This is sometimes called direct bilirubin, bilirubin that has been 'processed'. It is water-soluble.

Unconjugated bilirubin
This is sometimes called indirect bilirubin, and is protein-bound bilirubin. It has not yet been 'processed' by the liver.

Haemolysis
This is the destruction of red blood cells.

Bilirubin

Bilirubin is the broken-down (catabolised) product of haem, the red protein of the erythrocyte and is processed in the liver, spleen and in tissue macrophages as a result of cellular (microsomal) activity. In newborn infants, the circulating level of bilirubin is increased owing to the shorter lifespan of foetal erythrocytes, the greater proportion of red cells to body weight and to the immaturity of the liver.

Bilirubin is conjugated in the liver by converting insoluble unconjugated bilirubin to water-soluble bilirubin. Each molecule of unconjugated bilirubin is conjugated with two molecules of glucuronic acid and is then catalysed by the enzyme glucuronyl transferase. Conjugated bilirubin is excreted into the bile and then into the duodenum and small intestine.

In older children the process ends there, with the conjugated bilirubin further reduced to stercobilinogen by bacteria in the bowel. However, in the newborn infant, a second pathway exists and bilirubin can rebound back. This is due to the sterile uncolonised bowel and slow clearance of meconium, the bowel contents, because of poor peristalsis. Conjugated bilirubin is hydrolysed by glucuronidase back to unconjugated bilirubin, which is reabsorbed and transferred, via the enterohepatic blood circulation, for further hepatic metabolism.

The foetal liver is a fairly inactive organ; it is the maternal liver that processes the bilirubin from spent erythrocytes. If haemolysis is excessive, this could be obvious from birth, as the cord and the amniotic fluid may be stained yellow by the excess pigment. Blood production (haemopoiesis) may have failed to keep pace with the infant's need for erythrocytes, and secondary anaemia, and even heart failure, can result.

Neonatal jaundice is important because of the risk of Kernicterus, which occurs when bilirubin crosses the blood-brain barrier. The term comes from the discovery that, in dead infants who had been severely jaundiced, the brains were yellow (Schmorl, 1903). Although very rare, Kernicterus is fatal in 75% of cases.

Infants who do survive suffer fits, learning difficulties, and postural and behavioural disability.

Hyperbilirubinaemia is a toxic condition (Augustine, 1999) and has been incriminated in infants with poor feeding, hypotonic, lethargic states (Maisels, 1994) and hearing impairments (Vohr *et al.*, 1989). There is significant debate relating to the unconjugated bilirubin levels that will become pathological, as this varies with the maturity, weight and health of the infant. Large term infants can tolerate greater levels than small, sick, premature infants. Units throughout the UK vary tremendously in their practice as to when therapy should be instituted (Hansen, 1996; Coe, 1999).

Jaundiced infants who are otherwise well

The neonatal nurse does not see many well term infants. These infants are thought to tolerate much higher levels of bilirubinaemia but many jaundiced infants are not being screened as a precaution, owing to changes in care patterns. There is a preference for early discharge and some cases are no doubt going undetected (Maisels and Newman, 1998). If they are detected, there is sometimes a reluctance to medicalise and to admit the infant to hospital for therapy (Newman and Maisels, 2000). There is a need for a neonatal team in the community to monitor blood levels and administer home phototherapy when appropriate (Hamelin and Seshia, 1998). For guidelines on how to manage the jaundiced infant who is otherwise well, *see* Augustine (1999).

Jaundice timetable

Because there are so many possible causes of jaundice the infant could be subjected to a battery of unnecessary investigations. One fortunate aid to diagnosis is the time when the jaundice appears, and its pattern.

- Early jaundice is apparent at birth or appears within 24 hours. It requires urgent investigation.
- Prolonged jaundice appears by day two/three of life but fails to clear after 10 days.
- Re-occurring jaundice is jaundice which has cleared and then returns.
- Profound jaundice or jaundice with a greenish tinge should always be investigated immediately, regardless of time of onset.

INVESTIGATIONS

The investigations performed will reflect the manner in which the jaundice occurred and the severity of the condition. The rarer the cause of jaundice, the more profound the investigation.

Bilirubin measurement

Bilirubin measurement is the first and most obvious investigation. Non-invasive transcutaneous bilirubinometry methods exist (Schumacher, 1990). These are increasingly useful, correlate well with serum levels (Knudsen and Ebbesen, 1996), and may in time replace serum estimation. Most neonatal units have a bilirubinometer to measure bilirubin from the serum of a centrifuged sample of blood. More sophisticated tests, which split the levels of conjugated and unconjugated bilirubin, require laboratory testing. If phototherapy is in progress at the time of blood harvest, the light should be temporarily switched off.

Coombs test

This detects the presence of antibodies coating the erythrocytes. A reagent is used to cause the cells to agglutinate, which results in a positive Coombs.

Full infection screen

A full infection screen will vary from unit to unit. It may include a chest X-ray, blood samples for TORCH culture (toxoplasmosis, others [for example, syphilis], rubella, cytomegalovirus, herpes, hepatitis), lumbar puncture, urine for culture, gastric aspiration, and endotracheal aspirations. Suspicious-looking sites may also be swabbed.

Blood and urine tests

- The ethnic group and the family history will indicate if blood is appropriate, for specific investigation of sickle cell or G-6PD.
- Blood and urine tests should be undertaken for specific investigation of metabolic disorders such as galactosaemia.
- Urine should be tested for conjugated bilirubin.
- The infant's blood group should be established.
- The mother's blood group should be known.
- Haemoglobin, blood film and reticulocytes should be tested.

Other tests include:

- thyroid function tests;
- liver function tests;
- liver ultrasound;
- cholangiogram;
- liver biopsy;
- exploratory laparotomy.

TREATMENT FOR JAUNDICE

Conventional treatment to reduce unconjugated bilirubin levels will be either phototherapy or exchange transfusion. The method used will depend on the actual level of bilirubin, the rapidity with which the jaundice occurred, and the clinical condition and weight of the infant. Exchange transfusion gives rapid results whereas phototherapy takes longer.

Pharmacological methods of reducing bilirubin levels are possible (Valaes *et al.*, 1990), as many chemicals bind to bilirubin, but such methods are not currently popular. Phenobarbitone has been therapeutically used but has to be metabolised and has side-effects such as sedation. For the sick small infant, drug metabolism can be a problem. Even for the larger, fitter infant, sedation at such a critical time, when relationships need to be formed and breast-feeding established, would be counter-productive. A breakthrough may come with the clinical success of haem oxygenase inhibition (Rubaltelli, 1998; Steffensrud, 1998).

Phototherapy

Phototherapy, initially used in the late 1950s (Cremer *et al.*, 1958), is the first-line method of management. The equipment consists of a number of fluorescent light tubes, which emit light in the blue-green band of the visible spectrum at 420–470 nanometers (Ennever, 1990). Phototherapy works in a number of ways:

- by changing the structure of unconjugated bilirubin so it can be excreted through bile and urine without the need for conjugation;
- by photo-oxidation, which occurs when the bilirubin absorbs light, and is oxidised, producing water-soluble products that can be excreted in urine;
- by photo-isomerisation, converting unconjugated bilirubin into a soluble isomer that is harmless and slowly excreted into bile.

Phototherapy is never given for raised conjugated bilirubin levels as it results in Bronze Infant Syndrome, owing to the different photo-degradation products produced. This is harmless but daunting for the staff and parents.

There may be a few complications with phototherapy (see below), however, it is not invasive and is very effective, usually within a couple of days.

Risk of eye damage

Radiation from this band of light has been shown to cause retinal damage in animal models. Infants having this therapy must have eye protection, using a tinted screen or eye shields. Exposed infants are extremely mobile and can wriggle out from under a tinted screen. If eye shields are used, the eyes should be checked for corneal abrasion; this sort of damage is rare but should be avoided.

Risk of hypo/hyperthermia

Light at this wavelength does not emit much heat and the exposed infant can get cold. Incubators should be set in the correct thermo-neutral range and the infant's temperature monitored constantly – some need more help to maintain their temperature than others.

Risk of dehydration

Phototherapy may decrease the bowel transit time and result in diarrhoea, probably as a result of irritation in the bowel wall, caused by the presence of photo-isomers of bilirubin. Jaundiced infants are commonly drowsy and may not wake for feeds. Some units recommend a 25 per cent increase in fluids.

Risk of skin irritation and damage

Deposits of bile salts in the skin can cause irritation and itching. Strong term infants can scratch and traumatise themselves. Redness and inflammation can occur from a photosensitive reaction, resulting in the release of histamine from mast cells. This condition is exacerbated if lotions are used or if the nappy area is not thoroughly cleansed of urine and excreta prior to commencing therapy. Skin care using warm water should be performed every 4 to 6 hours to maintain skin integrity.

Risk of genetic changes

The gonads, which contain genetic materials, are vulnerable organs. There have been concerns regarding genetic damage from high-intensity light. Although maximum exposure is desirable for quicker resolution of the jaundice, the pelvic areas ought to be covered (Edwards, 1995) until further research can inform practice.

Information for parents

The greatest disadvantage of phototherapy is the impact that the treatment can have on the parents. New mothers, especially at about the third day, are in a vulnerable position; having a very jaundiced infant means extra blood tests, which may result in the infant's distress and increased maternal anxiety. With flexibility in today's care, the infant need not be admitted to the NNU solely for phototherapy, providing they are otherwise well. Such infants can be managed adequately on the post-natal ward, where the mother can remain the primary care-giver and have continuous contact. A detailed explanation, given to both parents and perhaps backed up with a written supplement, can help reduce anxiety.

Exchange transfusion

Exchange transfusion was first used in 1951 and the procedure is rarely seen these days. It is not undertaken lightly as it has several potentially hazardous complications. It is usually used in conjunction with phototherapy. It is effective, not only removing excess bilirubin but also, in the case of rhesus disease, removing antibody and correcting anaemia. The amount of blood to be exchanged will depend on the condition of the infant, but commonly about 90–95% of blood volume is replaced.

Transfusion can be performed by continuous removal of the infant's blood from the umbilical vein, balanced by continuous transfusion of donor blood into another limb. This has the advantage of ensuring that there is no serial fluctuation in the circulating volume. Flow rates can be difficult to manage and, if catheter complications occur in one line, the procedure should stop immediately so as not to lose track of the fluid balance.

An alternative is serial withdrawal and replacement of aliquots of 5, 10, 20 mls of blood, preferably using the umbilical vein. The volume removed and replaced with each cycle depends on the condition and weight of the infant, and its tolerance to the procedure. It is very time-consuming as it is performed slowly. It is often difficult to maintain concentration during such a repetitious procedure so various types of chart have been designed to ensure that the fluid balance is correct.

Both methods are equally efficient and both have the potential for serious haemodynamic, metabolic and mechanical complications. Whenever the umbilical vein is used, the position of the cannula is always checked by X-ray. For an excellent review of the procedure, *see* Yeo (1998).

Haemodynamic alterations

The infant's vital signs should be continuously monitored to detect changes from the baseline or progressive subtle alterations. Removal or replacement of blood that is too rapid can result in disastrous haemodynamic complications. All emergency equipment and drugs should be checked and available.

Metabolic alterations of exchange

In the past, walking donors were used, but, owing to the difficulties involved in screening these donors, fresh, banked blood is now used. Hyperkalaemia and arrhythmia can occur in infants more than two days old who have received blood. The citrate that is present in banked blood, to prevent it clotting, can cause hypocalcaemia in small infants who have had comprehensive exchanges. Blood gas, glucose and electrolyte levels should be monitored regularly, to ensure tight control of the metabolic status.

Mechanical complications of exchange transfusion

As with any invasive procedure, there is a risk of introducing infection, so an exchange transfusion should be performed under aseptic conditions. There should be close observation of the lines going to the infant, to prevent air emboli.

Other medical complications

- Thrombosis of the aorta and of the portal vein has been reported. Exchange transfusion via the umbilical vein has also been incriminated in necrotising enterocolitis.
- There is a risk of hypothermia.
- Infants undergoing exchange transfusion need continuous monitoring of temperature. If the incubator doors are likely to be open for a long period, the infant is best nursed under a radiant heat source. This ensures maximum visibility and optimal control of temperature. If the infant is unstable and already in an incubator, the desirability of a radiant warmer needs to be balanced with the undesirable effect of extra handling. A heat shield (which restricts access) or bubble wrap (which restricts visibility) may need to be considered.

- Cold blood will chill the infant, so blood should be given through a specialised blood warmer. Blood should never be left out to warm up.

CAUSES OF JAUNDICE

The causes of jaundice in the neonatal period can fit into a number of categories:

- Haemolytic jaundice occurs when excess haemolysis of red cells results in a level of bilirubin that overloads clearance mechanisms.
- Hepatocellular jaundice occurs when the infant's liver cells are unable to fulfil the normal functions.
- Obstructive jaundice occurs when the biliary tree is blocked and drainage of bilirubin cannot occur.

Causes of jaundice at birth or occurring within 24 hours

Haemolytic jaundice often appears in the first 24 hours of life and always needs investigating. The causes include:

- rhesus haemolytic disease;
- ABO incompatibility;
- congenital infection;
- severe overwhelming acquired infection;
- abnormality in shape or composition of red cells, such as hereditary spherocytosis, alpha thalassaemia, G-6PD and sickle cell anaemia.

Erythroblastosis foetalis
This is a severe, antibody-mediated haemolytic destruction of erythrocytes, resulting in profound anaemia, causing cardiac failure and generalised oedema. It occurs when the mother had been sensitised to an antigen present on the foetus's erythrocyte and subsequently produces antibodies to this antigen. An Rh– mother carrying an Rh+ infant is the most common but other antibodies can be involved. This sensitivity can result from the birth of a previous infant, a spontaneous miscarriage, termination of pregnancy and small antepartum haemorrhages. A detailed history may alert the obstetric and neonatal team to an infant at risk. Other risks are obstetric procedures such as chorionic villus sampling or amniocentesis.

The rhesus status of every pregnant woman is obtained. Rh– women should be given injections of anti D with every risk incident. Antenatally, serial antibody measurements are taken and, if these rise, intervention may be necessary. In a severely affected foetus the risk of early delivery versus the risk of a hostile uterine environment needs to be balanced. Occasionally, the dramatic step of giving an intra-uterine transfusion is taken.

Such infants demand a high level of care and expertise. Initial management of a severely affected infant includes the following:

- resuscitation;
- correction of acidosis;
- drainage of effusions;
- immediate exchange transfusion;
- administration of diuretics;
- sensitive handling of the family.

Successful resuscitation means that intensive care and support of the family will be required as will the management of repeated exchange transfusions and small top-ups, to relieve anaemia.

Congenital infection

Congenital infections, as causes of jaundice, include cytomegalovirus (CMV), rubella, herpes, toxoplasmosis and syphilis, etc.

Trans-placental transmission of the virus, parasite or spirochaete has important and long-term ramifications for the infant. Maternal infection with herpes may influence the mode and timing of delivery, to avoid vaginal contact. CMV, rubella and herpes are potentially infectious so, as well as treatment and management of the presenting condition and the jaundice, universal precautions will need to be applied. The jaundice may be a mixed haemolytic and hepatocellular type.

Abnormality in shape and structure of the red cell

Glucose-6-phosphate dehydrogenase deficiency (G-6PD) is an inherited enzyme defect rendering the erythrocyte prone to haemolysis when exposed to environmentally determined trigger factors such as infection, drugs and some foods. Alpha thalassaemia is a genetically transmitted cause of an abnormal red cell protein structure, causing serious haemolytic disease. Hereditary spherocytosis and sickle cell disease are abnormalities in shape and structure of the red cell; if severe haemolytic disease is present in the neonatal period, jaundice will occur.

Jaundice occurring from day two–five

Physiological jaundice may occur from day two–five. Causes of jaundice occurring at this period include the following:

- excessive bruising;
- infection;
- drugs;
- metabolic diseases such as galactosaemia;
- a few rare genetic syndromes such as Gilbert's or Crigler-Najjar.

Physiological jaundice

Physiological jaundice is an accepted deviation from normal. The pathology results from the imbalance between bilirubin production and excretion. Physiological jaundice may be exacerbated by dehydration and poor feeding. It arises on day three and is resolved by day 10, causing no damage and not requiring active treatment. Parental anxiety can be encountered, so sympathetic explanation and reassurance may be appreciated.

The jaundice resulting from excessive bruising is similar in origin as it occurs from the haemolysis of extravascular blood loss, caused by severe trauma, for example, a difficult breech extraction. The effects can be compounded if the infant is premature. Some of these infants need phototherapy.

Infection

Infected infants are always actively treated and many will need phototherapy. Bacterial infection causes erythrocyte destruction, liberating bilirubin. Infection causes the infant to be severely ill and shut down, subsequently impairing the ability of the liver to handle this extra load.

Drugs

Drugs such as oxytocin used during labour compete with bilirubin for bonding sites. As a consequence, the free bilirubin level is raised, sometimes enough to warrant phototherapy.

Metabolic disorders

These are numerically very rare and not all cause a rise in unconjugated bilirubin; phototherapy may not be indicated. These disorders may occur in the same period as physiological jaundice but may be initially mild then gradually deepen and fail to resolve, resulting in investigation.

Prolonged jaundice

One type of prolonged jaundice, occurring in breast-fed infants, is termed 'breast milk jaundice'. Other causes of prolonged jaundice include:

- the endocrine disorders of hypothyroidism and hypopituitarism;
- neonatal hepatitis;
- biliary atresia;
- other obstructive causes.

Breast-feeding and jaundice

Some studies have suggested that there are significant differences in the proportion of breast-fed infants developing jaundice when compared with those who are artificially fed (Salariya and Robertson, 1993). The causes are probably a combination of dehydration and a delay in passing first stool, as there is less stimulus and bulk in the neonate's intestine to promote peristalsis. This type of jaundice is harmless although more frequent access to the breast would probably be beneficial. There is, however, a phenomenon of prolonged jaundice in breast-fed infants, which is unfortunately termed 'breast milk jaundice'.

The cause of breast milk jaundice is probably due to enzymes in the milk splitting conjugated bilirubin back to unconjugated bilirubin and the increased levels of this in blood circulation colouring the infant's tissues. It is a diagnosis, almost by default, once other causes are ruled out. Usually the levels, although unconjugated, are not high enough to warrant treatment and it is regarded as harmless – although there may be trauma to the mother's esteem. Sadly, many of these mothers tend to give up breast-feeding, which is unnecessary but effective in clearing up the jaundice.

Hypothyroidism
Although this can result in prolonged jaundice, owing to sluggish metabolism, there are usually sufficient clues to aid diagnosis prior to this. Treatment is with thyroxine and, if diagnosed quickly, prognosis is good.

Hypopituitarism
This is very rare. If suspected, management is best in a specialist unit.

Neonatal hepatitis
This results in severe, prolonged, conjugated jaundice. Other indications are often non-specific and diagnosis may be delayed. Phototherapy is unnecessary and management is best in a specialist unit as over half of these infants will go on to develop cirrhosis or chronic liver failure.

Biliary atresia
This causes obstructive jaundice owing to the absence of the bile ducts, which means that bile produced cannot drain. It is a rare condition and may not present in the neonatal period. However, it is a diagnosis that should not be missed; clinic nurses and health visitors are well placed to alert the family to an intractable problem and direct the infant to medical attention. Stools are pale, owing to the absence of stercobilin, and the jaundice has a greenish tinge. Prognosis depends on how quickly repair can be attempted. The aim of repair is to establish bile drainage into the small intestine. With no intervention, diminished bile flow results in biliary cirrhosis, portal vein hypertension, varices, ascites and chronic liver failure (Kedzierski, 1991). With uncorrectable disease, transplantation becomes necessary, usually during the second year of life. Recent advances in liver reduction have made the outlook better but problems in tissue typing and insufficient organ donors remain.

Other causes of obstructive jaundice include inspissated bile, cystic fibrosis, rare tumours and cystic lesions.

SAMPLE EXAMINATION QUESTIONS

Question 1
What are some of the most common reasons for an infant suffering jaundice? (*70 marks*)
How can the infant/mother bond be promoted while the infant is having therapy for a raised bilirubin level? (*30 marks*)

Question 2

What are the complications of phototherapy? (*20 marks*)
What nursing strategies can be used to help overcome these? (*80 marks*)

REFERENCES

Augustine, C. (1999) Hyperbilirubinaemia in the healthy term newborn, *The Nurse Practitioner* 24(4), 24–41

Coe, L. (1999) Pathology and physiology of neonatal jaundice, *British Journal of Midwifery* 7(4), 240–3

Cremer, R. *et al.* (1958) Influence of light on the hyperbilirubinaemia of infants, *The Lancet* 1, 1094

Edwards, S. (1995) Phototherapy and the neonate, *Journal of Neonatal Nursing* 1(5), 9–12

Ennever, J. (1990) Blue light, green light, white light, more light, treatment of neonatal jaundice, *Clinics in Perinatology* 17(2) 467–81

Hamelin, K. and Seshia, M. (1998) Home phototherapy for uncomplicated neonatal jaundice, *Canadian Nurse* 94(1), 39–40

Hansen, T. (1996) Therapeutic approaches to neonatal jaundice; an international survey, *Clinical Pediatrics* 35(6), 309–16

Kedzierski, M. (1991) Liver disease in babies and children, *Nursing Standard* 5(43), 30–3

Knudsen, A. and Ebbesen, F. (1996) Transcutaneous bilirubinometery in neonatal intensive care units, *Archives of Disease in Childhood* 75(1), 53–6

Maisels, M. (1994) Jaundice. In: Avery, G., Fletcher, M. and MacDonald, M. (eds) *Neonatology, Pathophysiology and Management of the Newborn*, (4th edition), Lippincott-Raven Publications, Philadelphia, PA, pp. 630–708

Maisels, M. and Newman, T. (1998) Jaundice in the full-term and near-term babies who leave hospital – the pediatrician's nemesis, *Clinics in Perinatology* 25(2), 295–302

Newman, T. and Maisels, M. (2000) Less aggressive therapy of neonatal jaundice and reports of Kernicterus; lessons about practice guidelines, *Paediatrics* 1(3), 242–5

Rose, F. (2000) Monitoring bilirubin, *Journal of Neonatal Nursing* 6(5), 158

Rubaltelli, F. (1998) Current drug treatment options in neonatal hyperbilirubinaemia and the prevention of Kernicterus, *Drugs* 56(1), 23–30

Salariya, E. and Robertson, C. (1993) Relationships between baby feeding types and patterns, gut transit time of meconium and the incidence of neonatal jaundice, *Midwifery* 9, 235–42

Schmorl, G. (1903) Zur Kenntniss des Ikterus Neonatorum, insbesondere der dabei auftretenden Gehirnveranderungen, *Verhandlung Deutsche Pathology Gesellschaft* 6, 109

Schumacher, R. (1990) Noninvasive measurement of bilirubin in the newborn, *Clinics in Perinatology* 17(2), 417–35

Steffensrud, S. (1998) Tin metalloporphyrins – an answer to neonatal jaundice, *Neonatal Network* 17(5), 11–17

Valaes, T. *et al.* (1990) Pharmacologic approaches to the prevention and treatment of neonatal hyperbilirubinaemia, *Clinics in Perinatology* 17(2), 245–73

Vohr, B. *et al.* (1989) Abnormal brain stem function and acoustic cry features in term infants with hyperbilirubinaemia, *Journal of Pediatrics* 115, 303–8

Yeo, H. (1998) Nursing the neonate (Chapter 12). In: *Nursing Management of the Jaundiced Baby*, 241–59 Blackwell Science, London, pp. 241–59

FURTHER READING

Marieb, E. (1992) *Human Anatomy and Physiology*, (2nd edition), Benjamin Cummings Publishing Company, USA

Yeo, H. (1998) *Nursing the Neonate*, Blackwell Science, London

7 Nursing care of an infant with a disorder of the respiratory system

Doreen Crawford and Jill Fairhurst

Aims of the chapter

This chapter introduces the basic development of the respiratory system and considers the changes at birth. Supportive management and treatment strategies are reviewed and the care of an infant with some of the most common conditions found on the neonatal unit is discussed.

Introduction

Respiratory problems are the commonest cause of morbidity and mortality in the neonatal period. Each infant has an individual difference in its rate of respiration, although the average is about 40 breaths per minute. Efficient and effective respiration, with adequate gas exchange, will never result in laboured respiration.

What constitutes tachypnoea may be defined differently between units. Locally, we regard a respiratory rate of 60 breaths per minute or over as tachypnoeic.

The collection of clinical symptoms, indicating respiratory difficulties, remains fairly constant across a wide range of diseases and disorders. The main ones are as follows:

- The extra effort required in meeting the infant's respiratory needs causes retraction of intercostal and subcostal muscles. This makes the infant look as if the sternum is about to collapse.
- The use of accessory muscles makes the nose flare.
- Combined use of the neck and shoulder muscles may give the infant a tense and distorted look. The chest may look large and out of proportion.
- Hypoxia will lead to pallor or cyanosis of the skin and mucous membrane tissues.
- Respiratory muscle failure, mainly affecting the diaphragm, will rapidly lead to exhaustion and apnoea, especially in the premature infant.
- Initially, the infant may be restless, but the sicker the infant, the more lethargic it will become, conserving all its energy in a desperate struggle to breathe and stay alive.

Anatomy and physiology of the respiratory system

Knowledge and understanding of normal foetal development of the lungs and the respiratory tract, and of the transition from uterine to extra-uterine life, has

thoracic pressure exerted on the baby's chest wall by the maternal birth canal. The fluid remaining in the lungs, under normal circumstances, is removed by increased lymph drainage and swallowing after coughing and sneezing. Occasionally, in an otherwise well, mature term infant, these mechanisms fail to clear the lungs and the infant suffers a temporary respiratory problem called transient tachypnoea of the newborn.

The first breath does not expand both lungs fully. It is probable that hours or even days elapse until the lungs are well ventilated and evenly expanded. Vital capacity and residual volume will increase as the pattern of breathing becomes established. Chest circumference has a rapid increase in the first 24 to 48 hours after birth. It may take several months for the pulmonary anatomy to adapt and the pulmonary vessels to function in a mature way. These changes are sometimes delayed in infants who are born pre-term, in infants with cardiac abnormalities and those living at high altitude (MacGregor, 2000).

STRUCTURAL DIFFERENCES IN ANATOMY BETWEEN THE INFANT AND THE MATURE

Differences exist in the anatomy of the infant's respiratory system compared to that of the adult. The main differences are:

- The infant's airway has a smaller diameter.
- The infant's lungs are relatively immature and inelastic.
- Cough reflex is absent until 32–34 weeks gestation.
- An infant has a high larynx, protected by the epiglottis. This has the effect of producing a direct airway from the nasal cavity to the lungs. The infant is therefore an obligatory nose breather.
- The ribs of the newborn are positioned horizontally and the intercostal muscles are weak.
- The thoracic wall in the infant is compliant. The net effect of this is that the mode of lung ventilation is essentially a diaphragmatic one and, if difficulties occur, the thoracic wall may 'cave in' and give rise to sternal and intercostal retractions with the extra strain of breathing.
- The premature and sick newborn is highly susceptible to diaphragmatic fatigue and, up to a point, compensates for this by increasing the rate of respiration rather than the tidal volume. This is, in effect, a vicious cycle, as the sick newborn comes closer to respiratory failure.

Although foetal breathing movements are clearly seen on scans, the lungs are inactive during foetal life. They have no role to play in keeping the infant oxygenated because, prior to birth, the placenta and the membranes perform the functions of protecting, respiring, nurturing and excreting for the infant until an independent status is reached. Without an efficient system for the above functions, there would be severe foetal insult and death.

Maternal and foetal circulation, under normal circumstances, never mix and the foetus receives materials for transfer by courtesy of a difference in pressure between the high-pressure maternal side and the lower-pressure foetal side.

Table 7.1 Summary of respiratory tract development

Time from fertilisation	Developmental aspects
Day 15–21	Ectoderm, endoderm and mesoderm formation; lung buds appear below pharyngeal pouch; diaphragm development begins
Day 24	Laryngotracheal groove develops
Day 26–28	Bronchial buds form
Day 28+	Primary nasal cavity, tongue and pharynx formation; phrenic nerve originates
Day 35+	Pseudo-glandular phase lobar bronchi present, pulmonary artery and vein develop; lung bud into pleural canals
Day 42+	Arytenoid swellings (precursor to formation of larynx)
Day 49+	Oropharynx develops; tracheal cartilage; smooth muscle of bronchi present
Day 56+	Vocal cords develop
Day 63+	Bronchial arteries develop; secondary palate forms; mucous glands appear
11 weeks	Lymphatic tissue appears; cilia develop; tracheal cartilage
13 weeks	Goblet cells appear
16 weeks	Canalicular phase begins; pre-acinar bronchial branches complete
22 weeks	System for synthesis of lecithin
24 weeks	Alveolar phase begins; respiratory bronchioles develop; terminal sacs develop
26–28 weeks	Alveolar-capillary surface now sufficient to support life
36 weeks	Mature alveoli present
After birth	Additional conductive airways form (respiratory bronchioles, alveoli ducts and sacs)
Age 8 years	Respiratory tract now complete

Oxygen (O_2) and carbon dioxide (CO_2) are transferred by simple diffusion and the high concentration of foetal haemoglobin has a greater affinity to oxygen and so makes the most of a limited saturation. Certain maternal factors also limit the saturation of oxygen available to the foetus. Active or passive smoking is incriminated in a birthweight that is smaller than would otherwise be expected. Excessive maternal blood pressure causes damage to the placenta and maternal hypotensive incidents limit the placental circulation and therefore the circulation available to the foetus.

CARE AND SUPPORT OF THE INFANT WITH BREATHING DIFFICULTIES

Some causes of infant breathing difficulties are:

- meconium inhalation;
- congenital pneumonia;
- aspiration pneumonia;

- pulmonary hypertension;
- transient tachypnoea of the newborn;
- respiratory distress syndrome;
- chronic lung disease;
- hypoplastic lungs;
- choanal atresia;
- diaphragmatic hernia;
- tracheo-oesophageal fistula;
- tracheomalacia;
- drug-induced respiratory depression.

Many of the above require specific treatment strategies and a full review of the modes of ventilation support is beyond the scope of this chapter. The understanding of infant ventilation has progressed impressively over the past decade, and there is now a good awareness of how much damage can be done to the delicate lung tissue in the struggle to support the infant's life. To facilitate the understanding of ventilation techniques, the more common supportive strategies will be outlined and then applied to the care of infants with the following four of the more common conditions, which require different levels of support:

- transient tachypnoea of the newborn;
- severe respiratory distress syndrome;
- meconium aspiration syndrome; and
- diaphragmatic hernia.

Methods of respiratory support and oxygenation include:

- warm and humidified headbox oxygen;
- continuous positive airway pressure (CPAP);
- intermittent positive pressure ventilation (IPPV);
- intermittent mandatory volume (IMV);
- high-frequency ventilation (HFV);
- nitric oxide;
- continuous negative extra-thoracic pressure (CNEP);
- extra-corporeal membrane oxygenation (ECMO).

Headbox oxygen

Unless very obviously unable to self-ventilate or adequately oxygenate, most tachypnoeic infants are allowed time to settle and perhaps sort themselves out. The headbox is a clear plastic dome, which is placed over the infant's head. Into it flows oxygen and air that has been warmed and humidified by being passed through a hot water tank. The amount of gas needed is regulated by a flow meter. The concentration of oxygen that the infant is receiving is monitored by placing an oxygen analyser a safe distance from the face. Typically, the concentration is about 30–40%, but it may be more. A requirement for higher levels of oxygen may indicate a need for more support.

From a nursing perspective, it is important to ensure that there is a good flow of air, to prevent carbon dioxide being trapped and the infant re-breathing stale air. Increasingly, as incubator humidification, gas regulation and monitoring systems improve, this method of supplying oxygen enhancement is becoming less common. Oxygen is supplied directly into the incubator and is referred to as ambient oxygen.

CPAP

This is the administration of warm humidified gas by continuous positive pressure directly into the infant's airways. It can be given by nasal prongs, facial mask or by endotracheal tube. It supports the infant's own respiratory pattern and function and makes the work of breathing easier by increasing intrapulmonary pressure and 'splinting' open alveoli, which improves oxygenation. There are several very good pressure devices available, which are specifically designed to do this job. Most ventilators also have a CPAP setting, which will work with the same circuit. Developments and modifications of the CPAP equipment have allowed clinicians to try variable pressures so that pulses of higher pressures can be administered, to mimic the positive inspiratory phase of the ventilated infant breath cycle. Fixation of CPAP is critical for its success, and manufacturers supply various sizes of bonnet mask and prongs. Goggin (2001) has made some sound points as to the measurement, fixation and care of an infant on CPAP.

CPAP is routine in today's nurseries, but there are several disadvantages and potentially serious complications of nasal CPAP. More mature and recovering infants seem to tolerate it less well, often trying to wriggle away from it or remove it, so that pressures are lost – the system alarms and the infant has to be disturbed to reinstate it. An infant who is crying will also lose pressure, so a soother may be offered, both to placate the infant and to maintain a seal. Another disadvantage is the pressure that the system exerts on the nose; it is important to get a good seal to maintain the pressures, but the strapping securing the prongs must not be applied too tightly. Noses have become distorted and although the shape usually reverts to normal, damaged mucosa leading to infection and necrotic tissue damage could be much more serious. Feeding an infant on CPAP can be difficult as the stomach can get very distended with the constant flow of gasses. This has led to a trend of passing a nasogastric or orogastric tube and leaving this on free drainage. Enteral feeding is accomplished by giving small amounts continuously via a nasojejunum or orojejunum tube.

Endotracheal CPAP used to be a popular stage in the weaning-off process from ventilation. However, it was felt that this gave the infant too much dead airspace to cope with, altering pulmonary dynamics and leading to increased effort of breathing, which subsequently tired them out.

In all cases, neonatal care involves a balancing act and there may be a return to endotracheal CPAP, in an effort to avoid repeated traumatic reintubations as infants fail to maintain good blood gas levels on mask or nasal CPAP.

IPPV/IMV

Mechanical ventilation has gained acceptance and is a commonly used technique in the neonatal unit. As it is relatively routine, it may be easy to under-estimate the impact of the machinery on the infant and the family. Techniques and refinements are moving on so fast that IPPV/IMV have come to be accepted as conventional, without having been through proper clinical trials. Newer 'experimental' techniques may in fact do less damage to lung tissue, and today's ventilators are flexible, allowing the rate, ratio and pressures to be tailored to suit the individual.

Ventilators may be either volume-controlled or pressure-controlled. In volume control mode, a measured amount of gas is delivered to the patient. With a very small infant, this is not easy. The endotracheal tubes are not cuffed and this can result in a variable air leak. In addition, there is airway resistance and stiff lungs, causing the carefully measured volume to be lost without inflating the lungs. Most paediatricians use pressure-controlled ventilators, with the cycle being controlled by time. A set pressure of gas is given and maintained for a set time. This causes a rapid rise in pressure, which then maintains a plateau for the pre-set inspiratory (PIP) time. This gives the stiff lungs a chance to inflate and, once they are inflated, the inspiratory time allows gas exchange to occur by molecular diffusion across the alveolar membrane. In order to remove waste gas, the pressure is allowed to drop to a pre-set positive end expiratory pressure (PEEP), which prevents alveolar collapse. Displayed on a graph, this sequence would be seen as a series of square waves (Milner and Field, 1985).

The closed circuit of a continuous-flow ventilator ensures that fresh gas is always available with the start of each cycle. This is important, as many small infants, unless heavily sedated, will continue to make some respiratory effort between ventilator breaths and re-breathing used gas is not desirable. The continuous-flow ventilator is flexible and infants can be weaned off it by gradually decreasing the amount of ventilator support given to them.

There have been some useful modifications to IPPV. Trigger sensors can be attached or incorporated into ventilators, to detect and support the infant's own attempts at initiating a breath (Mehta et al., 1986). Ventilation is triggered by changes in the infant's abdominal expansion or changes in airway or oesophageal pressures, and works by either reinforcing the infant's inspiratory effort or synchronising with the infant while also delivering a predetermined number of breaths. These ventilator developments are proving valuable, especially for early weaning off the ventilator and in the clinical management of difficult, ventilator-dependent infants.

High-frequency ventilation (HFV)

High-frequency, positive-pressure ventilation techniques are gaining acceptance. The term 'high-frequency ventilation' covers a myriad of respiratory support strategies, which commonly involve ventilation rates in excess of physiological respiratory rates and may use tidal volumes, which approximate to the dead airspace volume.

The frequency of breathing is expressed as hertz (Hz). One hertz equals one breath per second or 60 breaths per minute. Frequencies of 10–15 hertz are commonly used, resulting in 'breathing' rates of 600–900 breaths per minute. The technique provides an alternative to ever-increasing (and damaging) inspiratory pressures in stiff resistant lungs that are proving difficult to ventilate. A high mean airway pressure is maintained without the conventional peaks and troughs of pressure, which damage the lungs.

Complete understanding of the way that these techniques work is yet to be achieved but the techniques have been efficient in oxygenating some infants who failed to respond with other therapy and may otherwise have died.

Nitric oxide

Nitric oxide is a powerful and selective vasodilator. Inhaled nitric oxide works on the endothelium to relax the smooth muscle and reduce vascular resistance, improving the pulmonary circulation. It is used for persistent pulmonary hypertension in newborn infants that have not responded to other methods of management. It also has fewer side-effects than tolazoline.

Special apparatus is required to deliver nitric oxide to the infant in small amounts; these amounts are measured in parts per million and there is some debate as to the most therapeutic range. For more on nitric oxide therapy, *see* pages 136–7.

Continuous negative pressure ventilation/respiratory support

This is modelled on the old 'iron lung' device, which supported polio victims during the 1950s and 60s. Extensive remodelling of the device has taken place and it is now much friendlier, both to the user and to the patient. It now looks similar to an incubator and those available for pre-term infants are efficiently heated. Its clinical application is currently under scrutiny.

Extra-corporeal membrane oxygenation (ECMO)

Extra-corporeal membrane oxygenation is now an accepted therapy. The infant's circulation is accessed via major vessels and a small amount of deoxygenated blood is removed and run through a circuit containing a membrane lung, which oxygenates the blood. This is then returned to the infant (Crawford, 1991).

There have been positive results in trials with ECMO for infants who were deteriorating on full ventilation and pharmacological support, but the method is not without risk, and the technique is not available in every NNU. An infant requiring ECMO would need to be transferred to one of the few centres where the facility is available, presenting an additional risk for an unstable infant. To ensure that the systemic and circuit circulation remains fluid, an infant on ECMO needs to be heparinised and this is not without risk, particularly following surgery, for example, for the repair of a diaphragmatic hernia. The risks and complications of circulatory bypass are considered in Chapter 9.

Liquid ventilation

This may be partial or complete. If it is partial, it can be administered using a modified ventilator circuit. Its use remains experimental and trials are required before adopting the therapy on a larger scale. It is an exciting therapy, which promises to be an effective method of management for the future. Potentially, the therapy could have fewer long-term effects on the lungs, as low-pressure delivery could be used. Theoretically, this would cause less scarring on the delicate lung tissue. Excellent oxygenation levels have been achieved using perfluorocarbons and, as the foetal lung is accustomed to the presence of fluid, it is well tolerated. With increasing confidence in the therapy, infants who are currently regarded as not viable could perhaps be maintained until lung development is sufficiently advanced to tolerate conversion to gas.

TRANSIENT TACHYPNOEA OF THE NEWBORN

Aetiology

This condition commonly affects the large term infant who is otherwise well, but it can also complicate the clinical picture of the premature infant. It is thought to arise from delayed clearance of foetal lung fluid. Typically, the infant develops increasing respiratory distress within an hour or two of birth. There may be grunting, nasal flaring and sternal and rib retractions, and the respiratory rate will be greatly elevated. Infants with this condition are satisfying to nurse, as they are quickly ill, demanding nursing skill for a period of about 48 hours, and then they are quickly better.

Differential diagnosis

It is difficult to distinguish the respiratory difficulties of transient tachypnoea of the newborn from pneumonia, other infections, or respiratory distress syndrome, especially in the early stages. Blood and (occasionally) gastric aspirates are cultured to exclude infection. Chest X-rays are performed but they are rarely helpful at such an early stage. Later, a chest X-ray may show large hyperinflated lungs and increased pulmonary vascularity. Free fluid may be present in the horizontal fissure. Because of the difficulty of distinguishing this condition from congenital pneumonia, these infants often earn themselves intravenous antibiotics until negative cultures come back from the laboratories.

Care of the parents

The sudden admission or transfer of such an infant to a neonatal unit will be a shock to the parents. They may feel less at ease on the unit, as their infant will usually be the biggest one there and look 'out of place' in an incubator, among the small and premature. Although these infants do look very ill, they are typically quickly better and the parents can be appropriately reassured. The mother can be encouraged to use a breast pump to establish her milk supply and to give her positive feelings, since this is something that only she can do for the infant.

Nursing care and management

The nursing diagnosis is one of breathing difficulties and distress. The aim is to support the infant, to provide oxygenation, to ease the work of breathing and to monitor the infant closely to detect signs of deterioration.

The care plan would take into account the infant's individual needs, but would always include the following.

Consideration of the infant's position

Infants should be positioned prone to splint the diaphragm or be supported on either side with the head elevated. Most units would use an apnoea mattress, which should be covered in a warm soft sheet, duvet or sheepskin, to provide tactile comfort, warmth and support.

Monitoring and observing the infant

Infants should be fully monitored to ensure continuous readings of cardiac trace, saturation of oxygen and rate of respiration. Non-invasive methods are used whenever possible (Paige, 1990) and, although pulse oximetery is gaining popularity, it has important limitations (Stoddart *et al.*, 1997). The advantage of continuous readings is that the infants are handled less and less stressed. They are able to rest, conserve energy and recover. The disadvantage is that parents focus on the monitors and may become very anxious. This is less likely if the reason for using the monitors is explained and reassurance given that they are temporary and will be removed as soon as possible.

Provision of oxygen according to the infant's needs

Warm and humidified oxygen should be given as prescribed, using a headbox. The amount of oxygen that an infant requires is determined by the blood gas result. As these infants are, typically, not very ill, intermittent radial artery samples are probably sufficient, on a 4–6-hourly basis, with the frequency decreasing as the condition stabilises. Arterial catheterisation is rarely warranted unless the infant is very unstable or there is serious doubt about the cause of the tachypnoea.

Once the infant is clinically stable – identified by a more, settled respiratory rate and improved blood gas results – the amount of oxygen should be weaned down in order to maintain a satisfactory level of oxygen saturation (SaO_2); this would be recorded by non-invasive pulse oximetery.

Warmth and comfort

Infants should be nursed exposed, for ease of observation, in an incubator or under an overhead heater, which is set at an appropriate temperature. A term infant typically needs less support in assisting temperature control and may become hot and sweaty due to the high environmental temperature of the unit. Skill is needed to keep the infant (and the parents) cool. An infant's basic hygiene needs are the same as for any big normal infant except that they will, initially, tolerate less handling.

Stable blood glucose

On admission, a blood glucose level should be checked by blood glucose stick. If this is satisfactory (4–6 mmol/l), random levels may be checked whenever the infant is disturbed. Normal blood glucose is maintained by intravenous dextrose until the infant is sufficiently stable to tolerate feeding by enteral means.

Hydration and nutrition

Infants need fluid and nutrition but are unable to suck owing to tachypnoea and respiratory distress. Typically, an intravenous line is established and the infant receives intravenous fluids, calculated according to its weight and local protocol. Fluid needs may vary as sick infants retain fluid and may not tolerate the calculated requirements. The disadvantage of keeping them 'nil by mouth' is that, once they start to feel better, they may become hungry and quite cross. With the parent's consent, a soother could be offered. A distressed, cross and hungry infant will result in a vicious cycle, with respiratory rate becoming elevated once again.

Feeding by nasogastric tube can be tried until the infant is able to feed by mouth. The nasogastric tube is passed and taped securely in place, then left for an hour to see if the placing of the tube and the narrowing of the infant's airway compromises the respiratory function. Once milk feeding is commenced and tolerated, the intravenous infusion is decreased.

Typically, these infants will improve rapidly and can be introduced to oral feeds by breast or bottle (whatever the parents choose) when it becomes apparent that they are ready to feed. Feeding techniques and management of hydration and nutrition are discussed in Chapter 15.

RESPIRATORY DISTRESS SYNDROME

Aetiology

Respiratory distress syndrome (RDS) is the commonest cause of admission to NNUs. It is primarily a disease of the pre-term, and smaller infants are more frequently affected. It is a major cause of morbidity and mortality in the UK. Improvements in mortality will depend on improved socio-economic factors to improve infant birthweight, as well as high standards of nursing care and medical treatment.

The disease is characterised by a typical 'ground glass' chest X-ray with air bronchograms. The clinical picture is one of multiple signs of respiratory distress:

- grunting – the sound of exhaling against a closed glottis, which maintains a high residual air volume in the lungs, preventing functional collapse;
- nasal flaring, tachypnoea and cyanosis may be present soon after birth or within 4 hours;
- severe rib and sternal retractions, which may be present in pre-term infants with a highly compliant chest wall.

Classically, RDS follows an acute course, with the infant deteriorating for the first two/three days of life, experiencing a period of supported stability and then, depending on gestation, often exhibiting a dramatic improvement.

RDS affects infants who are born too early and have immature lungs. Other causes include perinatal asphyxia, birth by caesarean section and maternal diabetes. The disease is not yet fully understood; some infants born at 28 weeks gestation do not develop the disease, while others born at 36 weeks do. However, it is clear that the level of surfactant plays a major role in the aetiology of the disease. The higher the surfactant levels before birth, the less likely it is that an infant will develop the disease. Infants with low surfactant levels are said to have 'stiff lungs' – the alveoli tend to collapse on expiration and a high inspiratory pressure is needed to re-inflate them (Bhutani et al., 1992).

Medical treatment of this condition includes the use of surfactants, and there are a number of preparations available, both naturally derived and artificially prepared (see Chapter 16). There is some debate as to the most effective preparation (Cummings et al., 1992), frequency and dosage to use (Speer et al., 1992), and whether to give it prophylactically or therapeutically (Hoekstra et al., 1991). Surfactant will, in many cases, support the infant until it can produce its own natural surfactant. Gortner et al. (1992) suggested that if infants are appropriately treated with surfactant, they are less likely to develop bronchopulmonary dysplasia (BPD). The expense of surfactant is often given as one reason for not using it, but the cost of caring for an infant with BPD may mitigate this argument. Production of the infant's own surfactant is impeded by cold, stress and metabolic disturbances such as hypoxia and acidosis.

The mainstays of treatment for RDS are the replacement of surfactant, support of the respiratory function, keeping the infant well oxygenated and providing time for the condition to improve, to allow for independent existence. Infants with severe respiratory distress are often ventilated soon after birth. In order to ventilate effectively, an endotracheal tube is passed, either through the nose or the mouth, into the trachea, and fixed securely. The use of an indwelling arterial line is highly desirable, as this allows easy access for blood gas sampling, with minimal disturbance. An umbilical arterial line allows continuous blood gas monitoring (Drucker and Hodgkinson, 1998).

Complications of ventilator therapy

The use of mechanical ventilation to care for sick infants with respiratory failure has been responsible for saving lives. However, the pressures that are sometimes needed have been associated with the development of severe barotrauma. Pulmonary air leaks and BPD are recognised as major consequences of conventional management (White et al., 1990).

Specific care of an infant who is mechanically ventilated

Some infants who are mechanically ventilated tolerate the treatment surprisingly well, while others 'fight' the ventilator. All infants who are being artificially ventilated should be sedated. Some may even need the introduction of a muscle relaxant to achieve good ventilator compliance. Diamorphine infusion has become popular and, if correctly titrated, the balance between optimum sedation and prevention of depression of the respiratory system can be achieved. The infant can be weaned slowly off sedation as the ventilation is reduced prior to extubation.

Synchrony with the ventilator can also be useful in helping infants to tolerate the treatment. This can be achieved by close observation of the respiratory rate and adjustment of the ventilator rate and rhythm.

Intubating an infant

Tracheal tubes can be inserted orally, nasally or, in some cases where long-term ventilation is being considered, via a tracheostomy. Each method has its advantages and disadvantages. Parents seem to prefer oral intubation but it is difficult to stabilise as movement can cause tracheal abrasion and dislodgement. The presence of a tube in the mouth encourages increased salivation (some more alert infants can be seen to suck). These secretions need to be removed to prevent them pooling and aspirating; they may also loosen sticky tape on the face if this is used to secure tubes. Long-term oral intubation can distort the soft palate, causing feeding and orthodontic problems.

The endotracheal tube is stabilised by being stitched or clipped on to an ET tube holder, which is supported in position by tying the distal ends of the holder to a small bonnet. Foam rectangles or dental rolls take the pressure of the holder and ties off the face. There are a number of other methods of fixation, but the best is probably the most familiar and secure.

Nasal intubation is more secure but can result in a lot of tape on the infant's face, which can distress the parents, who will not be able to see what the infant looks like. Pressure necrosis on the anterior nares (from a badly positioned tube) can result in quite severe deformity, necessitating plastic surgery. As the mouth is free an infant can use a soother but this can result in increased salivation.

In an emergency, such as an unexpected deterioration, intubation may have to be performed under stress, but the insertion or changing of a tracheal tube can often be planned in advance. At present, few NNUs use effective sedation to make the procedure easier for the infant. Premedication, muscle relaxants and rapid sequence induction is accepted practice for older children and adults; it may require more skilled personnel but as the need for tubes can largely be anticipated, there is time for these personnel to be contacted. With the increase in practising advanced nurse practitioners it is to be hoped that the situation will improve. There is good evidence of the physiological and practical benefits of sedation of an infant prior to intubation (Whyte *et al.*, 2000). Certainly, cold intubation is a distressing procedure for an infant and for the nurse having to hold the infant down. Seeing the infant in such obvious distress also raises child protection issues.

Care of an intubated infant

These infants are ventilated via endotracheal tubes (ETT), which allow effective access to the lower airways. Endotracheal (ET) intubation impairs the natural ability to clear lung secretions, owing to the impediment of the mucociliary function and an ineffective cough reflex (the result of a permanently open glottis).

Both nasotracheal and endotracheal methods of intubation can cause ear infection. The presence of an artificial airway can cause epithelial erosion and inflammation. The mucus and debris that build up on the tube provide an excellent culture medium, which can then be colonised by opportunistic pathogens and provide a focus for infection. This may subsequently track through the eustachian tube to the middle ear.

Tracheostomy has the advantage of cutting down dead airspace, making ventilation more efficient, but, like the other methods, it prevents the infant from communicating by crying. The longer the tracheostomy is present, the longer verbal skills are retarded; introduction to a speech therapist is recommended.

Suctioning and maintaining an artificial airway

There is controversy concerning the frequency and technique used in suctioning (White, 1997). Each unit has its own guidelines regarding suction method, frequency and instillation of irrigating fluid. There are no national recommendations to aid nurses. The purpose of endotracheal suctioning is to facilitate the removal of secretions and prevent obstructions. It is an important aspect of neonatal nursing care but should be carried out with caution as bradycardia, hypoxia and fluctuations in intracranial pressure, perhaps leading to intra-ventricular haemorrhage, may result.

Deep ETT suction can cause tissue damage to the trachea, so the length of the ET tube and the connector is measured (Table 7.2) and this is the length to which the suction catheter is inserted (Young, 1995; Wallace, 1998). Nurses should ensure that the catheter does not go beyond the distal tip of the ET tube. Suction is applied only during withdrawal of the catheter and should last approximately 5–10 seconds. The catheter design should be one of multiple side 'eyes', not single lumen tip, as this will cause less mucosal damage. Each catheter is only used once and a sterile or scrupulously clean technique prevents introduction of infection.

Table 7.2 Size of ETT related to weight and suggested catheter size

Weight (g)	Diameter of ET tube (mm)	Catheter size (FG)
<650	2.0–2.5	5–6
650–1500	2.5–3.0	6–7
1500–2500	3.0	7
2500–3500	3.0–3.5	7
>3500	4	7–8

Inappropriate size of catheter can result in the generation of a negative pressure when suction is applied. If the catheter is too large for the lumen of the tube it will occlude the entire artificial airway. Instillation of irrigation fluid is contentious (Ackerman, 1993) and arguments in favour of the use of saline instillation include inducing the cough response, thinning the mucus within the tube and making it easier to aspirate. How much to use is debated; the smaller the infant, the less it will tolerate (Shorten *et al.*, 1991) (see Table 7.3).

Table 7.3 Suggested suction pressures and volume of fluid instillation

Current weight (grams)	Suction pressure (mm Hg)	Saline instillation (mls)
1500	40	0.25
1500	60	0.50

Evidence on the deleterious effects of the procedure describes bradycardia and stress tachycardia (Shorten *et al.*, 1991), trauma to the delicate bronchial mucosa (Runton, 1992), fluctuations in cerebral oxygenation and increases in intracranial pressure (Shah *et al.*, 1992). Continuous observations of vital signs during suction are made and the infant allowed to recover between each pass.

Controversy also surrounds the use of pre-suction hyperoxygenation, hyperventilation and hyperinflation. It is suggested that these practices reduce the likelihood of dangerous fluctuations of the cerebral oxygenation during suctioning of the pre-term infant (Tolles and Stone, 1990), but they could be dangerous in unskilled hands. The science of infant ventilatory care is a fairly recent one and much study remains to be done. In the absence of guidelines and an extended nursing role towards that of a neonatal respiratory therapist, all changes to ventilation must be prescribed by the clinician. Infants need to have their care planned according to their unique needs.

Such controversy over suctioning leaves the neonatal nurse balanced between the need to keep the tube patent, to reduce repeated and traumatic tube changes, and the risks of suctioning.

Cool, dry gases desiccate the secretions and impair cilia activity causing stasis and pooling. Locally we have found that when the gas is warmed to body temperature at the point of delivery, by using a high humidification temperature and a circuit with a built-in heated wire, higher relative humidity is administered. As the gases being delivered are heavily saturated the secretions tend to be less viscid. Sticky secretions block tubes faster and need frequent removal. It is advisable to try not to interrupt the ventilation cycles when performing suctioning, and to use the smallest catheter and the minimal vacuum that will effectively aspirate the secretions. Catheters should allow a flow of gas around them and the tube should be accessed through the porthole on the ETT connector. Oral suctioning is performed frequently when there are visible secretions in the infant's mouth. Most commonly these are done with the infant's cares or prior to a position change, as the presence of a tube encourages salivation and the aim is to prevent the risk of inhaling saliva through the open glottis.

Physiotherapy

There is also debate over the appropriate timing, frequency and duration of physiotherapy, and discussion as to who should perform it. Over-vigorous physiotherapy has been incriminated in serious complications such as fractured ribs and intraventricular haemorrhage. Oberwaldner (2000) considered this client group to be more vulnerable to these complications as a result of reduced bronchial stability and a highly unstable chest. Physiotherapy has been regarded as a vital part of the care of an infant with breathing difficulties, as it was thought to loosen the secretions prior to suctioning, preventing the accumulation of secretions and reducing the risk of hypostatic infection. Preventing mucus build-up helps to maintain patent airways and prevents localised collapse and consolidation. Few units have full physiotherapy cover although such resources would be ideal. Neonatal nurses need to work in partnership with physiotherapists to become skilled in the techniques of chest physiotherapy.

The techniques of percussion and vibration to loosen secretions are the most favoured, with postural drainage to aid removal of secretions being selectively used and prescribed on an individual basis. Methods used include the following:

- laerdal face masks size 00;
- specially designed palm cups;
- electric toothbrushes for small infants.

These aids can be applied to the chest wall. Palm cups are used rhythmically, intermittently and gently. As face masks and palm cups make contact with the chest wall they trap air and provide the benefit of movement, force and contact, without the trauma of repeatedly hitting the infant's chest with a flat surface. With the electric toothbrush, vibration is continuous. The need for physiotherapy is assessed with each shift change and, whenever possible, the treatment is given to coincide with handling. For infants who are positioned on their side, physiotherapy starts at the anterior apex on the most accessible lung, working towards the base and gradually round under the arm to work on the posterior aspects of the lung fields. The infant is then turned and the treatment repeated on the opposite lung. Suction is applied to remove loosened secretions during or after treatment. Indications for suction would be visible or audible secretions (Runton, 1992). Fluctuations from the infant's physiological baseline may be an indication for suctioning but these could be a response to handling.

During treatment, the infant's condition is carefully observed, and there should be full emergency equipment (previously checked) on standby. Suction should be switched on and set at an appropriate, predetermined pressure.

Oxygenation is continually monitored and, if fluctuations occur, time is allowed for recovery. Pre-oxygenation may be prescribed, with or without manual bagging. There is a paucity of studies available for guidance (Downes and Parker, 1991). Wallis and Prasad (1999) call for more evidence to support its continued use in the NNU. Bertone (1988) gives a review of physiotherapy technique.

Nursing care plan

The nursing diagnosis would be failure to self-ventilate in room air. The aims would include the maintenance of a clear airway, and the provision of respiratory support and comfort, until the infant is able to self-ventilate in air with ease. The infant's individualised care plan would include the following.

Position of comfort and rest

Infants need to be supported on the side with the head elevated to prevent movement of the endotracheal tube, which has been incriminated in tracheal necrosis and sub-glottic stenosis. Anglepoise, sandbags, bean bags, rolled sheets and limb restraints all help to keep the tubing in the correct position.

Management of indwelling arterial line

Owing to the critical instability of an infant with severe RDS, an indwelling arterial catheter is necessary. Preferably this should be an umbilical line into the aorta, through which blood can be sampled, the PO_2 continuously monitored and blood pressure measured with minimal disturbance. Like other invasive procedures, the use of arterial lines is not without risk, which may include haemorrhage, local or systemic infection and vascular complications. Vascular complications may arise from trauma, thrombus formation, embolus formation, vasospasm and hypertension. The true incidence of umbilical line complications may never be known, as many remain asymptomatic.

Vasospasm is perhaps the most common vascular complication. It may be caused by the initial catheter placement, manipulation, sampling through the catheter or removal of the catheter. Vasospasm can cause blanching or cyanosis of the distal area. To prevent further damage when this occurs, the catheter will need to be removed (Bryant, 1990).

Thrombus formation in the umbilical artery is potentially very serious as it may result in emboli, which can lodge and occlude blood vessels, impairing the circulation and resulting in distal tissue hypoxia and necrosis. The loss of toes and necrotic patches on the infant's buttocks and limbs have been seen in NNUs throughout the world.

Care of an indwelling arterial line involves aseptic installation, secure splintage and ease of visibility of the catheter site and potentially affected extremities. An X-ray is used to confirm the location of the catheter. A high placement is between thoracic vertebrae eight and ten, above the level of the coeliac axis and renal artery origins. A low placement is between lumbar vertebrae three and four, below the origin of the inferior mesenteric artery – this ensures that the blood supply to those vital organs is not compromised.

Different policies exist regarding the infusion of fluids through these lines. Some are conservative, with the use restricted to slow infusion of heparinised saline and blood sampling. Others use the line to administer drugs and infuse all fluid requirements. Whichever policy is in force, the maintenance of strict fluid balance remains of primary importance.

There is some suspicion that the presence of an umbilical arterial catheter is associated with an increased risk of necrotising enterocolitis (*see* Chapter 8).

Feeding and nutrition

An infant with severe RDS cannot tolerate full enteral feeding, owing to a combination of factors, including instability of clinical condition and immaturity of the gastro-intestinal system. The pre-term infant has limited reserves. Intravenous hydration and correction of electrolyte imbalance is insufficient for longer than three days. If enteral feeding is not going to be introduced, or if there is doubt that it will be tolerated, a long feeding line should be placed and parenteral nutrition commenced. Infants with severe RDS will improve, gain weight and tolerate intravenous feeding for fairly long periods but its use can have complications (DoH, 2001). Ideally, the infant will also be given a small amount (0.5–1.0 mls) of expressed colostrum or breast milk every hour, to prime the gut.

Feeding is discussed more fully in Chapter 15.

Maintaining a thermoneutral environment

An infant with RDS needs warmth and there are two ways of maintaining optimal temperature: the closed incubator and the cot with a radiant heater. Other aids to maintain warmth include heat shields to cut down on the amount of heat loss, plastic bubble-wrap and clear cling film for insulation and good visibility. The very pre-term infant will need high humidity (*see* Chapter 5). As soon as the infant's condition improves, he or she should be dressed and warmly wrapped. This is satisfying for the parents, who can choose the clothing. It is equally satisfying for the infant, who feels more secure when cosily dressed. Once the condition is sufficiently stable and the temperature control is satisfactory, the infant can be transferred to a small crib in a low-dependency area, to establish feeding and grow.

Care of the family

The care of ventilated infants is a rewarding challenge, as both infant and family have multiple needs. So much information is given to the parents, in so short a time, that it is worth checking later that it has all sunk in. Locally we use support groups and counsellors to comfort the parents, and back up explanations of the infant's condition by the use of specially designed leaflets (Crawford, 1992).

Withdrawing care

For the majority of infants with RDS, recovery is assured. For some – usually the questionably viable – even support fails to bring improvement, and the infant may sink inextricably into a chronic state and multi-system failure.

Withdrawing care is a difficult ethical issue (Crawford and Power, 2001). The legal position is clear: no steps can be taken to hasten the demise of an infant but no officious measures need be taken to resuscitate in the event of a collapse. Between these two extremes there is a large and potentially dangerous minefield to negotiate – how much support should be offered to infants of borderline viability? The nursing perspectives include the viewpoint that this infant does not suddenly become unloved. As always, the family is nursed and not just the infant. The views and wishes of the family are extremely important.

For more on ethical issues in neonatal nursing, *see* Chapter 2.

MECONIUM INHALATION SYNDROME

Meconium is a thick, sticky, tar-like substance present in the foetal intestine, which is cleared and passed in the first few days following birth. Its release before or during birth can follow stress or asphyxial events, which both increases peristalsis and relaxes the anal sphincter. Meconium staining of the infant and the liquor is common – fortunately, meconium inhalation is not. The difference is probably due to the degree of asphyxia experienced. Severe cases will result in gasping and this will result in inhalation of the meconium into the airways.

Meconium inhalation can complicate the clinical course of other conditions such as birth asphyxia, gastroschisis, omphalus, and so on. Because of this it is commonly seen on the NNU and infants with it can be extremely ill. Meconium plugs in the airways cause obstruction and atelectasis. The presence of meconium in the alveoli may cause chemical pneumonitis, and impede gas exchange and production of surfactant. Such profound airway compromise and lung damage significantly alters the pulmonary dynamics and a severely affected infant can develop pulmonary hypertension, which often keeps the foramen ovale open and leads to right to left shunting.

In the past, such infants were often subjected to ferocious pressures in order to inflate stiff lungs and to improve the gas exchange; these pressures often resulted in pneumothorax. Fortunately, these techniques are seen less frequently as ventilation techniques have improved significantly. Infants with meconium inhalation may be extremely sick but respond extremely well to ECMO (Davis and Shekerdemian, 2001), although this is only available in a few units. To avoid the risky transfer of such an unstable infant, or as a holding procedure while awaiting the transfer team, other therapies such as nitric oxide or careful infusion of magnesium sulphate may be tried.

Inhaled nitric oxide therapy

Nitric oxide therapy is an effective treatment for persistent pulmonary hypertension in the newborn (Miller, 1995). Nitric oxide is a powerful substance already present in the body, where it has a vast number of roles and actions, including control of the circulation and maintenance of blood pressure. It has been recognised to be a potent smooth-muscle relaxant, acting on the vascular endothelium and promoting vasodilatation when inhaled into the lungs. It acts locally to improve the circulation to the lungs and reduces pulmonary pressures. As it is selective in its action there are no detrimental systemic side-effects.

To deliver nitric oxide therapy safely, a specially adapted ventilator circuit is used, in conjunction with a gas-blending system and an accurate analyser.

Exhaled gas is put through a scavenger to prevent occupational exposure. Minuscule amounts are used (calculated in parts per million); the strength used depends on the weight of the infant and the infant's response to it. There is a wide variation in prescriptions (Woodrow, 1997), which may range from a lower dose of 10 ppm (parts per million) up to 60 ppm.

Infants who have been stabilised on nitric oxide therapy will need to be weaned off slowly and gradually, to avoid rebound pulmonary vasoconstriction. Apart from the modifications to the ventilation circuit, and the additional monitoring and recording of the nitric oxide flow rates, the specifics of the nursing care of these ventilated infants remains much the same as those outlined above. For details on the care of the heavily sedated, *see* page 140.

CONGENITAL DIAPHRAGMATIC HERNIA

This condition occurs in approximately 1 in 2200 live births. It is not specifically genetically linked, although a family tendency is seen. More males than females suffer the condition and the incidence is higher in white infants than in other races (Juretschke, 2001).

Congenital diaphragmatic hernia remains one of the most serious challenges in neonatal surgery and neonatology. In the past, there was a 70–80% mortality rate, which was not evenly distributed geographically (Theorell, 1990). More recent developments have halved the mortality rate and it is possible that this may be reduced still further in the future (Shehata *et al.*, 1999; Yeo, 1999). The infants who do best are usually those who are diagnosed antenatally and have a planned delivery, with specialist staff available in the delivery room or theatre. Infants who collapse immediately after birth are the most seriously affected and are more challenging to care for. Infants who present days or weeks later, or are routinely found by chance X-ray, tend to do very well.

Aetiology

The anatomical defect is a simple one. The most common and the most severe is the left-sided defect, which results in a failure of the diaphragm to develop and fuse. Technically, this is described as a postero-lateral, Bochdalek-type hernia. The less severe and occasionally symptomless type is described as an anterior-medial Morgani-type hernia, where the defect is below the sternum.

A severe diaphragmatic defect results in herniation of abdominal contents through the gap in the diaphragm into the thorax, causing mediastinum shift, which in turn compresses the developing lung tissue. Although this defect is potentially surgically correctable, the hypoplasia of the lung tissue often makes the infant difficult to ventilate.

Initial resuscitation

An infant who has collapsed in the delivery room with a diaphragmatic hernia presents one of the most sudden and acute emergencies that the midwife or neonatal nurse will face. In the worst-case scenario, typically and sadly, these are term or near-term infants with whom no difficulty had been anticipated. The infant is born normally, gasps and then fails to establish a normal respiratory pattern, becoming cyanosed.

Diaphragmatic hernia should be suspected in the following cases:

• if heart sounds are heard on the right;
• if the abdomen appears to be scaphoid.

Definitive diagnosis is by chest X-ray, which shows bowel in the chest and a displaced heart. However, unless the infant is properly resuscitated, such a diagnosis is likely to be of academic interest. Resuscitation, by traditional methods of bag and mask inflation of the lungs, is undesirable as the misplaced abdominal contents also become inflated, compounding pulmonary embarrassment. Initial resuscitation includes the passage of a wide-bore oral/nasogastric tube, left on free drainage after aspiration. This decompresses the inflated bowel and allows expansion of existing lung tissue. The infant should be positioned head tilted up to allow maximum lung expansion and to reduce the weight of the bowel in the chest. Ventilation should be commenced via an endotracheal tube.

All senior midwives should be trained to perform emergency intubation (Whitten, 1989; Hancock and Peterson, 1992), as it can take time for expert paediatric help to arrive, especially in the middle of the night. The minimum possible pressures, which keep the infant pink, should be used to prevent lung damage. The infant will be shocked, so warmth, gentle handling and correction of metabolic abnormalities are important.

The workload of the NNU needs to be fully appraised and may have to be redistributed, as individual nurses need to be allocated to look after this critically ill infant. Because of this, the admission of such an infant has a knock-on effect for other staff on duty and also for the care of other infants. It can result in staff experiencing a disjointed shift and such shifts tend to be less satisfying. It is important to recognise the efforts that others, apart from the initial admissions team, make on this infant's behalf. This is where primary nursing and good team dynamics pay dividends. The parents have to forge links only with a small group of care-givers and unit morale is maintained, even though the workload and stress levels have increased.

Initial care of the parents

The culmination of an uneventful pregnancy and a normal labour should result in a beautiful healthy child. In contrast, the arrival of a pale, shocked infant who cannot breathe and is removed for resuscitation must seem the stuff of nightmares. At some point in the chaos of resuscitation, photographs of the infant should be taken, as tastefully as possible, as well as a hand/footprint. These should be sent to the parents as soon as possible, with an update on their infant's condition.

Unless they prefer it, the parents should not be left alone, and someone should stay and help them to keep a hold on the situation. This is difficult with the pressures on the staff of the NNU. A quiet, calm and sympathetic approach is ideal and there is a tendency to use infant care workers or nursery nurses for this important role. (Incidentally, team members who are good at being with people in times of stress tend to get over-used in this role, and there is some evidence that their own stress can be cumulative. When planning the off duty, time should be allowed for these people to be debriefed or befriended by their peers so that situations causing stress can be offloaded.)

As soon as possible, the parents should see their child and be offered honest explanations as to his or her condition by the team responsible for the care. The needs of every family are different and the management of the family is planned to meet those needs. Sometimes access to a telephone is all that is required.

Transfer

Many maternity units do not have the facilities for neonatal intensive care or surgery, and the infant will need to be transferred, away from the parents, to another hospital. The receiving centre will usually be responsible for the transfer. Transfer can sometimes be quite tricky. It is dangerous to move an unstable infant, but time is of the essence and it is vital to get the patient to a fully equipped hospital as quickly as possible, and in the best possible condition. The infant with diaphragmatic hernia is best transported with the contralateral lung upward, to avoid further compression of the lung by the weight of the bowel. General flying squad management is discussed in Chapter 13.

Traditional management

This is both medical and surgical. The decision on whether to go for early or deferred surgery is made on the clinical condition and the responses to treatment of each individual infant. The increasing trend is to delay surgery until the infant is more stable.

Observations of vital signs and clinical condition are constant. Ventilation management of a big term infant typically involves sedation and muscle relaxant, as large, vigorous term infants can be very difficult to ventilate. Hypoplastic lung tissue can be stiff and high inspiratory pressure may be needed to inflate the lungs; this means that a pneumothorax is a very real danger, especially if the infant is 'fighting' the ventilator. To prevent this, a muscle relaxant is used and the infant is effectively paralysed. This muscle relaxant is often based on curare and may be given by bolus, although continuous infusion is preferred. *Remember*: the immobile infant can still be frightened and in pain (Noerr, 1992), so sedation and analgesia should also be given.

Deliberate respiratory alkalosis may be induced by hyperventilation in order to break the vicious cycle of right to left shunting and pulmonary hypertension. A reduction in CO_2 levels may reduce shunting.

Pharmacological support may involve use of Tolazoline (Noerr, 1988) for the management of secondary pulmonary hypertension. Tolazoline is a direct peripheral vasodilator, which is effective by blocking alpha-adrenergic action. Owing to Tolazoline's ability to decrease peripheral resistance, systemic hypotension can result. Circulatory supportive measures may also include Dopamine and the infusion of human albumin or whole blood products. Major vessel access is preferable.

Specific nursing management of the paralysed infant

Transmission of nerve impulses, to muscles blocked by relaxant, prohibits movement and the infant becomes very dependent upon the nurse. Secretions build up in the oropharynx as the infant is unable to swallow, and gentle physiotherapy and frequent suctioning are required. The limbs can become over-stretched and sore if unsupported. Skin breakdown becomes a possibility because pressure reduces circulation. The bowel and bladder function may be impaired and the infant may require suppositories and catheterisation or manual expression of the bladder.

Oropharyngeal suction

Suction technique (*see* pages 131–2) should be carried out frequently to prevent aspiration of saliva.

Subluxation of limbs and skin care

Positioning and supporting the limbs in a neutral position of comfort is vital and the limbs should be moved through a full range of normal movement. This practice is called passive limb physiotherapy and should be performed when the infant has its cares. Following cares, the infant's position should be changed and pressure areas inspected. The frequency of this depends on how well handling is tolerated. If the level of toleration is limited, the nurse could make a net bed or a waterbed with part-filled litre bags of fluids. Pressure-relieving mattresses are commercially available. Moving mattresses, such as electric ripple versions, are an excellent idea but must be used with caution for fear of displacing the ETT.

Risk of urinary stasis and constipation

The paralysed infant may retain urine in the bladder. Apart from being uncomfortable, a large bladder containing stagnant urine may cause a urinary tract infection. In infants who do not have a catheter, supra-pubic pressure may be necessary to void this urine. Prolonged use of muscle relaxant may mean that the infant has to have a small suppository to evacuate the bowel.

Surgery

There are two approaches to surgical repair: transthoracic and transabdominal. Both are successful and each has particular advantages. The method of choice differs with the severity of the hernia, the experience of the surgeon and the condition of the infant. The transthoracic approach allows for the quickest decompression of the embarrassed pulmonary function and repair of the diaphragmatic defect from above. However, if there is insufficient abdominal space to contain the herniated bowel, an abdominal incision and formation of silastic pouch may have to be performed and the abdomen repaired in stages.

The transabdominal approach is felt by some to be less traumatic. The associated malrotation of bowel can also be repaired at the same time.

Usually, no attempt is made post-operatively to expand the compressed lung with suction decompression of the intrapleural space or selective intubation of the bronchi and positive pressure ventilation. The compressed lung naturally and gradually expands and the mediastinal shift will return to a midline position with passive management. Passive lung expansion and air leak is managed by underwater seal drainage.

Underwater seal drainage

Intercostal drains are sited to allow fluid and air to escape from the pleural cavity and to allow the lung to expand. This is a closed and airtight method of management. The drainage end of the system is submerged below a measured amount of sterile water. The water bottles are suspended below the level of the patient and never lifted above this level. Expansion of the chest wall, on inspiration, increases the intrapleural tension and there is reflux of the fluid from the bottle. On expiration, normal pressures are established and the level of fluid in the tube falls. These drains are said to 'swing'. Constant bubbling of the fluid in the drains suggests a continuing air leak. Intercostal drains are never routinely clamped off while active. Emergency clamping, as close to the chest wall as possible, is performed if accidental disconnection occurs.

Frequent observation of drain activity for patency is vital. Drains stop swinging if kinked, clogged or clotted. Excessive length of tubing can cause fluid to become trapped in bends, effectively blocking the flow of air down the tube.

Active drains will stop swinging when the lung is fully expanded and a chest X-ray will be taken to confirm this. Provided that the clinical condition is stable, the chest drains are removed and an airtight, occlusive dressing applied (Walsh, 1989).

Alternative methods of management

Pre-natal diagnosis of congenital diaphragmatic hernia is increasingly available as scanning techniques improve. It gives parents some control over the out-come and allows them to decide whether to continue with the pregnancy. It also means that an affected infant can be fully assessed and safely transferred while still in the uterus, for delivery in a unit with facilities to manage the condition.

In future, it is probable that early diagnosis will become even more important, as mid-trimester surgical techniques are improved; a diaphragmatic hernia could be repaired between 24 to 30 weeks gestation. Intra-uterine repair in some cases would have the advantage of allowing subsequent pulmonary development (Harrison, 1990; Mychaliska et al., 1996), but it has yet to be fully successful. As a holding procedure, Harrison and colleagues (1998) developed the technique of plugging the trachea, which seems to have a positive effect.

COMMON INVESTIGATIONS

Respiratory management would be impossible without some routine investigations that are taken for granted. Blood gas analysis has been available since the late 1950s, although exact interpretation varies between units (Askin, 1997). Current ventilator management would be unthinkable without it.

Blood gases explained

Homeostasis is of vital importance to the maintenance of life and operates within strict limits. If the body is subjected to repeated or prolonged deviation, serious organ damage or death can follow.

The transport of oxygen and carbon dioxide in the blood relies on healthy erythrocytes, good haemoglobin levels, and amounts of bicarbonate ions within the plasma. Blood gases can be defined as a measure of the oxygen and carbon dioxide level within the blood, which is commonly referred to as the partial pressure or PO_2 and PCO_2. A chain of reversible biochemical events finely maintains the balance of blood gas.

Oxygen diffuses across the alveolar membrane into the blood, and combines reversibly with haemoglobin. Only a small amount is dissolved in the plasma. The haemoglobin carries oxygen from the alveolar capillaries to the tissue capillaries, where it is released and diffuses across the cell membranes. The tissue cells use this oxygen. During aerobic respiration, carbon dioxide is released as a waste product. The carbon dioxide diffuses from the cells into the capillaries and is carried, dissolved in the plasma, in combination with haemoglobin or as bicarbonate ions (*see* Figure 7.1).

$$CO_2 \text{ (Carbon dioxide)} + H_2O \text{ (Water)} \xleftrightarrow{\text{Carbonic anhydrase}} HC_2O \text{ (Carbonic acid)} \longleftrightarrow H^+ \text{ (Hydrogen ion)} + HCO^3 \text{ (Bicarbonate ion)}$$

Figure 7.1   The process of aerobic respiration

The respiratory system and the renal systems are both extensively involved in the regulation of the acid base balance of the body fluids. The respiratory system and the regulation of CO_2 have a direct effect on the pH of blood. This mechanism takes only minutes to respond. The renal response is the balance of hydrogen and bicarbonate through selective elimination or conservation – this takes hours to have an effect on the pH. The pH of a substance is a measure of its acidity or alkalinity. An acid is a substance that can donate hydrogen ions; a base is a substance that can accept hydrogen ions (the smaller the value, the more acidic the substance). When this is applied to blood gas, apparently small changes have major effects on the viability of the tissues and the efficiency with which cellular metabolic process can be carried out. This is due to the fact that the measurement is a logarithmic one, calculated to the power of 10. A change from pH 6 to 7 represents a ten-fold change in hydrogen. Acidosis is generally regarded as being below 7.25 and alkalosis as being above 7.45. Optimal cell function requires a balance between acids and bases.

Saturation monitoring explained

Approximately 97% of the oxygen carried in the blood is transported in combination with haemoglobin and the remaining 3% is dissolved in the plasma. The oxygen-haemoglobin dissociation curve demonstrates the percentage of haemoglobin saturated with oxygen at any given PO_2. Haemoglobin is saturated when an oxygen molecule is bound to each of its four haem groups. At any PO_2 above 70 mm Hg, nearly 100% of the haemoglobin is saturated with oxygen.

It is important to note that foetal haemoglobin changes to adult haemoglobin by about four months of age. At birth, an infant's Hb is approximately 16–20 g/dl. This is important because, when monitoring an infant's saturation and PO_2 levels, the oxygen dissociation curve shifts to the left. This means that, at a lower PO_2, the relative saturation is higher. Safe oxygen levels have yet to be determined (Tin *et al.*, 2001), but toxic oxygen levels must not be reached, due to the risk of retinopathy of prematurity (ROP) developing.

The pulse oximetery probe contains a light source, emitting both red and infra-red light sources and a light detector. This probe is placed round a peripheral pulsing arterial bed. The red and infra-red wavelengths of light are absorbed differently by oxygenated and deoxygenated haemoglobin. The monitor distinguishes the difference and calculates the proportion of oxygenated haemoglobin circulating. Neonatal nurses need to take care when positioning the probe, as environmental light can cause false readings. Movement also affects the reliability of the monitor as it causes artefact. Rotation of the probe maintains skin integrity and optimum circulation, enhancing accuracy.

Chest X-ray

The lung fields of a neonate have a uniform radiolucent appearance; the hilar and perihilar regions appear dense because of the bronchi and vascular structures (Grossglauser, 1992). The spine should lie in the middle of the chest X-ray, dividing the chest in two and there should be symmetry between each hemithorax. This is a useful guide to assessing whether or not there is significant rotation. Other useful landmarks are the nasogastric tube and the endotracheal tube, if in place.

It is possible to shoot a good film through the perspex hood of an incubator, however, shadows and artefacts are possible with open portholes and the hole in the top of an incubator. Care should be taken to avoid positioning the cardiac leads on the anterior of the infant's chest wall, which would occlude the view of the lung fields. Covering the cold X-ray film plate with soft tissue or cloth can enhance the infant's co-operation. To avoid lordotic positioning, the infant does not have to be stretched, as if on a rack, to give good position. Instead, it can remain comfortably supported, with a towel roll below the buttocks.

SAMPLE EXAMINATION QUESTIONS

Question 1
Describe the structural differences between the airways of the newborn infant and that of the mature child. (*50 marks*)
What transitions of the lungs are made at birth in order to facilitate post-uterine survival? (*50 marks*)

Question 2
What respiratory signs may the nurse observe that would indicate a degree of respiratory distress in the newborn? (*20 marks*)
How can the family be involved in the care of an infant who is ventilated? (*80 marks*)

Question 3
Jamal is a 30 weeks gestation infant and is being managed on CPAP for moderate respiratory distress. What are the complications of CPAP? (*40 marks*)
How may Jamal be weaned off the CPAP? (*60 marks*)

REFERENCES

Ackerman, M. (1993) The effects of saline lavage prior to suctioning, *American Journal of Critical Care* 2(4), 326–30

Askin, D. (1997) Interpretation of neonatal blood gases: disorders of acid-base balance, *Neonatal Network* 16(6), 23–9

Bertone, B. (1988) The role of physiotherapy in the neonatal intensive care unit, *Australian Journal of Physiotherapy* 34(1), 27–34

Bhutani, V., Abbasi, S., Walker, A. and Gerdes, J. (1992) Pulmonary mechanics and energetics in pre-term infants who had respiratory distress and were treated by surfactant, *Journal of Pediatrics* 120(2), 18–24

Bryant, B. (1990) Drug, fluid and blood products administered through the umbilical artery catheter; complication experiences, *Neonatal Network* 9(1), 27–43

Crawford, D. (1991) A boost to the chances of survival: extra-corporeal membrane oxygenation in neonatal care, *Professional Nurse* 6(8), 426–30

Crawford, D. (1992) Putting parents in the picture, *Nursing Times* 88 (2), 41–2

Crawford, D. and Power, K. (2001) Nursing infants on the edge of survival, *Paediatric Nurse* 13(5), 16–20

Crowley, P. (1994) Antenatal corticosteroid therapy a meta-analysis, *American Journal of Obstetrics and Gynaegology* 173(1), 322–35

Cummings, J. *et al.* (1992) A controlled clinical comparison of four different surfactant preparations in surfactant deficient pre-term lambs, *American Review Respiratory Diseases* 145(5), 999–1004

Davis, P. and Shekerdemian, L. (2001) Meconium aspiration syndrome and ECMO, *Archives of Disease in Childhood* 84(1), 1–3

Department of Health (2001) *Review of the Deaths of Four Babies due to Cardiac Tamponade Associated with the Presence of a Central Venous Catheter*, Department of Health, London

Downes, J. and Parker, A. (1991) Chest physiotherapy for pre-term infants, *Paediatric Nursing*, 3(2), 14–17

Drew, D., Jevon, P. and Ratby, M. (2001) Resuscitation of the newborn: a practical approach. Step-by-step guide, *Journal of Neonatal Nursing* 7(4) [central supplement]

Drucker, T. and Hodgkinson, J. (1998) Continuous blood gas monitoring, *Journal of Neonatal Nursing* 4(2) [centre insert]

Goggin, M. (2001) Developments in NCAP fixation, *Journal of Neonatal Nursing* 7(2), 58

Gortner, L. *et al.* (1992) Early treatment of respiratory distress syndrome with bovine surfactant in very pre-term infants; a multi-centre controlled clinical trial, *Pediatric Pulmonology* 14(1), 4–9

Grossglauser, L. (1992) Neonatal radiology; assessment of the quality of the neonatal X-ray film, *Neonatal Network* 11(7), 69–72

Hancock, P. and Peterson, G. (1992) Finger intubation of the trachea in newborns, *Paediatrics* 89(2), 325–7

Harrison, M., Mychaliska, G., Albanese, G. *et al.* (1998) Correction of congenital diaphragmatic hernia in utero. Fetuses with poor prognosis can be saved with temporary tracheal occlusion, *Journal of Pediatric Surgery* 33(7), 1017–23

Harrison, R. (1990) Correction of congenital diaphragmatic hernia in utero. Initial clinical experience, *Journal of Pediatric Surgery* 25(1), 47–57

Hoekstra, R., Jackson, J., Myers, T. *et al.* (1991) Improved neonatal survival following multiple doses of bovine surfactant in very premature infants at risk of respiratory distress syndrome, *Pediatrics* 88(1), 8–10

Juretschke, L. (2001) Congenital diaphragmatic hernia: update and review. Principles and practice, *Journal of Neonatal Gynaecological and Obstetric Nursing* 39(3), 259–68

Kolobow, T. (1988) Acute respiratory failure: on how to injure healthy lungs (and prevent sick lungs from recovery), *Transactions America Society Artificial Internal Organs*, Vol. XXXIV, 31–4

Kotecha, S. (2000) Lung growth; implications for the newborn infant, *Archives of Disease in Childhood* 82(1), 69–74

Langston, C., Kida, K., Reed, M. and Thurlbeck, W. (1984) Human lung growth in late gestation and in the neonate, *Am Rev Respiratory Dis* 129, 607–13

Liggings, G. and Howie, R. (1972) Controlled trial of antepartum glucocorticoid treatment for the prevention of respiratory distress syndrome in premature infants, *Pediatrics* 50(4), 515–25

MacGregor, J. (2000) *Introduction to the Anatomy and Physiology of Children* (Chapter 4), Routledge, London

Macklem, P. (1971) Airway obstruction and collateral ventilation, *Physiology review* 5(1), 368–436

Mehta, A., Callan, K. *et al.* (1986) Patient-triggered ventilation in the newborn, *Lancet*, ii, 706–12

Miller, C. (1995) Nitric oxide therapy for persistent pulmonary hypertension in the newborn, *Neonatal Network* 14(8), 9–15

Milner, T. and Field, D. (1985) Ventilation in the neonatal period, *Care of the Critically Ill* 1(6), 14–15

Mychaliska, G., Bullard, K. and Harrison, M. (1996) *In utero* management of congenital diaphragmatic hernia, *Clinics in Perinatology* 2(3), 823–41

Noerr, B. (1988) Pointers in practical pharmacology: Tolazoline, *Neonatal Network* 8(12), 74–5

Noerr, B. (1992) Pointers in practical pharmacology: pancuronium bromide, *Neonatal Network* 11(2), 77–9

Oberwaldner, B. (2000) Physiotherapy for airway clearance, *European Respiratory Journal* 15(1), 196–204

Paige, P. (1990) Non-invasive monitoring of the neonatal respiratory system, *American Association Critical Nursing* 1(2), 409–21

Resuscitation Council (2000) *Resuscitation at Birth: The Newborn Life Support Provider Course*, Resuscitation Council (UK), London

Runton, N. (1992) Suctioning artificial airways in children; appropriate technique, *Pediatric Nursing* 2 (2), 115–18

Shah, A., Kurth, C. *et al.* (1992) Fluctuations in cerebral oxygenation and blood volume during endotracheal suctioning in premature infants, *Journal of Pediatrics* 120(5), 769–74

Shehata, S., Mooi, W., Okazaki, O. *et al.* (1999) Enhanced expression of vascular epithelial growth factors in lungs of newborn infants with congenital diaphragmatic hernia and pulmonary hypertension, *Thorax* 54(5), 427–31

Shorten, D., Byrne, P. *et al.* (1991) Infant responses to saline instillation and endotracheal suctioning, *Journal of Obstetrics Gynaecology and Neonatal Nursing* 20(6), 464–9

Speer, C. *et al.* (1992) Randomised European multi-centre trial of surfactant replacement therapy for severe neonatal respiratory distress syndrome; single versus multiple doses of Cureosurf, *Pediatrics* 89(1), 13–20

Stoddart, S., Summers, L. and Ward, M. (1997) Pulse oximetry, *Journal of Neonatal Nursing* 3(4), 10–14

Theorell, C. (1990) Congenital diaphragmatic hernia; a physiological approach to management, *Journal of Perinatal and Neonatal Nursing* 3(3), 66–79

Tin, W., Milligan, D. and Pennefather, P. (2001) Pulse oximetry, severe retinopathy and outcome at one year in babies of less than 28 weeks gestation, *Archives of Disease in Childhood* 84(2), 106–10

Tolles, C. and Stone, K. (1990) National survey of neonatal endotracheal suctioning practices, *Neonatal Network* 9(2), 7–14

Vyas, J. and Kotecha, S. (1997) The effects of antenatal and postnatal corticosteroids on the pre-term lung, *Archives of Disease in Childhood* 77(2), 147–50

Wallace, J. (1998) Suctioning – a two-edged sword; reducing the theory practice gap, *Journal of Neonatal Nursing* 4(6), 12–17

Wallis, C. and Prasad, A. (1999) Who needs chest physiotherapy? Moving from anecdote to evidence, *Archives of Disease in Childhood* 80(4), 393–7

Walsh, M. (1989) Making sense of chest drains, *Nursing Times* 85(24), 40–1

White, C., Richardson, C. *et al.* (1990) High-frequency ventilation and extra-corporeal membrane oxygenation, *American Association Critical Nursing* 1(2), 427–44

White, H. (1997) Suctioning – a review, *Paediatric Nursing* 9(4), 18–20

Whitten, C. (1989) *Anyone Can Intubate; A Practical, Step-by-step Guide for Health Professionals*, Medical Arts Press, K-W Publications, San Diego, California

Whyte, S., Birrell, G. and Wyllie, J. (2000) Premedication before intubation in UK neonatal units, *Archives of Disease in Children* 82(1), 38–41

Woodrow, P. (1997) Nitric oxide: some nursing implications, *Intensive and Critical Care Nursing* 13(2), 87–92

Yeo, H. (1999) Congenital diaphragmatic hernia; lowering the mortality rates, *Journal of Neonatal Nursing* 5(5), 6–9

Young, J. (1995) To help or to hinder; endotracheal suction and the intubated neonate, *Journal of Neonatal Nursing* 1(3), 23–8

FURTHER READING

Aloan, C. (1987) *Respiratory Care of the Newborn*, JB Lippincott, Philadelphia, PA

Carlo, W. and Chatburn, R. (1990) *Neonatal Respiratory Care* (2nd edition), Year Book Medical Publishers, Chicago, IL

Tortora, G. and Anagnostakos, N. (1990) *Principles of Anatomy and Physiology* (6th edition), Harper and Row, New York

Williams, P. and Warwick, R. (1980) *Gray's Anatomy* (36th edition), Churchill Livingstone, Edinburgh

MacGregor, J. (2000) *Introduction to the Anatomy and Physiology of Children*, Routledge, London

8 NURSING CARE OF AN INFANT WITH A GASTRO-INTESTINAL CONDITION

Wendy Hickson

Aims of the chapter

This chapter provides a basic insight into the embryological development of the gut and the gastro-intestinal tract of the infant. This will help to provide an understanding of the congenital malformations and conditions that may affect the gastro-intestinal tract of the neonate. It introduces the care and management of infants in relation to the following topics:

- necrotising enterocolitis (NEC);
- gastroschisis and omphocele;
- tracheo-oesophageal fistula;
- malrotation; and
- gastric reflux.

The nursing care of these conditions in conjunction with the specific pre- and post-operative care is reviewed.

INTRODUCTION

With the advent of advanced scanning techniques and diagnostic expertise, the majority of gastro-intestinal disorders can be identified antenatally. This should enable comprehensive preparation of the parents and enhance communications between the entire multi-disciplinary team who will care for the infant after delivery. Controversy exists as to where a previously diagnosed infant requiring surgical intervention should be delivered. Some believe that delivery in the centre providing surgery will improve the outcome; the neonate will not have to endure the risks of a transfer and the expertise and services are on-site. Others believe that it is important for the mother to be delivered in the area where she has an established relationship with the obstetrician. Several studies illustrate no real difference in outcome following surgery (Nicholls *et al.*, 1993; Stoodley *et al.*, 1993).

The chosen method of delivery is also controversial and depends on the defect. Some advocate the use of a caesarean section, for example, to prevent trauma to the externalised bowel and to prevent colonisation with vaginal flora (Swift *et al.*, 1992). Stephenson and colleagues (2000) suggest that the infant should be delivered vaginally unless there are maternal indications for a caesarean section.

Not all malformations are identified from a scan (Roberts and Burge, 1990); in these cases, the delivery of an infant with a defect may come as a major shock for the parents. They may experience feelings of guilt, disbelief and anger, and time for adjustment to the condition may not always be possible, as immediate intervention may be necessary. Parents need regular communication, honest information and support from the nursing and medical staff to allay as much anxiety as possible at this traumatic time.

EMBRYOLOGY OF THE GASTRO-INTESTINAL SYSTEM

Gestational age

Table 8.1 Characteristics of the gastro-intestinal system

Day 21–24	Separation of gut from yolk sac
4 weeks	Stomach appears as dilation of foregut
5–6 weeks	Gall bladder forms; hepatic ducts appear; intestinal loops cause large swelling in umbilical cord; stomach structure is established
5–8 weeks	Circular muscle develops in small intestine
7–8 weeks	Fusion of pancreas
8 weeks	Gastric pits appear; development of the intestinal villi; anal membrane ruptures and rectum is formed
9–10 weeks	Formation of circular muscle in the colon
10 weeks	Formation of longitudinal muscle in the small intestine; intestine returns to the abdomen
12 weeks	Bile is formed by hepatic cells, takes on a green colour and can enter the gastro-intestinal tract; primitive parietal cells develop in the gastric mucosa; formation of Islets of Langerhans in the pancreas; complete innervation of ganglion cells of the myenteric plexus
14 weeks	Layers of muscle lining the alimentary tract
16 weeks	Meconium begins to fill the colon
20 weeks	Islets begin to secrete insulin; non-nutritive sucks begin; host defences are present in the intestine
22 weeks	Digestive enzymes such as amylase are present; gastric glands mature
24–30 weeks	Rapid elongation and maturation
28 weeks	Foetus developmentally capable of single 'sucks'; increase in gastro-oesophageal pressure
28–30 weeks	Peristalsis commences
31 weeks	Foetus able to sustain and repeat 'suck' (sucking bursts)
34 weeks	Mature 'sucks', developmentally able to co-ordinate with swallowing
34 plus weeks	Meconium present in distal colon; reactive anal sphincter
38 plus weeks	Rooting reflex combined with sucking and swallowing

Modified from Clark (2000)

EXAMPLES OF GASTRO-INTESTINAL (GI) MALFORMATIONS AND NEONATAL
DISORDERS

Upper GI disorders

- Malformation of face and oropharynx;
- Oesophageal pouch, atresia (with or without fistula to trachea);
- Reflux;
- Pyloric stenosis.

Middle GI disorders

- Diaphragmatic hernia;
- Small/large bowel atresia;
- Meconium ileus;
- Volvulus and malrotation;
- Necrotising enterocolitis (NEC);
- Gastroschisis and omphalocele;
- Duodenal/intestinal atresia, stenosis and obstruction;
- Intussusception.

Lower GI disorders

- Inguinal hernia;
- Imperforate anus;
- Necrotising enterocolitis (NEC);
- Anal fistula;
- Hirschsprung's disease;
- Meconium ileus.

NECROTISING ENTEROCOLITIS (NEC)

Aetiology

The incidence of NEC is common in pre-term infants, especially those of
extreme prematurity (Beeby and Jeffery, 1992) and very low birthweight
(VLBW). Mortality may be as high as 30% (Stephenson *et al.*, 2000). The actual
cause of NEC is unknown, however, factors thought to contribute to its likelihood include birth asphyxia, umbilical catheterisation, artificial milk feeding
and early feeding (Thomas and Harvey, 1997), particularly into the under-
developed or compromised gut. Other factors include blood transfusion, polycythaemia and patent ductus arteriosus (Pearse and Roberton, 1988). Bleeding in
the third trimester, multiple births and maternal diabetes have been linked to
NEC.

Pre-term infants respond to perinatal stress, hypotension and hypoxia by
shunting and redirecting blood to the vital organs. This reduces the mesenteric

circulation, causing necrosis and damage. Damaged intestinal mucosa allows the entry of gas-producing bacteria, which normally reside in the intestine. Bacterial proliferation is enhanced by formula milk, which acts as a food source. The bacteria in the submucosal wall form gas. This will cause the bowel to distend, the intralumenal pressure to increase and the blood flow through the mucosa to decrease. The result of these processes, if left undetected, will be bowel perforation or infarction, which may be localised or general (Pearse and Roberton, 1988; Koloske and Musemeche, 1989; Rushton, 1990).

Clinical features

Infants with NEC may have bile-stained vomits and increasing bile-stained naso-gastric aspirates as well as a distended abdomen. As the condition progresses the bowel may obstruct, causing a distended abdomen, which becomes red, hard and shiny, with loops of bowel identifiable. The infants will exhibit signs of infection such as apnoea, unstable temperature, mottling and pallor, and the blood gas analysis may identify a metabolic acidosis. With early presentation of the condition they may not have passed meconium, although this is not always a certain feature. They may pass bloody stools and, in extreme cases, tissue can be present in the stool. Abdominal X-ray will depict the presence of intramural bubbles of gas, resulting from the invasion of the bowel with gas-forming organisms (Thomas and Harvey, 1997), and thickened, dilated portions of bowel can also be apparent.

Nursing measures to help prevent NEC

The cause of NEC is most likely to be multi-factorial although a genetic pre-disposition cannot be ruled out. Certain precautions may be taken to reduce the risk.

- Early, small enteral feeds of expressed breast milk are recommended to stimulate gut motility. Secretion of the intestinal hormone necessary for adaptation to postnatal life may respond to the introduction of early feeds.
- High osmolarity milk and enteral (oral) drugs can be avoided.
- If there is evidence of perinatal hypoxia, withholding feeds and intravenous and subsequent long-line feeding are recommended (Stephenson et al., 2000).
- If bowels are not opened within 12 hours a suppository can be administered (Stephenson et al., 2000).
- Some studies have recommended the avoidance of plasma products for infants suspected of NEC (Squire et al., 1992).

Continuing studies researching the prevention of NEC include the use of prophylactic oral Vancomycin (Ng et al., 1988; Siu et al., 1998), and the detection of T and TK antigen activation in severe cases (Osborn et al., 1999). The results compare favourably, but both studies confirm the need for further work.

Medical and nursing care associated with conservative management of NEC

The aim of conservative management of NEC is to rest the gut, allowing the inflammation to resolve, while treating infection and maintaining the infant's life (Pearse and Roberton, 1988).

The role of nutrition in NEC

Enteral feeds should be withheld as the milk provides a growth medium for gut bacteria. Fluids should initially be given via an intravenous line and 24 hours later total parenteral nutrition (TPN) may be commenced via a long line (Stephenson *et al.*, 2000). All infusions should be carefully calculated, and rates and volumes should be monitored. A two-nurse aseptic technique is recommended for drawing up and connection of long-line fluids. The fluid balance needs to be carefully regulated to prevent fluid overload and the electrolyte levels of both serum and urine require daily analysis.

A nasogastric tube should be passed and left on free drainage. Frequent aspiration of the tube should be performed depending on the amounts being obtained. The aspirates are then discarded. If the total aspirate over 4 hours exceeds half of a 4-hourly amount of fluid, intravenous fluid replacement therapy of normal saline ml for ml is required.

Comfort, rest and monitoring

Infants should be nursed naked and supine in either an incubator or an overhead heated cot, to ensure adequate observation of the abdomen and overall appearance. This allows early identification of changes without disturbance. Positioning is important to reduce pressure on the abdomen. Skin probes and tape should be positioned away from the abdomen and blankets should not be placed over the abdomen. A minimal handling regime should be exercised to allow maximum rest for the infant.

It is essential that adequate analgesia, for example, intravenous diamorphine (according to unit policy), is administered to alleviate discomfort of the infant. Broad spectrum antibiotics – for example, Metronidazole, Gentamicin and Benzylpenicillin in combination – should be prescribed as per recommended regime. The administration is usually for 7–10 days, dependent on the resolution of symptoms.

An unstable infant should be continually monitored with hourly recordings of respiration, apex beat and oxygen saturations. Core and skin temperature measurements are simultaneously measured and this can be effective in detecting signs of early infection. A gap of greater than one degree may be indicative of clinical deterioration.

Although most units remove it at the merest suspicion of NEC, the umbilical arterial catheter may be left in situ, providing the position of the tip is satisfactory on X-ray and there are no signs of occlusion. Meticulous attention should be paid to the entry site of the catheter and to the perfusion of the lower limbs. If there appears to be impairment of the blood supply to the lower limbs, any difficulty in obtaining a blood specimen, or mottling and distension of the abdomen, the line should be removed immediately (Pearse and Roberton, 1988).

A peripheral arterial line will be required for easily obtaining blood specimens and for continuous recordings of blood pressure. Perfusion to the peripheries of the limb in which the line is situated requires constant observation. The cannula should be taped with the minimum of tape, to secure it but to allow for observation of the digits. Any blanching of the digits should be reported and the line removed immediately.

Extremes of blood sugar may occur as a result of stress, infection, dehydration and poor nutrition. Levels of less than 1 mmol or greater than 8 mmols are unacceptable and should be reported (Fleming et al., 1986). Initially, whilst unstable, 1-hourly blood sugar readings are warranted; once stable, the time between readings may be lengthened. All blood glucose specimens can be taken from the arterial line (providing the infusion is heparinised saline), to minimise discomfort of the neonate.

Assisted ventilation may be required owing to the very unstable condition of these infants. The effect of the disease may cause 'splinting' of the abdomen, making breathing difficult, and sepsis can cause recurrent apnoea and bradycardia (Pearse and Roberton 1988). In many units, continuous positive airway pressure (CPAP) is the preferred method of ventilatory support. However, due to the increased abdominal distension caused by CPAP, it may be preferable to use another method of supporting the respiratory function (see Chapter 7).

Dependent upon unit policy, abdominal distension can be measured with a tape measure around the area of maximum distension. The position should be gently marked with a pen so that the same area can be measured each time (usually 4- to 6-hourly) and recorded. A progressive increase may indicate perforation (Stephenson et al., 2000).

Haematological disturbances may occur and require intervention and anaemia may need to be corrected (Stephenson et al., 2000).

If the infant has a diminished urine output, a catheter may be passed under aseptic technique (size 4 NGT is suitable), to enable accurate monitoring of urine output, especially if output is less than 1.5–2ml/kg hour (Rushton, 1990), and colloids may be prescribed. Specimens of urine are sent for urea and electrolyte levels. Ward analysis is performed twice daily or as unit policy dictates.

Resolution and recovery

If infants respond positively to the medical and nursing measures (as shown by the reabsorption of gas in the bowel wall, reduction of abdominal distension and increasing stability of vital signs), milk feeds may be gradually reintroduced at 0.5–1ml/hour and increased slowly – for example, 12-hourly, with the intravenous infusion adjusted accordingly. Nurses need to be vigilant in detecting any deterioration in the infant, unstable vital signs, pallor, mottling, and must check by nasogastric aspiration that the milk is being absorbed. If any aspirates are bile-stained or there is an increase in aspirate, the feeds should be stopped immediately and total feeding via intravenous fluids commenced.

Surgical management of NEC

Surgery is indicated if infants show continuing signs of deterioration, or worsening acidosis, which may suggest necrotic bowel (Stephenson *et al.*, 2000), and/or an increase in abdominal distension, which may indicate perforation. Thomas and Harvey (1997) suggest that, in the acute stages of NEC, due to the high mortality rate associated with surgery, perforation is the only indication for laparotomy. When laparotomy is undertaken, resection of the necrotic bowel and anastomosis of both ends is performed. Alternatively, the two ends are sutured to the abdominal wall, forming an active stoma and a distal stoma.

Pre-operative nursing care

Adequate preparation (when time allows) is imperative for the parents of infants undergoing surgery. In the case of a life-threatening illness such as NEC, parents may display extreme anxiety and this will be combined with other emotions. Whenever possible it is important to allow time for questions concerning their infant's condition.

An accurate weight is required pre-surgery to assess fluids and drug dosage. However, due to the instability of the infant, the most recent weight measurement may have to suffice. Baseline observations of temperature, apex beat, respirations, blood sugar, blood glucose and blood pressure need to be documented, along with respiratory support, fluid balance and urine output. The infant's haemoglobin, urea and electrolyte status are assessed and recorded prior to surgery. Maternal blood is taken for cross-matching and it is important to ensure that blood is available for transfusion should the need arise. As these infants are 'nil by mouth', intravenous fluids are commenced, to maintain hydration and blood sugars. Blood sugar should be taken before surgery, from the arterial line.

Obtaining parental/guardian consent is the responsibility of the medical staff. The nurse's role is to check that consent for both the anaesthetic and the operation has been obtained. Nurses should ensure that the parents and doctors liaise to prevent any delay in surgery. If contact with the parents is not possible in the event of an emergency procedure, the responsibility for consent of the infant lies with two consultants. If the unit where the infant is admitted does not perform surgery, the infant is transferred to a surgical unit. Many of the principles of transport (reviewed in Chapter 13) apply to ensure the safety and warmth of the infant going to and returning from theatre.

Post-operative care

Initial ventilation is required due to the effects of surgery and the infant's unstable condition.

General hourly post-operative monitoring of vital signs and continuous monitoring will occur and post-operative hydration will comprise intravenous fluids.

Urine output will be accurately measured and charted. If infants are nursed with an overhead heater, or in a humidified incubator, weighing in nappies is not recommended, as these variables will affect the accuracy of the urine output measurement.

Infants may return from theatre with an abdominal wound and the formation of two stomas from the proximal and distal ends of the resected bowel. The type of stoma depends on the area excised; it will be either an ileostomy or colostomy. Initially, the wound and stoma may be dressed with gauze, which may be left in situ until it becomes soiled from any stoma discharge. Alternatively the infant may return from theatre with a bag covering the site. This should be left in position unless leakage occurs. It may need to be emptied of gas contents once a day, using clean technique. Easy access is necessary to check the stoma site during handling for cares, perhaps on a 6–8-hourly basis, to cause minimal disturbance. The stoma needs checking for colour, perfusion and activity. A healthy stoma may be initially quite dark and may bleed easily post-operation, then becomes red or pink in colour and is slightly raised above the skin.

The abdominal skin around the stoma should not show any signs of irritation from the stoma, sutures or the stoma appliance. With very small infants, non-adherent sterile gauze dressings may be all that is necessary until the stoma begins to function. The stoma should function within 5–7 days and if the stoma has healed then a stoma bag may be applied and kept in situ, provided there is no leakage and the stoma and surrounding skin are satisfactory. The bag is emptied 12-hourly and the amount, consistency and colour of the output is charted. Output from the stoma should be less than half of the enteral intake (Harjo, 1988) and any excessive loss will need to be replaced in order to prevent dehydration. A reducing sugar greater than 0.5% needs to be reported, as intolerance may occur due to damage of the intestinal mucosa and decreased intestinal absorption (Harjo, 1988).

A stoma created from the jejunum or first part of the ileum may result in excessive sodium and nutrient losses, which can result in a metabolic acidosis and failure to thrive (Bower *et al.*, 1988). Sodium supplements may be required and close monitoring is necessary.

Nurses should contact the paediatric stoma nurse, who will visit the infant and parents, in order to show them how to clean the stoma and apply the stoma bag, and to answer any anxieties that may arise. Closure of the stoma may occur at a later stage, particularly if it is formed from the jejunum (Bower *et al.*, 1988).

GASTROSCHISIS

Incidence

Gastroschisis is particularly common in the infants of young mothers (Sadler, 2000; Stephenson *et al.*, 2000) and appears to be increasing in frequency (Sadler, 2000; Stephenson *et al.*, 2000). There are no known genetic associations. There is some discrepancy over the underlying factors, but rupture of exomphalos or a developmental defect of the abdominal wall (Twining *et al.*, 2000) may be implicated.

Aetiology

Gastroschisis occurs when there is a defect in the anterior abdominal wall, resulting in herniation of the bowel into the amniotic cavity (Sadler, 2000; Stephenson *et al.*, 2000). The occurrence is usually to the right of the umbilicus. As the bowel is exposed and not covered by amnion or peritoneum, there is a risk of contamination from foetal urine. Due possibly to chemical peritonitis, the bowel wall may become thickened (Twining *et al.*, 2000). Infants with gastroschisis are usually associated with low birthweight (Boyd *et al.*, 1998) but rarely associated with other anomalies (Davies and Stringer, 1997; Twining *et al.*, 2000). Stenosis and atresia can occur if the bowel twists around the hole in the abdominal wall (Roberton, 1986; Meller *et al.*, 1989). Gangrene and perforation may occur if the bowel is damaged or becomes ischaemic (Fleming *et al.*, 1986).

Diagnosis

Accurate diagnosis of gastroschisis can be made in the second trimester of pregnancy (Boyd *et al.*, 1998). In a six-year review of antenatal diagnosis of abdominal wall defects by ultrasound, poor detection rates were highlighted (Roberts and Burge, 1990). Misdiagnosis may result occasionally due to scanning technique or if there is a multiple pregnancy.

The antenatal diagnosis of gastroschisis does not affect management as such but accurate diagnosis enables parental counselling and allows time to plan an in utero transfer to a surgical centre.

Pre-operative nursing care specific for gastroschisis

The parents must be allowed to see and touch their infant as soon as possible. Often the defect is perceived by the parents as being worse than it really is. If the gastroschisis has been detected prior to delivery, the parents should have the opportunity to speak to the medical/surgical team. Ample explanation needs to be given to the parents regarding the operation and what it entails.

Following delivery, the infant's lower body is encased in a sterile plastic bag. This is drawn up over the herniated bowel and secured underneath the arms. It is imperative to prevent infection in the exposed bowel and to reduce water and heat loss from evaporation. Recommended practice is to provide the mother with a sterile bowel bag should she deliver in a tertiary hospital (Stephenson *et al.*, 2000). The bag is not removed until the infant is in theatre.

A Replogle tube should be passed to deflate the bowel (Stephenson *et al.*, 2000) and the tube left in situ and low suction applied (no greater than 4–5 mmHg), to aid decompression. Alternatively, a nasogastric tube may be passed and left on free drainage with intermittent aspiration perhaps every 4 hours.

The infant should be nursed naked in an incubator set within the appropriate thermo-neutral range or in a cot with overhead heater. It is preferable to nurse them in an incubator, to reduce insensible heat loss, and the addition of humidity is recommended. The exposed bowel represents a large surface that will lose heat quickly. Additional cling film or bubble wrap can be placed over the abdomen to reduce the heat loss and preserve the central temperature.

The appearance of the bowel is assessed hourly. Nursing the infant in the lateral position allows good visualisation and reduces the pressure that the gastroschisis can have on the abdominal contents. If the circulation to any area is compromised the bowel may become discoloured and blue, and medical staff will need to be informed immediately. Broad spectrum antibiotics will be commenced immediately as these infants are at high risk of infection due to contamination of the exposed bowel.

Respiratory support may be needed if the infant is premature or if blood gases, vital signs or general condition indicate a need for respiratory assistance. Parenteral feeding should be commenced to supplement insensible fluid and protein loss from the bowel (Boxwell, 2000).

A chest and abdominal X-ray should be taken to detect any abnormalities and assess the status of the lungs prior to surgery. Pre-operative care includes accurate weighing, baseline observations, and measuring of blood glucose and blood pressure. A low blood pressure may result in the need for colloid due to large volume losses from the exposed bowel. The infant's haematological status will be assessed in the same manner for each surgical procedure (*see under* NEC, page 154). Consent for surgery is obtained in the same way as for NEC (*see* page 154).

Surgery should take place as soon as possible when the infant is stable. Recommendation is within 6 hours of birth due to the vulnerability of the exposed bowel (Meller *et al.*, 1989). The aim of the surgery is to return the bowel to the abdomen without comprising the abdominal circulation or functioning of the bowel. Primary and complete closure can be achieved if the abdominal wall will stretch over the bowel; in most cases this is possible (Stephenson *et al.*, 2000). In cases where this cannot be achieved a silastic patch is attached to the skin surrounding the bowel and primary closure is delayed until the skin has stretched and oedema of the bowel has resolved.

Post-operative nursing care

The infant will require post-operative care, including hourly observations of vital signs, care of intravenous nutrition, and adequate analgesic cover. Respiratory support may be required as a result of raised intra-abdominal pressure or the diaphragm being displaced upwards. In addition the silastic patch may embarrass respiration and analgesic infusions or paralysing agents will further compromise respiratory effort (Meller *et al.*, 1989; De Lorimier *et al.*, 1991). Support for the parents is also required.

The suture line is inspected daily for signs of infection (redness, inflammation, tenderness), septic areas or tissue breakdown. Abnormal findings are recorded. Likewise if there appears to be any infection or ischaemia of the encased bowel, this is recorded.

If the infant has a silastic patch, the suture line may be treated with a topical, antibacterial agent and dressed daily using an aseptic technique, with dry gauze to absorb serous drainage (De Lorimier *et al.*, 1991). The amount and colour of the drainage is recorded on the fluid balance chart.

If a silastic patch has been created, it is then suspended from the incubator using the ties (attached in theatre), so that tension is placed on the skin; in this way it is stretched, so that it will eventually cover the bowel. The size of the pouch is reduced daily over the next week, until the skin has stretched suffi- ciently and all of the bowel can be returned to the abdomen (De Lorimier *et al.*, 1991). When handling the infant, the tension on the silastic pouch needs to be maintained by another person.

Intra-abdominal pressure can be increased with the repair of the defect (De Lorimier *et al.*, 1991). The lower limbs should be exposed so that the legs may be observed for signs of discolouration, oedema and impaired perfusion (decreased pulses, blanching, coolness and capillary return can be tested by applying slight pressure to the feet). Central venous pressure may be monitored to detect inadequate venous return or impaired intra-abdominal perfusion (De Lorimier *et al.*, 1991).

Renal impairment and poor urine production may occur due to hypotension, and large fluid and plasma losses may occur from the herniated bowel (Stringer *et al.*, 1991). Urine production needs to be greater than 1 ml/kg/hr (De Lorimier *et al.*, 1991). Output should be measured and urinalysis performed and recorded. A specific gravity of greater than 1.015 may indicate dehydration.

Fluid balance is important and extra fluids may need to be prescribed. Gastric losses from the nasogastric tube may require intravenous replacement and plasma expanders may be necessary to maintain the systolic blood pressure.

OMPHOCELE

Incidence

Incidence of omphocele is put at between 1 and 2.5 in 10 000 births (Sadler, 2000).

Aetiology

During the 6th to 10th week of embryonic development, the intestine rotates and returns to the abdomen. Failure of this process results in omphocele, whereby the abdominal contents herniate through a defect in the umbilicus. Herniation may vary in size, from a relatively small defect that will require straightforward surgical closure on the first day of life, to a major defect where the liver, intestine, spleen or bladder may be involved (Sadler, 2000). The herniation is covered with peritoneum and amnion. This is a feature that distin- guishes omphocele from gastroschisis. With omphocele there is a high asso- ciation with congenital abnormalities, including cardiac, bowel (Thomas and

Harvey, 1997), trisomy 13, trisomy 18, trisomy 21 and Beckwith Wiedmann Syndrome (Kelnar *et al.*, 1995; Stephenson *et al.*, 2000).

As with gastroschisis, the defect can be detected on scan as early as 12 weeks and the place of delivery is dependent upon the medical staff involved. Rupture of the omphocele may occur, resulting in a life-threatening situation. The infant may be delivered in a surgical unit. There is no reason why the infant should not be delivered by the vaginal route if other complications do not appear to be evident.

Pre-operative nursing/medical management

Safety and comfort
Surgical repair should be done as soon as possible (Berseth, 1998). Following delivery it is imperative that the sac is protected and that the infants are commenced on antibiotics, as they are extremely prone to infection. Following the same procedure as for infants with gastroschisis, they should be placed in a sterile plastic bag to the armpits, to limit insensible fluid loss, reduce heat loss and protect against rupture of the omphocele (Stephenson *et al.*, 2000). A nasogastric tube is passed and aspirated 4-hourly and left on free drainage or low flow suction to aid decompression. Infants are nursed naked in a humidified incubator in the supine position to aid observation and to prevent further discomfort. At this stage analgesia is not normally prescribed, as opiates depress the respiratory drive and they may show no signs of distress.

Nutrition
Parenteral feeding is recommended as there may be increased fluid loss due to the lesion, and hypoglycaemia may be present, particularly if the omphocele is an element of Beckwith's Syndrome, which occurs in 10% of the cases (Twining *et al.*, 2000). Blood sugar should be monitored 6- to 8-hourly and necessary action taken if it is not within the normal limits.

Psychological care
When omphocele is detected antenatally the parents should have ample opportunity to ask questions and address issues with the combined medical team, comprising obstetrician and surgeon. As there is a high association with other anomalies, all aspects of the infant's care need to be discussed with the parents. X-rays and scans need to be arranged with the parents' consent, awareness and understanding. Due to chromosomal abnormalities being common (Roberton, 1986), foetal karyotyping is recommended (Stephenson *et al.*, 2000). The parents may need counselling and adequate guidance.

Following delivery, the parents should have a chance to see and touch their infant prior to admission to NNU. At all stages the parents should be encouraged to be involved with the care of their infant.

Post-operative care of the infant

Safety and comfort

Primary closure of the omphocele is the preferred method of treatment (Boxwell, 2000). Following surgery there is a high likelihood that these infants will require mechanical ventilation. They should be nursed supine and hourly observations made of the wound site. General post-operative care comprises hourly observation of vital signs, urine output, and oozing or inflammation of the wound site. Any signs of infection should be monitored and any deviation from the norm immediately reported to the doctor.

Analgesia should be prescribed intravenously, diamorphine or morphine being a standard choice. A minimal handling policy should be adhered to in order to prevent further discomfort. Antibiotics should be continued for 7–10 days post-operatively.

When larger lesions are present it may not be possible to return the viscera to the abdominal space. One method used is to suture a silastic pouch to the wall of the abdomen so that gradual reduction occurs of the herniated contents into the abdominal space. The silastic pouch is reduced on a daily basis by a series of suture lines until the contents are gradually forced into the abdomen (Holland *et al.*, 1998). This normally takes approximately 10–14 days. Complications include infection of the silastic pouch and respiratory depression as a result of the diaphragm being splinted. Additional problems include impairment of the bowel function, stenosis or atresia, and decreased venous return caused by increased abdominal pressure (Holland *et al.*, 1998). The nurse needs to observe very closely for signs of infection and deterioration by hourly monitoring and clear observation of the silastic pouch.

Conservative management of an infant with omphocele is to stimulate the epithelial growth of the sac to prevent rupture. A mercury-based topical agent was once the preferred choice, however, following the detection of high levels of mercury in the organs and blood (Fagan *et al.*, 1977), alternatives such as 65% alcohol or silver sulfadine are now used (Holland *et al.*, 1998). Several months later there may be further surgical reduction of the hernia.

Nutrition

Prolonged parenteral feeding is recommended to reduce the incidence of necrotising enterocolitis, which is present in these infants. Other potential problems include gut stenosis or atresia. There should be a gradual introduction to enteral feeds when the surgical decision allows.

OESOPHAGEAL ATRESIA AND TRACHEO-OESOPHAGEAL FISTULA (TOF)

Aetiology

Tracheo-oesophageal fistula occurs when there is a failure in the differentiation of the foregut into the trachea and oesophagus during the 4th to 5th week of development. Oesophageal atresia may occur in isolation, but this rare. This occurs during the 8th week of foetal development as a result of the oesophagus not cannulating. The incidence of TOF is approximately 1 in 3000–4500 live births and males are mostly affected (Moore and Persaud, 1998). The incidence is higher in twins and in infants of parents who themselves have had the condition (Holland *et al.*, 1998). The infant is frequently of low birthweight and an additional feature may be the presence of 13 pairs of ribs (Roberton, 1986).

The majority of infants present with oesophageal atresia (Moore and Persaud, 1998) and 50–70% of infants display further congenital anomalies collectively known as the VACTERL association. These defects include vertebral, anal, cardiac, TOF, oesophageal atresia, renal and limb (Sadler, 2000).

There are five variations of this condition (Holland *et al*, 1998; incidence in brackets):

1   A fistula between the distal oesophagus and trachea (86%);
2   Oesophageal atresia only (7.7%);
3   H-type TOF without oesophageal atresia (4.2%);
4   Oesophageal atresia with a proximal fistula (0.8%);
5   Oesophageal atresia with proximal and distal fistulae (0.7%).

Diagnosis

Diagnosis can be made antenatally due to polyhydramnios (the foetus is unable to swallow due to the oesophageal atresia), but the condition is usually noticed in the newborn, which has copious frothy saliva that is constantly regurgitated. The infant's prognosis is better if identification occurs before the first milk feed.

To confirm the diagnosis, a large radio opaque nasogastric tube (size 8 or 10 FG) is passed gently through the nostril as far as possible and, once resistance is met, secured into position. When oesophageal atresia is present the catheter will not advance more than 5–10cm from the mouth (Kelnar *et al.*, 1995). An urgent X-ray is taken, encompassing the neck, chest and abdomen, to confirm the diagnosis and to identify the level of the atresia. On X-ray the NGT will be viewed in the upper oesophagus, as advancement is not possible. The abdomen needs to be included as the presence of air in the stomach determines a distal fistula. Contrast medium is contra-indicated because of the risk of aspiration into the lungs, intensifying the risk of pneumonia (Kelnar *et al.*, 1995).

Signs and symptoms

If the condition is not identified before the infant is fed, coughing and choking will occur as a direct result of feeding. The infant is at an increased risk of aspiration and pneumonia if allowed to continue feeding and may become cyanosed if milk is aspirated into the lungs.

Immediate nursing care

Immediate treatment is to free the airway of secretions and reduce the risk of aspiration. A double lumen or Repogle tube is passed into the pouch or oropharynx and continuous low suction is applied. Suction should be no greater than 50 cm of water. The tube needs to be flushed with 1–2 mls normal saline every 15–30 minutes to free the secretions from the tube. The suction tubing needs to be checked to ensure that it has not become overloaded with secretions and therefore lost its efficiency. If oral suction is needed it should be performed very gently. The infant should be nursed with the head elevated to an angle of 45 degrees (Boxwell, 2000), to prevent milk aspiration and gastro-oesophageal reflux.

Hydration is maintained by the commencement of a 10% dextrose infusion. Regular monitoring of blood sugar is necessary in the initial phase of treatment, as these infants are more prone to hypoglycaemia (Roberton, 1986).

Pre-operative care

The infant needs to be in optimum condition for surgery. Antibiotics will be prescribed prophylactically. Surgery may occur within 24 hours on a term infant with an early diagnosis (Kelnar et al., 1995). This may extend to a period of many weeks for an infant who is either unstable, or if growth of the oesophagus is necessary.

If surgery is withheld, the infant may be fed via a gastrostomy. Gastric feeds need to be given slowly, to prevent gastric distension, vomiting and aspiration. It is imperative that the sucking reflex is not lost. Locally our policy is to give a small amount of water orally (10 mls 4–6-hourly) if the infant becomes distressed. No adverse effect has been noted as the water is suctioned from the tube preventing aspiration.

A chest X-ray and abdominal scan should be taken to ascertain whether there are further anomalies. An echocardiogram should also be obtained to enable the surgeon to identify the side of the aortic arch so that the thoracotomy may be performed from the opposite side (Stephenson et al., 2000).

The parents should be kept informed of the various investigations and given the opportunity to voice any anxieties.

Surgical procedure

Surgery is usually performed by a right thoracotomy and access is gained to the trachea by deflating the right lung. The fistula is ligated and an anastomosis of the oesophagus performed. Sometimes the gap is too wide for anastomosis and surgery has to be halted until there has been more growth of the infant. In extreme cases the gap never shortens and a graft may be the only form of treatment. This may entail serious complications and recovery may be severely affected.

Post-operative care

The infant may be ventilated post-operatively. Muscle relaxants are recommended to prevent dislodging of the endotracheal tube and extubation as reintubation will put tension on the anastomosis. If reintubation is necessary, a skilled practitioner should perform the procedure (Stephenson et al., 2000).

The infant will continue on antibiotic therapy for at least 5 days and intra-venous fluids of 10% dextrose will be continued, to provide hydration. Intra-venous analgesia should be prescribed immediately post-operatively.

Following surgery, a trans-anastomostic tube will be passed into the stomach to prevent stenosis of the oesophagus. It is crucial that the tube is secured firmly in place as reintroduction may lead to serious damage of the anastomosis. The tube is left on free drainage to aid gastric decompression and is aspirated 4-hourly. The colour, consistency and amount of drainage are recorded. Large amounts of drainage may need to be replaced intravenously. If the tube should become dislodged, the surgical team needs to be informed. A doctor should replace the tube, as there is a potential risk of injury to the repair. If suction is required, this should be done very gently and the catheter should not be passed through the repair.

An extrapleural chest drain is inserted to aid re-inflation of the lung, and the underwater drainage bottles from the chest drain are suspended securely below the level of the chest. The amount and colour of any drainage should be noted, along with any bubbling or swinging in the reservoir. In case of accidental disconnection, a spare pair of forceps should be kept near by. The chest drain is removed when there is no drainage apparent and the water has stopped swinging and bubbling – usually 48–72 hours post-operatively. The tubing may be clamped for 2 to 3 days prior to the removal of the drain.

A barium swallow is performed before the infant begins breast- or bottle-feeding to assess the efficiency of the anastomosis. Any leaks or presence of a stricture will be identified. If the results from the X-ray are satisfactory, then oral feeds may commence. If the gastric aspirate is minimal then nasogastric feeds may be commenced, with the surgeon's permission.

Complications

Gastro-oesophageal reflux is a common problem and may persist for a long time. Methods of alleviating the condition include thickening of the infant's feeds, giving the feeds slowly, elevating the cot head 35–45 degrees, and placing the infant in the prone posture (Holland *et al.*, 1998). In severe cases a fundopli-cation may be required.

Stricture may form at the anastomosis and regular dilatation may be necessary. When oral feeding is not possible, due to stricture, severe gastro-oeso-phageal reflux or inability to perform a primary repair, a gastrostomy is created to enable feeding.

Breakdown and leakage of the anastomosis may occur. The initial mode of treatment is adequate antibiotic cover, intravenous feeds and insertion of a chest drain (Stephenson *et al.*, 2000). Frequently, the leak will resolve. If the leak remains, surgical intervention may be necessary.

Long-term complications associated with the mechanics of respiration may include cough, wheeze, aspiration pneumonia and near-death episodes (Agrawal *et al.*, 1999).

Psychosocial care

An infant with TOF is potentially very sick, not only requiring surgery but also at high risk of being diagnosed with further anomalies or a chromosomal disorder. The parents need much support throughout this period and indeed in the future, as the infant may have ongoing complications. Support groups may be recommended and contact addresses of other families who have been through similar experiences may be supplied.

MALROTATION AND VOLVULUS

Aetiology

Herniation of the midgut occurs at approximately 6 weeks of development (Holland et al., 1998); by the 10th week, the primitive midgut rotates 270 degrees and fixates within the right side of the abdominal cavity. If during the return to the abdominal cavity this rotation does not occur, the result is a malrotation. If the mesentery does not fixate to the upper left and lower right side of the abdomen there is a risk of the gut twisting (volvulus) and occluding the blood supply, which may lead to necrosis and ischaemia of the gut (Roberton, 1986). Malrotation may occur in isolation or may co-exist with defects such as gastroschisis, omphalocele and diaphragmatic hernia (Holland et al., 1998).

Signs and symptoms

Initially, an infant with malrotation may exhibit no signs or symptoms. Following feeds they may have bile-stained vomits and abdominal distension. If volvulus has developed, the infant will be seriously ill and will present with a similar clinical picture, including the passage of bloody, mucousy stools. The infant may be mottled in appearance, be lethargic, apnoeic, and have an unstable temperature, hypovolaemia and dehydration.

Diagnosis

The characteristic 'double bubble' may be present on an abdominal X-ray. The gas in the stomach may extend beyond the duodenum (Levene et al., 1987). Contrast studies of the upper gastro-intestinal tract and a barium enema are needed to determine where the occlusion has occurred in the gastric tract.

Pre-operative care

Infants with volvulus are in a life-threatening situation and emergency laparotomy is required. A size 6 nasogastric tube is positioned and placed on free drainage, with intermittent aspiration to aid abdominal decompression. They will be 'nil by mouth'.

These infants may be dehydrated. Intravenous fluid therapy and the necessary additives to correct any electrolyte imbalance will be commenced. If they are shocked, volume expanders and inotropes may be necessary. Full monitoring will be required to detect any further deterioration.

Consent will need to be obtained. It is important to remember that volvulus is a surgical emergency and there may not be much time to contact the parents. Within 4 hours the bowel of the infant with volvulus becomes irreparably damaged (Holland *et al.*, 1998).

Broad spectrum antibiotics will be prescribed, as it is imperative that the infant has some protection from the impending infection.

Surgical procedure

A laparotomy is performed and the volvulus is untwisted. Sometimes this is sufficient as corrective surgery. However, Ladds bands may be present causing duodenal obstruction and surgery will need to incorporate the division of these. Positioning of the bowel into the abdomen involves the colon to the left and the small bowel to the right (Holland *et al.*, 1998). The base of the mesentery is widened to prevent further twisting (Roberton, 1986). Appendectomy is also performed, as a future diagnosis of appendicitis may be difficult and the appendix could form the focus of further twisting.

Post-operative care

Immediately post-operatively infants may be ventilated so nurses should follow the rules of general care of ventilated infants. Adequate analgesia is required to ensure that the infant is kept comfortable. Antibiotic cover is continued for 5–7 days post-operatively. The wound site is inspected regularly for signs of redness, oozing or inflammation.

If there has been major resection of ischaemic bowel, the infant may have had a colostomy formed, to enable the gut to rest. *See* pages 154–5 for the principles of the care of the stoma. Full monitoring is carried out and any deterioration immediately reported to the medical staff.

Nutrition initially is via intravenous fluids and gradual regrading of milk feeds is implemented. If the surgical procedure was straightforward then a vast improvement will occur very quickly. If there was a large amount of bowel resected, the infant may require long-term total parenteral nutrition.

GASTRO-OESOPHAGEAL REFLUX (GOR)

Gastro-oesophageal reflux (GOR) is commonly seen on the neonatal unit and can present in a mild or severe form. Milk may reflux from the stomach into the oesophagus as a result of immature development, weakness or slackening of the oesophageal sphincter. Premature infants are most likely to be at risk for several reasons:

- a shortened oesophagus, which can allow the contents of the stomach to reflux back, and reduced oesophageal motility (Ewer *et al.*, 1996);

- the large volumes of milk that are fed to the very low-birthweight infant in order to catch up on growth (Stephenson *et al.*, 2000);
- delayed gastric motility owing to immaturity or perhaps a result of some types of formula milk (Ewer *et al.*, 1994);
- pre-term infants are more likely to be treated with caffeine for apnoeas or bradycardias, which causes an increase in the secretion of gastric acid and a decrease in the tone of the circular muscle of the oesophageal sphincter.

If left untreated, GOR can have serious detrimental effects upon the infant. Aspiration pneumonia, severe apnoea and respiratory distress may be complications of GOR.

Signs and symptoms

The infant with GOR is very likely to vomit following feeds. A severely affected infant may appear mottled at times and may have spells of apnoea. It is important to eliminate the suspicion of infection, as the symptoms are very similar to those of GOR. When associated with GOR, apnoea and bradycardia will usually present following the infant's feed.

Management

A simple but effective measure is to position the infant in such a way as to encourage gastric emptying. The recommended position is with the cot mattress elevated so that the infant is placed prone with the head tilted. The findings of a recent study determined that the prone position or the left lateral position significantly reduced the symptoms of gastro-oesophageal reflux (Ewer *et al.*, 1999). A further study supported the theory of left lateral positioning but concluded that head elevation may not be beneficial (Tobin *et al.*, 1997).

Feeding the infant with GOR

It is common practice on the NNU to add food thickeners such as Gaviscon or Carobel to the feed. If the infant is very small and a size 4 nasogastric tube is used, blockage of the tube may occur. The feed needs to be given immediately following the addition of the thickener, and at room temperature.

The method of tube feeding the infant with GOR promotes much discussion. The variants include naso/orogastric, transpyloric, continuous or bolus feeding. Each method will be discussed taking into consideration the advantages and disadvantages.

Nasogastric feeding (NGT)

When an infant has a nasogastric tube passed, it is important that that there is no trauma to the nostril, oropharynx or oesophagus. The nurse should confirm the position of the tube by careful aspiration and litmus testing of the aspirate. This mode of feeding is commonly seen on the NNU as an alternative method of feeding the compromised infant.

Laing *et al.* (1986) studied the effectiveness of nasogastric feeding and recommended it as the preferred method of feeding low-birthweight infants. Feeding the large volumes of milk required by the pre-term infant for growth may further exacerbate the symptoms of GOR and affect the gastric emptying time. Ewer *et al.* (1996) stated that gastric emptying is not a variable in relation to GOR.

If an infant is bolus-fed, the nurse needs to give the feed very slowly. Fast administration may result in bradycardia, vomiting or, in the worst scenario, aspiration. This may also occur if the continuous method of feeding is adopted and the tube becomes misplaced.

Transpyloric feeding (nasoduodenal, nasojejunal)

The passing of a transpyloric tube to feed the infant and a naso/orogastric tube (in order to aspirate stomach contents) may be the recommended method of management when an infant has marked GOR. The milk is passed directly into the jejunum or duodenum. This may aid gastric motility and reduce the incidence of vomiting.

Nurses need to be competent in the technique for passing a transpyloric tube. Force should not be exerted as this could cause damage to the stomach, duodenum or oesophagus. The correct procedure includes the very slow advancing of the tube and X-ray to determine the position. This is the only definitive confirmation of the exact site of the tube, but it may result in the infant being exposed to several X-rays if there is uncertainty about the position of the tube.

Concerns have arisen regarding the poor weight gain of infants fed nasojejunally. Studies determined that the weight gain of infants fed by this method was significantly reduced when compared with infants fed by the nasogastric route (Macdonald *et al.*, 1992).

Oral drugs

Oral drugs are frequently used to treat infants who present with GOR, when food thickeners and careful positioning of the infant are not effective. Cisapride, a prokinetic agent responsible for the stimulation of gastro-intestinal motility, has been popular, but its effectiveness has come under close scrutiny. It has been shown to affect the QTc interval in term neonates (Semama *et al.*, 2001). Currently it should not be used in the treatment of GOR. Trials determining its efficacy concluded that food thickeners were equally effective (Greally *et al.*, 1992), and showed that Cisapride did not aid gastric motility (McClure *et al.*, 1999). Domperidone, a prokinetic agent acting upon upper gut motility, is an alternative drug used in the treatment of GOR. This also needs to be used with caution and should not be prescribed in an over-zealous manner.

SAMPLE EXAMINATION QUESTIONS

Question 1

What are the characteristics of an infant's stools in the first week of life? (*30 marks*)

What nursing observations should be made on a 28-week gestation infant who has not opened his bowel for a week and who has a distended abdomen? (*70 marks*)

Question 2
What is understood by the term GOR? (*10 marks*)
For what reasons may an NGT be passed in a pre-term infant? (*30 marks*)
What assessments and precautions must a nurse take prior to feeding via an NGT? (*60 marks*)

Question 3
Mrs Chan has delivered twin girls at 28 weeks gestation. She would really like to breast-feed them. How can the neonatal team help her to achieve this ambition? (*100 marks*)

REFERENCES

Agrawal, L., Beardsmore, C. and MacFadyen, U. (1999) Respiratory function in childhood following repair of oesophageal atresia and tracheoesophageal fistula, *Archives of Disease in Childhood* 81(5), 404–8

Beeby, P.J. and Jeffery, H. (1992) Risk factors for necrotising enterocolitis: the influence of gestational age, *Archives of Disease in Childhood* 67(4), 432–5

Berseth, C.L. (1998) Disorders of the umbilical cord, abdominal wall, urachus and omphalomesenteric duct (Chapter 76). In: Taeusch, H.W. and Ballard, R. (eds) *Avery's Diseases of the Newborn* (7th edition), WB Saunders, New York

Bower, T.R., Pringle, K.C. and Soper, R.T. (1988) Sodium deficit causing decreased weight gain and metabolic acidosis in infants with ileostomy, *Journal of Paediatric Surgery* 23, 567–72

Boxwell, G. (2000) *Neonatal Intensive Care Nursing* (Chapter 15), Routledge, London

Boyd, P., Bhattacharjee, A., Gould, S. *et al.* (1998) Outcome of prenatally diagnosed anterior abdominal wall defects, *Archives of Disease in Childhood, Fetal Neonatal Edition* 78(3), 209–13

Clark, David A. (2000) *Atlas of Neonatology*, WB Saunders, Philadelphia, PA

Davies, B.W. and Stringer, M.D. (1997) The survivors of gastroschisis, *Archives of Disease in Childhood* 77(2), 158–60

De Lorimier, A.A., Adzick, N.S. and Harrison, M.R. (1991) Amnion inversion in the treatment of giant omphalocele, *Journal of Pediatric Surgery*, July, 26(7), 804–7

Ewer, A.K., Durbin, G.M., Morgan, M.E. and Booth, I.W. (1994) Gastric emptying in pre–term infants, *Archives of Disease in Childhood, Fetal and Neonatal Edition* 71(1), 24–7

Ewer, A.K., Durbin, G.M., Morgan, M.E. and Booth, I.W. (1996) Gastric emptying and gastro-oesophageal reflux in pre-term infants, *Archives of Disease in Childhood, Fetal and Neonatal Edition* 75(2), 117–21

Ewer, A.K., James, M.E. and Tobin, J.M. (1999) Prone and left lateral positioning reduce gastro-oesophageal reflux in pre-term infants, *Archives of Disease in Childhood, Fetal and Neonatal Edition* 81(3), 201–5

Fagan, D.G., Pritchard, J.S., Clarkson, T.W. and Greenwood, M.R. (1977) Organ mercury levels in infants with omphaloceles treated with organic mercurial antiseptic, *Archives of Disease in Childhood* 52, 962–4

Fleming, P.J., Spiedel, B.D. and Dunn, P.M. (1986) A *Neonatal Vade-Mecum*, Lloyd-Luke (Medical Books) Ltd, London

Greally, P., Hampton, F.J., MacFadyen, U. and Simpson, H. (1992) Gaviscon and Carobel compared with cisapride in gastro-oesophageal reflux, *Archives of Disease in Childhood* 67(5), 618–21

Harjo, J. (1988) Alterations in the gastro-intestinal system. In: Kenner, C., Harjo, J. and Brueggemeyer, A. (eds) *Neonatal Surgery: A Nursing Perspective*, Harcourt Brace Jovanich, London, pp. 121–90

Holland, R., Price, F. and Bensard, D. (1998) Neonatal Surgery (Chapter 27) In: Merenstein, G. and Gardner, S. (eds) *Handbook of Neonatal Intensive Care* (4th edition), Mosby, St Louis, IL

Kelnar, C.J.H., Harvey, D. and Simpson, C. (1995) *The Sick Newborn Baby* (3rd edition), Ballière Tindall, London

Koloske, A.M. and Musemeche, C.A. (1989) Necrotising enterocolitis of the neonate, *Clinics in Perinatology* 16(1), 97–111

Laing, I., Lang, M., Callaghan, O. and Hume, R. (1986) Nasogastric compared with nasoduodenal feeding in low-birthweight infants, *Archives of Disease in Childhood* 61(2), 138–41

Levene, M., Tudehope, D. and Thearle, J. (1987) *Essentials of Neonatal Medicine*, Blackwell Science, Oxford

Macdonald, P.D., Skeoch, C.H., Carse, H. *et al.* (1992) Randomised trial of continuous nasogastric, bolus nasogastric, and transpyloric feeding in infants of birthweight under 1,400g, *Archives of Disease in Childhood* 67(4), 429–31

McClure, R., Kristensen, J. and Grauaug, A. (1999) Randomised controlled trial of Cisapride in pre-term infants, *Archives of Disease in Childhood, Fetal and Neonatal Edition* 80(3), 174–7

Meller, J.L., Reyes, H.M. and Loeff, D.S. (1989) Gastroschisis and ompalocele, *Clinics in Perinatology*, 16(1), 113–22

Moore, K.L and Persaud, T.V.N. (1998) *The Developing Human: Clinically Oriented embryology* (6th edition), WB Saunders, Philadelphia, PA

Ng, P.C., Dear, P.R. and Thomas, D.F. (1988) Oral vancomycin in prevention of necrotising enterocolitis, *Archives of Disease in Childhood* 63(11), 1390–3

Nicholls, G., Upadhyaya, V., Gornall, P., Buick, R. and Corkery, J. (1993) Is specialist centre delivery of gastroschisis beneficial? *Archives of Disease in Childhood* 69(1), 71–2

Osborn, D.A., Lui, K., Pussell, P. *et al.* (1999) T and Tk antigen activation in necrotising enterocolitis: manifestations, severity of illness, and effectiveness of testing, *Archives of Disease in Childhood, Fetal Neonatal Edition* 80(3), 192–7

Pearse, R.G. and Roberton, N.R.C. (1988) Infection in the Newborn. In: Roberton, N.R.C. (ed.) *Textbook of Neonatology*, Churchill Livingstone, Edinburgh, pp. 753–9

Roberton, N.R.C. (1986) *Textbook of Neonatology*, Churchill Livingstone, Edinburgh

Roberts, J.P. and Burge, D.M. (1990) Antenatal diagnosis of abdominal wall defects: a missed opportunity? *Archives of Disease in Childhood, Fetal and Neonatal Edition* 65(7), 687–9

Rushton, C.H. (1990) Necrotising enterocolitis, Part 2: treatment and nursing care, *Maternal and Child Nursing* 15, pp. 309–13

Sadler, T.W. (2000) *Langmans Medical Embryology* (8th edition), Lippincott Williams and Wilkins, London

Semama, D., Bernardini, S., Louf, S. *et al.* (2001) Effects of Cisapride on QTc interval in term neonates, *Archives of Disease in Childhood, Fetal and Neonatal Edition* 84(1), 44–6

Siu, Y.K., Ng, P.C., Fung, S.C.K. *et al.* (1998) Double blind, randomised, placebo-controlled study of oral vancomycin in prevention of necrotising enterocolitis in pre-term, very low-birthweight infants, *Archives of Disease in Childhood, Fetal and Neonatal Edition* 79(2), 105–9

Squire, R., Kiely, E., Drake, D. and Lander, A. (1992) Intravascular haemolysis in association with necrotizing enterocolitis, *Journal of Paediatric Surgery* 27, 808–10

Stephenson, T., Marlow, N., Watkins, S. and Grant, J. (2000) *Pocket Neonatology*, Churchill Livingstone, Edinburgh

Stoodley, N., Sharma, A., Noblett, H. and James, D. (1993) Influence of place of delivery of outcome in babies with gastroschisis, *Archives of Disease in Childhood, Fetal and Neonatal Edition* 68(3), 321–23

Stringer, M.D., Bereton, R.S. and Wright, V.M. (1991) Controversies in the management of gastroschisis: a study of 40 patients, *Archives of Diseases in Childhood*, 66(1), 34–6

Swift, R.I. *et al.* (1992) A regime in the management of gastroschisis, *Journal of Paediatric Surgery*, Jan, 27(1), 61–3

Thomas, R. and Harvey, D. (1997) *Neonatology, Colour Guide* (2nd edition), Churchill Livingstone, Edinburgh

Tobin, J., McCloud, P. and Cameron, D. (1997) Posture and gastro-oesophageal reflux: a case for left lateral positioning, *Archives of Disease in Childhood* 76(3), 254–8

Twining, P., McHugo, J. and Pilling, D. (2000) *Textbook of Fetal Abnormalities*, Churchill Livingstone, Edinburgh

9 NURSING CARE OF AN INFANT WITH A DISORDER OF THE CARDIOVASCULAR SYSTEM

Doreen Crawford and Jill Fairhurst

Aims of the chapter

This chapter introduces the basic development of the heart, and then goes on to consider the transitions at births. Elements of general nursing care and specific investigations are reviewed, then pre- and post-operative care are explained and applied to specific conditions.

INTRODUCTION

Few branches of nursing can be as challenging as neonatal cardiology. Nursing an infant with a cardiac defect requires limitless creativity and skill as well as excellent nursing standards. Small deviations from the infant's usual baseline may herald a significant deterioration in condition. Nurses are uniquely placed to monitor these deviations by close observation and, using their intuition based on their experience, can then alert the medical team. Early intervention is often the key to a successful outcome.

Statistics relating to the incidence of congenital heart disease vary depending on the study and the source, ranging from 1 in 100 (Children's Heart Foundation, 2000) to 8–12 in 1000 live births (Witt, 1997). The risk is not shared equally among the population. Some lower socio-economic groups are more at risk than others (Vrijheid *et al.*, 2000), while children with conditions such as Down's Syndrome are at much greater risk.

RELATED ANATOMY AND PHYSIOLOGY

Embryogenesis

In order to comprehend cardiac anomalies, it is useful to have an understanding of early development. The cardiovascular system is the first major system to function in the embryo. It begins to develop in the 3rd week of gestation and is functioning by week eight. This explosive early development may be the reason why congenital heart disease is so prevalent in the newborn.

It is beyond the scope of this text to give anything more than the most basic introduction to the miracle of embryogenesis. For a more detailed understanding the reader is referred to several excellent texts (*see* References and Further Reading).

The human heart derives from the mesoderm, which forms two endothelial tubes that quickly fuse to form a single functioning chamber by about 22 days gestation (MacGregor, 2000). In the subsequent weeks this chamber will grow, twist and contort, causing major structural changes, eventually creating four chambers and becoming recognisable as the heart. These changes are all the more remarkable because the 'primitive' heart is a functional organ during this time.

Development of the atria and the ventricles

The precursors to these structures arise from the dilations, forming hollows in the heart tube. The development of the atria is slightly ahead of the ventricles. The folding of this tube on itself allows the structures, which will become the atria, to be positioned 'on top' of the forming ventricles. Developing tissue between the right and left sides and the atria/ventricles is called the endocardial cushion. The tissue thins and changes to become the cuspid valves. The developing tissue between the two ventricles becomes thick and muscular and, with the development and downward spiral of the great arteries, all communication between the ventricles is normally closed by the 7th week.

Any malformation, interruption or adverse developmental occurrence, such as maternal infection, during the early stages, may lead to defects, which will result in life-threatening cardiac lesions. For example, failure of the endocardial cushion to grow or fuse would result in abnormal formation of the cuspid valves or atrioventricular/ventricular septal defects. Disorders this early in development can then have a cascading effect, leading to increasingly complicated malformations (Witt, 1997). Amazingly, not only does the heart form and function for the period of foetal life, it is also able to plan ahead to cope with the changes that occur when birth forces the anatomical transition to an independent structure and function (Sansoucie and Cavaliere, 1997).

Foetal circulation

The purpose of foetal circulation is to supply oxygen and nutrients and remove carbon dioxide and waste. This is done via the maternal circulation and the placenta (Figure 9.1). The foetus is always hypoxic, with oxygen saturations running at between 60–70% (MacGregor, 2000). However, to maximise available oxygen and bypass non-functioning organs, the following modifications (circulation bypass shunts) are present.

- The oxygenated blood from the placenta enters the foetal circulation from the umbilical vein. Much of this bypasses the liver via the ductus venosus to flow to the inferior vena cava.
- The foramen ovale, a flap in the septum between the two atria, allows most of the oxygenated blood flow to bypass the right ventricle. This delivers the most highly oxygenated blood to the brain and heart.
- The ductus arteriosus connects the pulmonary artery with the aorta. This allows most of the blood to bypass the non-functioning foetal lungs.

Changes at birth and subsequent adaptations

The foetal circulation has to adapt, at birth, to support extra-uterine existence and these changes result in a recognisably mature circulatory pattern. The first few breaths are of vital importance and initiate the alteration of the circulation.

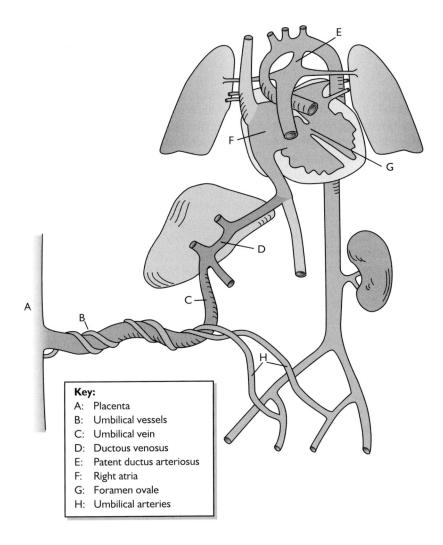

Key:
A: Placenta
B: Umbilical vessels
C: Umbilical vein
D: Ductous venosus
E: Patent ductus arteriosus
F: Right atria
G: Foramen ovale
H: Umbilical arteries

Figure 9.1 Foetal circulation

These changes are brought about by the following:

- the onset of respiration in air;
- loss of lung fluid and decrease in pulmonary vascular resistance;

- an increase in capillary oxygen;
- increased extra-thoracic pressure and blood pressure.

The changes are as follows:

- The ductus venosus closes soon after birth and becomes the ligamentum teres.
- The foramen ovale closes at or within hours of birth and forms a complete septum between the two atria. Complete anatomical closure is usually within 3 months.
- The ductus arteriosus constricts after birth and usually closes within 3 weeks to become the ligamentous arteriosus.

Infants with very severe congenital heart malformations are able to survive in utero because of the parasitic relationship with the mother and the architecture of the cardiovascular system. This arrangement is not compatible with survival in the post-natal state (Sansoucie and Cavaliere, 1997). There are many types of congenital cardiac malformations, only a few of which cause immediate distress in the newborn period (Paul, 1995). Infants with severe lesions can sometimes survive past this period owing to the time it takes to complete the transition from foetal to self-sustaining circulation; the ductus arteriosus and foramen ovales can sometimes take time to close. Altered pressures within the heart may maintain the presence of intra-cardiac shunts and preserve life-sustaining oxygenated circulation (Schindler, 1999).

CAUSES OF CONGENITAL HEART DISEASE

The exact cause of most heart defects is not known as the heart has already undergone major development, usually before the woman realises that she is pregnant.

Possible aetiology

Congenital heart disease can develop as a result of:

- genetic inheritance;
- poor diet;
- environmental factors;
- smoking;
- excess alcohol;
- some drugs;
- foetal/maternal infection;
- maternal diabetes;
- maternal age;
- gestational age.

Congenital heart disease, by convention, is divided into two categories: cyanotic and acyanotic. The difference is the result of blood mixing, and it is an imprecise classification.

Cyanosis can be the result of blood shunting from the pulmonary circulation to the systemic circulation without having circulated through the lungs to be oxygenated. With acyanotic lesions, the lung perfusion and blood oxygenation may not be affected.

The difference between the two broad groups of heart defects is not rigid. Conditions such as Fallot's tetralogy and hypoplastic left heart may initially present as acyanotic but may become cyanotic later, owing to a change in the haemodynamics.

An abnormal heart can be recognised by certain investigations. An electro-cardiograph (ECG), for example, shows abnormalities by deviations in the normal patterns of iso-electric line, displayed on a monitor or on graph paper. Other non-invasive investigations that may suggest abnormalities include ultra-sound scan, chest X-ray and nitrogen wash-out. The invasive cardiac catheteri-sation procedure will confirm the diagnosis. (For more on these procedures, *see* pages 178 and 190–1.)

Cyanosis

Central cyanosis occurs when venous blood bypasses the lungs so that the arterial oxygen saturation remains low even when high inspiratory oxygen fractions are given. Severe lung disease can present with the same features and a differential diagnosis must be made.

Peripheral cyanosis is fairly common in the neonate and is evidenced by blueness of the lips, hands and feet with good perfusion and pink colour of the warm parts of the body such as the mucous membranes. Arterial oxygen satura-tions are normal. Peripheral cyanosis may be caused by poor circulation and is often associated with hypothermia, polycythaemia and shock.

Acrocyanosis is a very common phenomenon. The characteristic blueness of the palms of the hand and soles of the feet is typically of short duration in the newborn during transition to extra-uterine life and may last a couple of hours.

The infant presenting with cyanosis needs to have its respiratory pattern observed and noted so that lung disease can be excluded as a diagnosis. The heart rate should be continuously monitored and oxygen saturations measured.

Further investigations will need to be performed; many of these are discussed later. An infant with no apparent respiratory distress who remains cyanosed in 100% oxygen needs urgent referral to a cardiac unit. Prostaglandin E may be prescribed as immediate therapy to maintain an open ductus arteriosus until diagnosis and correct medical or surgical treatment can be given (Rikard, 1993).

Congestive Cardiac/Heart Failure (CCF)

Detecting congestive heart failure (CHF) in the neonatal period is more difficult than at any other time (Furdon, 1997). The signs and symptoms are directly related to the inability of the heart as a pump to meet the output and perfusion needs of the body. The cardiac function is dependent on circulatory loads and cardiac contractility. The preload is the amount of blood distending the ventricles immediately prior to contraction. Stroke volume is the amount of blood pumped by the ventricle and the afterload is the arterial pressure against which the heart has to pump. Neonates in cardiac failure suffer a circulation backlog and higher pressures. For example, in heart failure the venous return is compromised and the back pressure in the hepatic vein leads to liver enlargement. Backlog of blood in the pulmonary circulation causes serious fluid shift and the lungs become 'waterlogged'. The infant can compensate up to a point, as the lymphatic system can drain off some of the excess fluid in the lungs, but when this ability is exceeded, alveolar oedema will occur and gas exchange will be compromised.

The infant in cardiac failure may present with breathlessness when recumbent and during feeding, and may become increasingly lethargic. At rest, the infant may have a characteristic bounding tachycardia of over 180 beats per minute, owing to ventricular overload. In addition, these infants may also have copious, frothy secretions, which require frequent suction, and often have a respiratory rate of more than 60 breaths per minute. The feeds taken by the infant may be inadequate for their growth and metabolic needs or may take longer than 30 minutes to complete. The struggle to feed may leave the infant looking exhausted, pale and sweating. Despite this poor feeding, weight gain may be in excess of 20–30 grams per day. Hepatomegaly and oedema may be detectable on examination.

In later infancy, pulmonary oedema causes a dry cough and leads to respiratory infections. The infant is either lethargic or irritable and is cold, pale and sweaty, with grunting, indrawing and possible cyanosis.

Cardiac failure may be rapid in onset and if it presents early in life, the cause is often quite sinister. Medical therapy may succeed in controlling heart failure for a short time and surgical correction of the cardiac defect, where applicable, may be urgently required. Delays in recognising and treating heart failure may lead to a rapid deterioration and cardiogenic shock. Cardiac shock may resemble early septicaemia, pneumonia and meningitis.

In full-term infants, from birth to 1 week, left ventricular failure is more common than right ventricular failure. Cardiac failure in later infancy often involves combined right- and left-sided failure.

Nursing care of an infant with CCF

Working as a partner with the parents

The purpose of the monitoring equipment should be explained to the family and a verbal explanation of CCF should be given in simple terminology, and backed up with written information. The British Heart Foundation produces a set of excellent leaflets that may help. In cardiac care, as in other specialist branches of neonatology, the parents are partners in care and should be made fully aware of any changes in the infant's condition. Changes in the management of a child's care must be made with the consent of the parents.

Maintenance of optimal temperature

The infant should be nursed in an incubator or under an overhead heater to help maintain a thermo-neutral environment. Large infants may not require this, but the temperature should be regularly monitored and they should be kept warm and adequately dressed. Traditionally, neonatal nurses have used a core/peripheral temperature differential as an indication of good circulation. However, in this group of patients, such data must be interpreted with caution (Tibby *et al.*, 1999).

Administration of medication

Medication should be administered as prescribed and where possible timed to coincide with feeds so that there is minimal disturbance of the infant. Some medication, such as Digoxin (*see* page 198), can be toxic and its effects may be cumulative. Prior to administration, the heart rate and rhythm should be checked; if these are slower than the infant's usual baseline, or if the beats seem to come together, the nurse should withhold the drug until the infant has been assessed by the medical team.

Comfort and rest

Invasive procedures should be kept to a minimum, as rest and sleep periods are sacrosanct. The mother is encouraged to nurse her infant, cuddling and feeding as required to keep the infant settled. Generally speaking, excess crying is detrimental to the care of cardiac infants and they can be offered a soother with the parents' consent. The infant's daily care will include a daily or twice-daily weighing, preferably done when the infant is already being handled, for example, first thing in the morning, before the bath or with a nappy change. These daily rituals can often become a focus for anxiety and the parents should be encouraged to be realistic about small fluctuations, as the general trend and clinical condition is more important.

Adequate hydration and nutrition

Small, frequent feeds are offered, to avoid over-tiring the infant and, if the feed is taking longer than 30 minutes or the infant is becoming dyspnoeic, the feed may be completed via a nasogastric tube. Should the mother wish to breast-feed, she should be encouraged to express until she can feed normally; alternatively, the infant can have a short comforting and closely monitored nuzzle at the breast while the nurse delivers the nasogastric feed. Breast milk can be given instead of formula, and may have lower levels of sodium (Quan *et al.*, 1994), which can help prevent oedema. An intake and output chart should be kept, with the nappies being weighed and measurements made of the specific gravity of the urine.

Provision of oxygen according to needs and prevention of orthopnoea

Administer O_2 therapy if prescribed and measure saturations regularly, if possible continuously, in addition to making regular recordings of vital signs. It is important to note the trend of oxygen requirements and, if this is increasing, to alert the medical team. In cardiac nursing the infant's comfort, and the need for boundaries and security, need to be balanced by the functionality of a position. To relieve the weight of the abdominal contents and to allow maximum expansion of the diaphragm, a head-up position is often adopted, with the infant supported on the side. When awake, the infant may enjoy, from an early age, a cradle chair with suitable support for the back.

Safe environment and prevention of cross-infection

The neonatal nurse will assist with any tests and investigations necessary and these may include cardiac catheterisation. Stringent hygiene and a limit on the number of carers will help to prevent cross-infection, which could delay vital operations or retard growth.

Care of an infant undergoing diagnostic investigations

Cardiac enzymes

Nurses caring for adult cardiac patients are already familiar with blood being taken to measure cardiac enzymes as these tests have become key aids in the estimation of cardiac damage (Verklan, 1997b). Other conditions occasionally seen in the neonate also release enzymes, and these would need to be eliminated, but the measurement of cardiac enzymes is increasingly being used to assess neonatal myocardial stress. Unfortunately, it requires blood to be drawn and, in order to achieve the most meaningful results, the blood may need to be drawn frequently, so that a serial picture can be drawn up. Frequent blood sampling can compromise the small infant both because of the loss and the handling. As confidence grows in the interpretation of the analysis of these enzymes, based on knowledge of how the neonate's physiology handles and eliminates these enzymes, the investigation will be increasingly useful.

Nitrogen wash-out or hyperoxia test

This test is used as an aid to confirm suspected cyanotic heart disease. The test involves measuring the PaO_2 in air and again after 10 minutes of the infant breathing 100% oxygen. If the post-ductal PaO_2 fails to rise above 19.5 kPa, a suspected right to left shunt is more likely to be due to congenital heart disease rather than severe respiratory disease.

Before the test begins, the neonatal nurse must calibrate the oxygen analyser and, if a headbox is to be used to deliver the oxygen, ensure that a tight seal is achieved around the infant's neck. The infant should be fully monitored throughout the procedure and details and explanations given to parents.

The nitrogen wash-out test is not without risk. If the infant is dependent on a patent ductus arteriosus to maintain the circulation the sudden hyperoxia may cause the ductus to spasm, with serious consequences.

Chest X-ray

Many anomalies have a typical heart shadow, with an abnormal cardiac outline clearly defined. Some have very descriptive names – the 'boot-shaped heart' is suggestive of Fallot's tetralogy, while the 'egg on its side' is said to be indicative of transposition of the great arteries.

No special preparation of the infant for chest X-ray is necessary, but they will need to be held in a suitable position to maximise the quality of the film and prevent unwanted rotation. In addition, there should be adequate protection for the nurse and the infant's reproductive organs, using lead shields. ECG monitoring leads should not be placed on the chest wall in a position to occlude the view of the heart and lungs. Any radio opaque fasteners on the infant's clothing should also be removed from direct vision.

Ultrasound scan

This non-invasive technique is used to enable visualisation of the heart. In the hands of experienced personnel it can be very informative and in some cases may save the infant from cardiac catheterisation. No special preparation is needed. Many ultrasound scanners, although large, are portable and it is possible for the infant to have the scan while on the unit. If this is not possible the transport incubator system or a converted pram could be used to transport the infant to the department. The infant's co-operation and chances of immobility during the procedure can be enhanced if the conductive jelly is warmed prior to application. Some commercial jellies are very difficult to remove once dried on so every attempt should be made to remove the excess while it is still damp.

Cardiac catheterisation

This may be performed to confirm X-ray findings and assist in diagnosis, or may be used as part of a therapeutic process. Serial catheterisation may be used to evaluate the progression of a severe lesion or both pre- and post-operatively. For guidance on the nursing care of an infant undergoing this invasive and occasionally risky procedure, *see* pages 190–1.

Nursing care of an infant with an abnormal heart rate, rhythm or pressure

Monitoring the heart rate

An electro-cardiogram is a tracing of the different stages of the heart's electrical activity (Figure 9.2). To get good assessment of rhythm, wave complexes and intervals between waves there must be simultaneous recordings over all three surface leads. To decrease the skin resistance to the flow of electricity, and improve contact, the sites can be prepared with mild pH neutral soap or alcohol wipes (Verklan, 1997a). The normal ECG comprises of a P wave, a Q wave, an R and an S wave (QRS complex) and a T wave. The P wave represents electrical activity associated with atrial contraction. The QRS complex represents electrical activity associated with ventricular contraction. The T wave represents electrical activity associated with ventricular relaxation. The rest period between these waves is known as the refractory period.

Abnormalities of the heart rhythm can be detected when monitoring the heart rate on a cardiorator or monitor, but a five or 12-lead ECG is required for definitive diagnosis. It is very important to chart all abnormalities in rate and rhythm carefully. As with all equipment, alarms should be set within suitable ranges, responded to if triggered and always switched on.

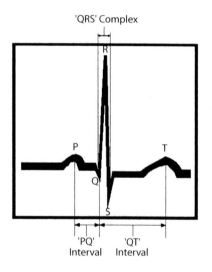

Figure 9.2   An electrocardiogram

'Normal' parameters vary tremendously. In the neonatal unit, alterations of rate may be influenced by gestational age, handling and clinical condition so each infant should be individually assessed. Massin and colleagues (2000) studied heart rate and variability during the circadian cycle and, although further studies are required to confirm applicability to the pre-term and to neonates, the results demonstrated the huge variation in rate over the 24-hour period. Guidelines for the normal parameters are shown in Table 9.1.

Table 9.1   Normal parameters of the heart's electrical activity

	Term infants	**Pre-term infants**
Normal	80–160	100–180
Tachycardia	160 >	180 >
Bradycardia	80 <	100 <

Bradycardia

Bradycardia is very common in the premature infant. Many bradycardia are transient and self-resolving, including those which occur when the infant is in a deep, restful sleep, and require no further action except charting and observation by the neonatal nurse. If the bradycardia is profound (less than 50 bpm), prolonged (lasting more than 15–30 seconds), or is accompanied by apnoea, cyanotic attacks, desaturations or unresponsiveness, then immediate action must be taken. Gentle stimulation such as auditory stimulus, gentle touching, stroking is given first, followed by squeezing the heel and patting the bottom. If these interactions have no effect, more drastic action must be instituted. The infant should be turned supine and the heart rate counted using a stethoscope. If the position change and invariably cold stethoscope fail to revive the infant and the infant remains bradycardic, shallow oral, nasopharyngeal or endotracheal suction should be given, and resuscitative measures commenced. Assistance in the form of nursing and medical personnel should be summoned as necessary and the infant's response to nursing interventions recorded.

Any inferences that can be made pertaining to the bradycardic episode must be documented. These might include the following:

- passing an NGT or tube feeding;
- regurgitation or aspiration of feed;
- vomiting;
- vasovagal stimulation caused by deep suctioning or a build-up of secretions;
- bad positioning and insensitive handling during certain procedures (for example, lumbar puncture).

Other possible triggers of bradycardia include airway compromise, such as a blocked endotracheal tube or a misplaced nasogastric tube, a cerebral event such as an intraventricular haemorrhage, infection, toxicity, and hyper or hypothermia. If there appears to be no associated cause then bradycardia of prematurity can be suspected.

Rarely, a sinus bradycardia can be the result of congenital heart block. It carries a high mortality rate and requires a pacemaker. It is caused by the abnormal development of the conduction system of the heart or by the presence of maternal auto immune disease destroying foetal tissue (Klassen, 1999). The clinical presentation will depend on the extent of the bradycardia and the diagnosis could be complicated by the need for resuscitation.

Tachycardia

Tachycardia is less common than bradycardia but can be associated with pain and distress, temperature instability, hypovolaemia, caffeine or a cardiac dysfunction. A visibly agitated infant, thrashing around the cot, or one returning from a traumatic procedure or surgery may have an increased heart rate related to distress. Measures to reduce discomfort should be instigated (see Chapter 12). In the case of an otherwise settled infant, the tachycardia is more likely to be caused by an anomaly of the conduction system regulating the heart rate.

There is no one single defective mechanism responsible for the condition termed supra-ventricular tachycardia (SVT), although the conditions are generally rare and may be intermittent, benign and unrecognised. However, they may be prolonged, associated with episodes of tachypnoea, pallor and poor feeding, as well as the abnormal cardiac rate and rhythm (Page and Hosking, 1997). These infants may have a structurally normal heart but should be fully monitored. All tachycardia incidents must be noted and a multi-lead ECG performed.

Tachycardia can be reverted by vagal stimulation, either by unilateral massage of the carotid sinus or by initiating the diving reflex. An extreme method involves wrapping the fully monitored infant in a blanket or towel and then immersing the face for 5 seconds in iced water. Apnoea and bradycardia will occur as a reflex and resolve when the infant's normal rhythm returns. Pharmacological intervention may be necessary to maintain an acceptable heart rate. Digoxin or Adenosine may be used to slow down the conduction in the A-V node or calcium channel blockers.

Cardioversion may be indicated in some situations. This requires a general anaesthetic and administration of a shock of 0.5–1.0 J/kg (Sreeram and Wren, 1990).

Wolf Parkinson White syndrome can occur after reversion of SVT in some infants, characterised by ventricular pre-excitation. This lesion is a conductive problem, stemming from an accessory bundle between the atria and the ventricles. This causes an abnormal heart rhythm. Wolf Parkinson White Syndrome can be a congenital disorder and is also associated with cardiac malformation such as tricuspid atresia or Ebstien's anomaly. It can also occur following the repair of a transposition of the great vessels (Page and Hosking, 1997).

Measurement of blood pressure

In the infant, blood pressure can be monitored invasively and continuously as well as intermittently and non-invasively and some studies have indicated good levels of correlation between the two (Moniaci and Kraus, 1997). In general, the sicker and more unstable the infant, the less well they will tolerate handling and the more precise the measurement needs to be. In such cases, the invasive route and the attachment of a transducer to an arterial line will be the preferred option, but this is not without problems. If a small-bore peripheral cannula is used, a dampened trace may be apparent and the readings may not be reliable; some readings are up to 20 mmHg higher than central blood pressure readings.

Accurate, non-invasive monitoring can be performed using doppler techniques, wrapping an appropriately sized cuff neatly around the limb and locating the pulse. Doppler techniques allow assessment of the systolic blood pressure only. Oscillometry can measure both systolic and diastolic pressure and some monitors can be programmed to repeat reading at set time intervals. If the cuff is left on the infant to ensure minimal disturbance it needs to be repositioned every

4–6 hours, to prevent skin damage, nerve palsies and limb ischaemia. The size of the cuff is important – too large a cuff can give falsely low readings and a cuff that is too small can give falsely high readings.

The blood pressure in the neonate can vary according to the state of arousal of the infant as well as birthweight and post-natal age. The lowest average blood pressure readings are recorded in the sleeping infant. Wakefulness, suckling, crying and agitation all cause an increase in measurable blood pressure. The effect of extremes of birthweight on blood pressure needs further study but it is known that the low-birthweight infant has lower readings than the full-term infant. Trends are much more important than a one-off recording.

Four limb blood pressures are performed when coarctation or divided aorta is suspected. It is important that the infant is relaxed and settled for this procedure, which is best performed after a feed. It is probably preferable to apply four cuffs matched to the size of the limbs and the blood vessel. If the upper arm is used, it makes sense to use the upper leg. Table 9.2 shows mean arterial blood pressures.

Table 9.2 Mean arterial blood pressure

BW (kg)	<1.0	1.0 – 1.5	1.5 – 2.0	>2.5
	Blood pressure mmHg			
Birth	32.9 ± 15.4	39.1 ± 18.2	42.4 ± 19.6	48.8 ± 19.4
7 days	41.4 ± 15.4	47.2 ± 18.2	50.4 ± 19.6	60.2 ± 19.4
14 days	44.6 ± 15.4	50.1 ± 18.2	53.2 ± 19.6	64.2 ± 19.4
28 days	47.6 ± 15.4	53.0 ± 18.2	56.1 ± 19.6	68.3 ± 19.4

Modified from Stork et al. (1984)

Acyanotic cardiac malformations

Obstructive lesions
Problems in the development of the heart valves or major arteries may lead to obstructive lesions; the severity and the presentation will depend on the extent (Table 9.3). Pulmonary stenosis restricts blood flow from the right ventricle, while aortic stenosis and coarctation of the aorta both restrict blood flow from the left ventricle. Coarctation of the aorta is a constriction of the aorta, and may present as an isolated defect. In infancy, it may be associated with a patent ductus arteriosus. Obstruction of the flow from the left ventricle may present as cardiac failure. Although some of the more frequently seen and recognised lesions are detailed below, some of the lesions are not easy to categorise, as they are unique to the affected infant.

Table 9.3 Some of the recognised congenital cardiac malformations

Acyanotic	Cyanotic
• Patent/persistent ductus arteriosus	• Tetralogy of Fallot
• Pulmonary stenosis	• Transposition of the great vessels
• Coarctation of the aorta	• Tricuspid atresia
• Aortic valve stenosis	• Truncus arteriosus
• Atrial septal defect	• Severe pulmonary stenosis or atresia
• Ventricular septal defect	• Total anomalous pulmonary venous drainage
	• Hypoplasic left heart

Pulmonary stenosis

This may describe any obstruction from the right ventricle. It may be classified as being valvular, sub-valvular or affecting the pulmonary arteries themselves (Wood, 1998). The symptoms are proportional to the degree of obstruction. A mild degree is generally asymptomatic in the neonatal period but, with severe obstruction, the infant may have dyspnoea, and may develop general cyanosis. Symptoms resemble those associated with Fallot's tetralogy (Spilman and Furdon, 1998). Hepatic enlargement may appear with right ventricular failure and the defect can be associated with tricuspid regurgitation. There may be serious tachycardia and low cardiac output.

Sudden death is a great risk with severe and untreated stenosis. Active treatment involves prostaglandin to maintain the ductus arteriosus, a valvotomy, possible further surgery and, if necessary, aggressive medical management of CCF.

A pulmonary atresia would be a cyanotic defect as blood would not be getting to the lungs for oxygenation. With an intact septum these infants are duct-dependent with a right to left shunt for survival (Harris *et al.*, 1997).

Coarctation of the aorta/interrupted aortic arch/aortic stenosis

These can occur at any level and their presence obstructs the flow from the left ventricle (Wood, 1998). In the newborn period they are often asymptomatic unless very severe. The most common sign to be discovered is the reduction in volume or absence of femoral pulses and pedal pulses. Other later signs include failure to thrive, tachypnoea, dyspnoea, peripheral oedema and severe congestive cardiac failure.

Coarctation of the aorta can be defined as a discreet narrowing of the aorta, most commonly the aortic arch in the region of the ductus arteriosus. It may be associated with a host of other defects (Wood, 1998). Complications can be life-threatening, including rupture of the aorta. Vigorous management of congestive cardiac failure is essential and surgery is offered to infants who present early with heart failure. An infusion of prostaglandins E_1 or E_2 may be started to maintain the patency of the ductus arteriosus and increase the perfusion to the lower body. Surgery depends on the lesion and involves the resection of the coarctation and an end-to-end anastomosis or graft performed under partial cardio-pulmonary bypass.

Interrupted aortic arch can be defined as atresia of the aortic arch. These patients are critically ill, with poor systemic perfusion causing metabolic acidosis. The poor circulation may cause cerebral ischaemic seizures as well as affecting the kidneys and the gut. Prostaglandin infusion needs to be commenced and when the infant is stabilised a single-stage repair is the preferred option (Wood, 1998).

Aortic valve stenosis

The presentation of this condition varies depending on the severity. It may be classified as valvular, subvalvular or supra-valvular. It may be an asymptomatic finding or crashing CCF and shock. With the milder form there may be a murmur, poor feeding, weak peripheral pulses and subtle heart failure. In the more extreme form the infant may be duct-dependent. If the cardiac failure is severe and peripheral perfusion is poor, a prostaglandin infusion should be started to try to open the ductus and immediate surgical referral made. Initial treatment is with an aortic valvotomy.

Bacterial endocarditis is a severe hazard to the child with untreated forms of this condition, as it can turn an asymptomatic aortic stenosis into gross aortic regurgitation with severe cardiac failure. Antibiotics to prevent the onset of infection should cover any invasive procedure. Medical management with Digoxin and diuretics should be tried and, if unsuccessful, valvotomy or valve replacement should be performed (Schindler, 1999).

Abnormal mixing and shunting of blood

Atrial septal defect (ASD)

This is an abnormal opening in the septum between the right and left atrium of which there are several types (Wood, 1997). The ostium secundum defect is located in the centre of the atrial septum and is one of the most common defects to occur in isolation. The ostium primum is a large gap at the base of the septum and is often associated with deformities of the mitral and tricuspid valves. Occasionally, a ventricular septal defect (VSD) also occurs as an abnormal opening in the septum between the right and left ventricles. The sinus venosus occurs high in the atrial septum near the junction of the superior vena cava and the right atrium. There may be an associated anomalous right pulmonary vein to the right atrium. An ASD may be initially asymptomatic, even if the defect is large but its presence imposes a volume overload on the right side of the heart. The chambers of the right side of the heart become dilated with the chronic overload and there will be chronic changes in the pulmonary vascular bed (Wood, 1997).

In affected infants, there may be slow weight gain, CCF, tiredness, dyspnoea with exertion and severe respiratory infections. If the infant is very sick and suffering frequent infections and/or regular bouts of failure, surgical closure is advocated, with cardio-pulmonary bypass. The defect is repaired with a suture or patch.

Ventricular septal defects (VSD)

A ventricular septal defect results from the incomplete division of the right and left ventricles; they are classified according to their anatomical position (Wood, 1997). They may be asymptomatic and many close spontaneously (Turner *et al.*, 1999). VSDs vary in size, from small (as in Roger's defect) to large, and may occur in either the membranous or muscular section of the ventricular septum. Large VSDs may develop symptoms as early as 1–2 months of age. There may be poor weight gain, failure to thrive and feeding difficulties. Often these are pale, delicate-looking infants who have frequent respiratory infections. Other symptoms may include tachypnoea, excessive sweating or congestive cardiac failure. Congestive cardiac failure should be actively treated. If this fails, surgical closure is indicated.

As with ASDs, one of the most significant problems is back-pressure to the lungs. Infants with significant pulmonary arterial hypertension may need early surgery or a palliative pulmonary banding to avoid irreversible pulmonary bed changes. If necessary, the definitive repair will be performed under bypass.

Patent ductus arteriosus (PDA)

This is the persistence of the foetal connection between the aorta and the pulmonary artery. In the foetus the flow is from right to left, bypassing the lungs. It normally closes in the first week in response to the high blood oxygen levels. Patency is common in infants with respiratory distress syndrome because of the lower oxygen tensions. The flow through a patent duct can be bi-directional, depending on pressures, and a considerable and variable blood flow can occur through this channel. As the systemic circulation generates greater pressures, the flow through this open duct is in the reverse direction of foetal blood flow. If undetected or untreated, it may result in heart failure.

Usually, a PDA is detected by the presence of a loud murmur and bounding pulses. The incidence of isolated PDA in term infants is 1 in 2000, but it is much higher in the pre-term, at 8 in 1000 (Wood, 1997). It is the most common defect seen on the NNU – this is largely an indicator of success, as improved supportive technology has kept alive infants who would previously have died.

If small, a PDA may be asymptomatic. Larger ones may develop symptoms in early infancy and in premature neonates may be the reason for the infant's failure to wean from the ventilator or oxygen. In infants who are supporting themselves there may be bounding pedal pulses, low weight gain, feeding difficulties, frequent respiratory infections or congestive cardiac failure.

Medical treatment can be prescribed and is the treatment of choice for many neonates. Indomethacin can be prescribed 8-hourly for up to six doses but, to be effective, it needs to be given early; preferably in the first 8 days after birth. It is less effective in the very premature (less than 30 weeks gestation) and in those, irrespective of gestation, who are more than 3 weeks old. Administration of Indomethacin is not without complications and as infants on the drug will have their fluids restricted, they will need to have their urinary output closely monitored. Blood samples will need to be taken for clotting studies. Surgical ligature or insertion of a device causing occlusion performed during catheterisation under scan control is recommended for those who do not respond to Indomethacin.

Cyanotic cardiac malformations

Tetralogy of Fallot – right-to-left shunt
This comprises four abnormalities:

1   Pulmonary stenosis or atresia;
2   Ventricular septal defect (VSD);
3   Over-riding aorta;
4   Right ventricular hypertrophy (gradual onset, not always present at birth).

Occasionally, pathology is found which has all of the above, plus an atrial septal defect. The degree of pulmonary stenosis and the size of the ventricular septal defect often determine the severity of the condition. The presence of cyanosis depends on the direction of the shunt. A large amount of blood shunted from the right to the left, so bypassing the lungs, may cause cyanosis from birth.

Infants who are not cyanosed from birth may become so as they grow and as the stenosis increases in severity. Untreated infants can experience acute hypoxic spells, particularly if they are left crying for long periods of time, feeding, passing stool or pyrexial. This can be due to spasm of the right ventricular outflow tract causing right to left shunting. These infants may need to be placed in the knee to chest position to increase systemic resistance and improve circulation to the lungs (Spilman and Furdon, 1998).

The infant may be slow to gain weight and be dyspnoeic on exertion. The objective of any treatment is to improve oxygenation of arterial blood, and this can be either palliative or a total correction. The palliative creation of a shunt, for example, could be an anastomosis between the posterior lateral aspect of the ascending aorta and the right pulmonary artery, or an anastomosis between the right or left subclavian artery and the right pulmonary artery. This improves blood supply to the pulmonary artery.

Total correction would involve cardio-pulmonary bypass and the removal of the palliative shunt (if one has been performed previously), then the ventricular septal defect would be repaired and the right ventricular outflow obstruction relieved.

Transposition of the great arteries (TGA)
This is one of the more common forms of cyanotic heart lesion in infancy. It occurs when there is an early developmental failure of the great heart vessels to spiral down and attach to the developing septum dividing the ventricles. This results in the aorta rising from the right ventricle and the pulmonary artery from the left. There are two main forms. In the more common simple transposition, the heart anatomy is normal, and the main arteries are quite simply transposed, resulting in two parallel circulations. With L- transposition there are frequently

other abnormalities and the intra-cardiac circulation is altered radically by the position of the great arteries, resulting in oxygenated blood being returned to the left atria entering the right ventricle to reach the systemic circulation (Witt, 1998).

In TGA cyanosis develops shortly after birth and can be very profound. Survival may depend on early diagnosis and/or associated malformations such as a patent ductus arteriosus or a defect in the septum of the heart and effective mixing of pulmonary and systemic blood. An infusion of prostaglandins will be given to maintain patency of the ductus arteriosis to allow blood mixing. Surgery can either be palliative or corrective. In palliative management there is the formation of an ASD with a balloon catheter, which will be performed during a cardiac catheterisation, or the surgical formation of an ASD. To protect the lungs a pulmonary artery banding procedure may be performed, especially for infants who have VSDs with large pulmonary outflow.

Corrective surgical techniques have been developed that mean in effect a direct switch of the transposed vessels and reimplantation of the coronary arteries. One of these is called the Jatene procedure. Results to date have been promising and this may become the preferred surgical technique replacing the Mustard and the Senning techniques (Schindler, 1999).

Tricuspid atresia

A complete atresia of the tricuspid valve would mean that there was no passage between the right atrium and the right ventricle. For survival, this condition has to be associated with other anomalies such as an interatrial septal defect or a ventricular septal defect allowing a right to left shunt.

Survival depends on a large atrial septal defect for blood to reach the left side of the heart and on the VSD, a PDA or bronchial collaterals for blood to reach the lungs. In a few rare cases, transposition of the great arteries occurs and there may be coexisting anomalies, which balance each other.

It presents with very severe cyanosis in the neonatal period. There is also respiratory distress, hypoxic spells, delayed weight gain and, possibly, right-sided heart failure. Clubbing of fingers and toes are later signs that are not evident during the neonatal period. Because of the complexity a satisfactory complete surgical correction is not possible at present but there are palliative procedures to improve the quality of life experienced:

- an anastomosis between the ascending aorta and right pulmonary artery;
- the Glenn procedure – side-to-end anastomosis of the superior vena cava to the right pulmonary artery or a total cardiopulmonary connection.

Persistent truncus arteriosus

This is a rare, complex and serious condition. It occurs when the developing embryo's truncus arteriosus (a single tube-like structure) fails to partition and divide into the aorta and pulmonary arteries from about the 5th week of gestation (Witt, 1997). Because of this, a single large vessel rises from the ventricles and strives to serve as the heart's own blood supply as well as the systemic (via the aorta) and pulmonary circulation. The situation is further complicated by the presence of a poorly formed valve and a VSD (Witt, 1998).

Cardiac surgeons recognise subdivisions of the abnormality. Because of the high pulmonary blood flow infants present with heart failure within a few weeks of birth (Schindler, 1999). Treatment is both medical and through complicated surgical procedures, although pulmonary hypertension may persist after repair. There is a significant risk to the infant during surgery.

Anomalous venous drainage

This is a 'catch-all' term for a variety of defects, describing an abnormality of pulmonary venous return. Without treatment it carries a high and early mortality risk (Ruth-Sanchez, 1998). Essentially, this defect occurs very early from the 3rd week of embryonic formation; the early development of drainage from the lungs, rather than connecting to the left atria, will attach to a range of other systemic blood vessels. The defect can be partial or total. If the obstruction is total, survival depends on associated abnormalities such as a patent foramen ovale or prompt medical intervention and administrations of prostaglandin to sustain life.

Treatment may be a surgical emergency and ideally involves reattachment of the pulmonary venous return to the left atria. It is performed under bypass.

Hypoplastic left heart

The heart is a muscular structure. During embryonic and foetal life, the type and amount of work it has to do determines its ultimate shape and function (Witt, 1997). The condition referred to as 'hypoplastic heart' is usually a collection of abnormalities with a weak and under-developed left ventricle unable to support the heart's own circulation as well as the rest of the body. Hazinski (2000) outlines three treatment options:

- tender loving care – the lesion will be fatal;
- palliative creation of a shunt so the effort of the right ventricle will support that of the left as a systemic pumping chamber;
- a cardiac transplant, although for neonates the transplantation option is an emotive issue and the opportunities are few.

Complications of cyanotic heart lesions

Congestive cardiac failure (CCF) can present during the newborn and neonatal period; for guidance on the care of cardiac failure, *see* pages 176–8. Infective endocarditis is an infection of the endocardial surface of the heart. It is a rare condition, which is usually found with pre-existing cardiovascular disease (congenital or rheumatic), but can develop in a normal heart during an episode of septicaemia. The infants who are most at risk are those with:

- VSD, especially a small VSD;
- surgically created shunts;
- patent ductus arteriosus;

- semi-lunar valve stenosis;
- coarctation of the aorta;
- tetralogy of Fallot.

The signs and symptoms are much like any acute infection but a chest X-ray may reveal vegetative growth within the heart. This may be difficult to detect in a small infant due to the size of the heart but, if an infection is suspected, treatment must be started immediately. The medical management involves the administration of large doses of intravenous antibiotics over a 4–6-week period.

Nursing care should include the regular recording of vital signs, and the infant should be encouraged to rest as much as possible. The parents should be encouraged to visit or stay if possible during the long hospitalisation. Stringent infection control is essential to both parents and staff.

The cardiac infant is also at risk of cerebral vascular accident due to thrombosis, severe hypoxia or emboli. Brain abscess can be a later complication for a child with a cardiac problem. The cause of these abscesses is incompletely understood but they are probably related to episodes of bacteraemia and reduced cerebral circulation and perfusion.

Disability and death may ensue if the condition is impossible to treat, difficult to treat or remains undetected.

Nursing care of an infant undergoing cardiac catheterisation

This is an invasive procedure, which has a changing role in the management of cardiac care owing to the increased use and skilled interpretation of ultrasound (Verklan, 1997b). The procedure is not without risk as it involves the introduction of a radio-opaque catheter into a vein or artery in the groin or in the arm, either by direct insertion as in venepuncture or by cutdown. Venous access (via the groin) is preferred as it allows examination of all four heart chambers. The catheter is passed up into the cardiac chambers and vessels, where pressures are measured and oxygen saturations can be directly obtained.

This procedure has various functions, both as a diagnostic tool in investigating cardiovascular anomalies and the severity of the defect, and also to evaluate the effects of the defect on the cardiovascular system. As a therapeutic approach, cardiac catheterisation can be used to carry out palliative procedures (balloon septotomy) and to locate and close a patent ductus arteriosus using an umbrella device (this prevents the need for surgery and in older children can be done as a day case).

The procedure can be done in conjunction with angiography, which is the injection of radio-opaque material into the chambers of the heart. This makes it easier to identify anomalies.

Pre- and peri-operative care

Parental anxiety
Parents should be given a detailed explanation of surgery. It is good practice to check back with them to assess their level of understanding, as informed

consent is vital. The nurse administers any sedation that had been prescribed for the infant. Ensuring a calm and relaxed environment is nursing priority, to avoid the infant becoming tense and irritable. The parents should be given as much time and privacy with their infant as possible and be given all the support they need.

Hydration, nutrition and maintenance of blood glucose

The infant needs to be kept well hydrated prior to the procedure and the investigation should be timed to avoid interruption of the infant's feed regime. If feeds are going to be missed, a dextrose infusion is set up to maintain blood glucose; glucose levels are closely monitored. The nurse should check that the infant has been cross-matched and has blood available. All pre-operative fluids should be charted and the infant's charts sent to theatre to ensure continuity of the fluid balance.

Optimal condition and temperature

Baseline observations are also sent to theatre with the infant. A warm transport incubator is made available, with oxygen and ventilator attached. All monitoring equipment must be functional. The temperature of a small infant can drop quickly and preventing cold stress in theatre is a nursing priority (Verklan, 1997b). Suitable clothing, such as a warm bonnet, mitts and boots, should be sent to theatre; quick-release babygrows, tops and bottoms, fastened by studs or poppers allow for rapid undressing and redressing. The appropriateness of such clothing depends on the insert site of the catheter line.

Post-operative care following a cardiac catheterisation

Safe environment and close observation

All emergency equipment must be available and functioning. Arrhythmias can occur because of cardiac irritability, so vital signs need to be monitored frequently. The puncture site is visually inspected for any signs of bleeding. Occasionally, damage can be done or infection introduced to the entry vessel, and the site may show signs of redness or swelling. The limb is kept exposed and checked frequently; with frequent monitoring, signs of pallor, decreased temperature, decreased activity, cyanosis or any mottling are accurately recorded. Pulses in the affected limb should be compared with the unaffected limb, as thrombus formation can be a complication. Absent pulses or a white limb must be reported and acted upon immediately.

Maintaining the infant's temperature and hydration

The infant must be kept warm, comfortable and suitably wrapped to maintain temperature, and avoid hypothermia; an incubator or an overhead heater may be used. The infant will need to rest for several hours after the procedure in order to recover. Adequate hydration is maintained via an IV infusion and blood glucose is checked as necessary to avoid hypo/hyperglycaemia. The infant should be fed as soon as it is sufficiently recovered and hungry.

Assessment of urine output

An overloading of contrast medium can cause renal damage, so urine output must be recorded and if no urine has been passed within 4–6 hours post surgery, the doctors should be informed. Sodium overload has been reported as a complication of flushing the catheter with saline. If electrolyte levels may need to be frequently assessed an indwelling line may be the kindest option.

General nursing care of an infant undergoing cardiac surgery

Parental anxiety

Parents of an infant undergoing cardiac surgery are often very vulnerable. Many will be away from home, perhaps living in accommodation provided by the hospital in order to be near their infant. They may be without the usual support of family and friends and may be worried about other children at home. This is a very emotive time for parents. They often feel very guilty and angry about what is happening to their infant. It is important to help them feel involved and understand that they are doing the right thing. There needs to be full and free discussion of many issues, not least the possibility of their infant dying during or after the procedure. All facts, however unpleasant, must be presented in order to avoid conflict later. The neonatal nurse needs to be both compassionate and knowledgeable. Counselling is vital at this point.

The nurse should discuss with the parents what they will do while their infant is in surgery; the time may pass very slowly when they are anxious and frightened. Some parents clearly want to be left alone with their thoughts, while others may welcome support, particularly by those who have been through this process themselves. The parents' support network may be useful for these parents. Locally, the cardiac hospital has a private, pleasant and peaceful all-weather garden for parents.

For many parents, one of the major worries is the degree of pain that will be felt by the infant. The nurse is in a position to give reassurance about the use of analgesics. Some parents worry about the place where the infant will be nursed, and a trip to the intensive care unit, with an introduction to the staff who will be involved in their infant's care, is often appreciated. With the correct emphasis on individual variation and needs, a description of how their infant may look after theatre may be helpful in some cases; other parents may prefer to handle one thing at a time.

Pre-operative – warmth and hydration

The infant should be kept warm and well hydrated with an IV infusion. A warm, checked and functional transport incubator should be made available, with all monitoring equipment and pumps safely secured, and oxygen cylinders full.

Prevention of infection

Antibiotic cover is usually given at the start of the procedure to try and prevent sepsis. The most recent weight of the infant should be on the prescription chart and sent to theatre with the infant. If the infant is fit, the parents can enjoy giving the pre-theatre bath. Special skin preparation is usually done in theatre.

Safe environment

The correct hospital number bracelets must be attached to the wrist and ankle. To avoid last-minute anxieties, all vital documentation should be gathered together. Consent forms, observation charts, notes, X-rays, and results of any investigations such as blood tests, ECG, nitrogen washout, and cardiac catheterisation, should all be sent to theatre with the infant.

There should be sufficient blood, cross-matched and ready, should the infant need a transfusion. This might be an issue with some religious groups. If parents do object, ensure that all staff are aware of this and make alternative arrangements; advance donations from the mother or close family may be acceptable. Counselling can often encourage parents to do what is right for their child, regardless of beliefs or convictions.

Peri-operative cardiac surgery management – cardio-pulmonary bypass (CPB)

As surgery on tiny infants becomes increasingly sophisticated, cardio-pulmonary bypass (CPB) is used to facilitate surgical procedures that need direct access to the heart, and to ensure a still and 'bloodless' field. Blood is drained from the right atria, passed through a membrane to allow the exchange of gases, and then returned to the body via a pump to maintain perfusion and organ viability. To prevent coagulation in the circuit the blood is thinned (the risks of this are discussed below). During bypass the heart and lungs are isolated from the body and the heart is artificially stopped. To reduce the risk of ischaemic injury the heart is cooled sometimes to 15–18 degrees centigrade and the time the heart is stopped is ideally limited to about an hour (Schindler, 1999).

The infant on bypass will need careful fluid management and will need adequate crystalloid and colloid infusions according to the acid-base balance and circulatory pressures. In infants the estimated circulating volume is calculated according to weight as 80 mLs/kg. Not surprisingly there are risks with this process and these include severe systemic inflammatory response, multi-organ failure, embolisms and shock.

Coagulation and haemostasis

To facilitate bypass or post-surgery extra corporeal membrane oxygenation (ECMO), anticoagulation is used to try and prohibit the normal clotting mechanisms. Heparin is infused at 300 units/kg to try to maintain an activated clotting time of greater than 200 seconds (normal about 80 seconds). Under normal circumstances, factors which prolong clotting times are unwelcome during surgical procedures, but in these circumstances it is a case of balancing and managing the risks. As the infant is weaned off bypass, the prolonged clotting times are reversed with an infusion of protamine sulphate (Jones and Steer, 2000).

Hypothermia

Hypothermia may be used to support cardio-pulmonary bypass or in isolation for a quick procedure. In future it may also be used selectively to protect vital structures such as the brain when at risk of oxygen fluctuations. Cooling reduces oxygen requirements; at around 22–24 degrees centigrade cardiac asystole occurs, which will allow surgery to be performed on a non-pulsating heart (Jones and Steer, 2000). Up to a point, the more profound the cooling, the longer the surgeon has to perform the work required. Temperatures of lower than 15 degrees are not yet used as there is a risk of cold damage to the tissues that the surgeon is trying to preserve.

When hypothermia is used in addition to cardio-pulmonary bypass, the reversal process can include gradual re-warming via the heat exchanger, which is built into the circuit. This allows the surgeon the luxury of enough time to evaluate the effectiveness of the work and to make an assessment for bleeding. As the infant's core temperature begins to rise, the heart will begin to function normally and the infant can then be taken off bypass.

Rebound pyrexia can occur following cooling, perhaps because of hypothalamic reaction to the cooling process, or owing to neonatal immaturity. Pyrexia is unhelpful in these circumstances as it increases the oxygen consumption required and the risk of arrhythmias. Temperature control air blankets may be useful as may muscle relaxants, to prevent shivering. The use of vasodilators to increase circulation to the extremities and the resulting heat loss from the periphery would depend on the infant's blood pressure as well as the overall clinical picture. Cool peripheral temperatures may be an indication of circulation instability, low circulation volume or poor cardiac output.

Cardiac transplant

This remains rare in neonates as the need for organs significantly outweighs the number of donors and this is perhaps the single largest factor in preventing an increase in the procedure. Acceptance on to a transplant programme is no guarantee of a donor organ being available and more patients die on the waiting list than have the operation.

If an organ is available, the infant has to be in a stable physical condition and infection-free. The closer the match the better the outcome, although the infant will only be matched on blood group and heart size. Following the operation the infant needs to be attached to a pacemaker, as the nerves normally controlling the heart rate and rhythm are severed. The infant needs to be on considerable amounts of anti-rejection immuno-suppression drugs, which have many side-effects.

Post-operative assessment and management

Most infants are ventilated following cardiac surgery as this allows excellent management of the airway, effective lung expansion and facilitates the manipulation of the blood gases. Should pulmonary hypertension be a post-operative problem, full ventilation would allow the inhalation of nitric oxide to reduce the pulmonary vascular resistance. Ventilation also allows for substantial pain relief to be given, without compromising the respiratory drive, and muscle relaxants to be administered to protect the repair and suture line from excessive movement. On the negative side, the infant is unresponsive to the parents and neurological assessment is difficult.

Assessing blood loss and coagulation after surgery

Constant observation of post-operative drainage is required. Post-operative loss is regarded as abnormal if the blood loss for mediastinal drains is in excess of 3 mls/kg hour for longer than 3 hours, or is incessant. Bleeding greater than 10 mls/kg hour may need an urgent surgical review (Schindler, 1999). Post-operative bleeding may be the result of heparin loading and may respond to a protamine infusion. Cardio-pulmonary bypass or large-volume replacements may dilute the infants' clotting factors and post-operative bleeding following this may respond to fresh whole blood, fresh frozen plasma or platelets. To avoid the infant enduring further surgery to explore for bleeding, fibrinolysis inhibitors may be tried.

Specific complications following cardiac surgery include arrhythmia, diaphragmatic paralysis and chylothorax. The arrhythmia may be transient owing to electrolyte imbalance, cold or vagus stimulation, or a response to handling of the heart. Should the arrhythmia be prolonged or anticipated by the surgeon, a pacemaker may be fitted. These can be used temporally or incorporated into long-term cardiac management.

The diaphragmatic paralysis may be temporary or longer-term. It can occur with the chilling of the heart and resolve with the re-warming of the infant, or it can result following the surgical process and the severance of the phrenic nerve. The infant has a highly compliant chest wall and is dependent on the function of the diaphragm. Respiratory function would be unequal and compromised and weaning off the ventilator would be difficult. There would be radiological evidence of an elevated diaphragm. The nerve action can be replaced by the use of a diaphragmatic pacer or the diaphragmatic action made equal by division of the opposing nerve. There may be spontaneous recovery in the majority of patients within 2 years.

Another surgical accident may be the division of the lymphatic drainage channels. This is more likely with some types of surgery than others, with the bi-directional cavopulmonary anastomosis having some of the highest risk factors. Treatment is initially by drainage and the infant's feeds are changed to medium chain triacylglyceride formulas, which are more completely digested, bypassing the lymphatic system. If this does not work, long-term total parenteral nutrition should be considered (Schindler, 1999). Spontaneous resolution occurs in the majority of cases but surgery may be considered for intractable cases.

Due to the small size of the infants being worked on, it is perhaps surprising that these complications are not seen more often.

Care example – specific pre-operative care of an infant with PDA

A PDA can pose significant problems to a pre-term neonate with respiratory disease and particularly one who is ventilated on intermittent positive pressure ventilation. For this reason it is desirable to close the ductus as soon as clinically possible. In an infant who is ventilated, the clinical signs are a progressive increase in carbon dioxide and an increasing inspired oxygen requirement. There is also the need for higher inspiratory and expiratory pressures, on IPPV. For oxygen-dependent premature infants who are not ventilated, the ductus arteriosus presents with increasing dyspnoea, increasing oxygen requirements and/or apnoeic episodes.

On auscultation, loud, machine-like murmurs can be heard and the rhythm is galloping in nature. This murmur may come and go from day to day, and neonatal nurses will often hear it when checking the air entry in ventilated infants.

Nursing care in the pre-operative stage involves keeping the infant warm and stable using the techniques described above. The fluid restriction should be maintained as prescribed and the input continuously balanced with output. In an infant who is not catheterised, the nappies can be weighed pre- and post-use to give an estimation of amount voided. This is important, to detect any signs of CCF, and should be recorded on the appropriate chart.

Post-operative care following ligation of PDA

During the immediate post-operative period the infant may be critically unstable and need full ventilatory support and skilled intensive care. Typically, these infants get better quickly. Many are weaned rapidly from the ventilator and do very well once extubated and supporting themselves in headbox oxygen. Vital signs should be charted as appropriate and blood pressure accurately measured. Any deviation from the infant's norm should be promptly reported to the medical team.

Specific observation

The neonate is nursed with the left side uppermost as the surgical approach is via a left thoracotomy. The lung is collapsed to allow the PDA to be reached and, when it is re-inflated, there is a possibility that a pneumothorax, haemothorax or chylothorax can occur. The PDA lies very close to lymphatic vessels and, very rarely, a vessel may be punctured, leading to large amounts of fluid being lost into the thoracic cavity. Chest drains must be kept patent and the colour and quantity of any loss charted. With the wound uppermost it is easier to see any bleeding or oedema developing and the lung is more likely to remain inflated.

Physiotherapy

If physiotherapy is needed, it should be very gentle and a non-vibration technique should be used, as vibration could induce a collapse of the lung. The chest drain is usually removed after 24–48 hours, when a chest X-ray confirms re-inflation and a short period of clamping does not result in reaccumulation.

Pain control

This is vital. A thoracotomy is a very painful incision and post-operative recovery will be far quicker if the infant's pain is controlled. Most NNUs use continuous morphine infusions and then wean the infant down slowly. This is very effective and keeps the infant very comfortable.

Fluids and blood glucose levels

All intake and output should be noted. The IVI may be reduced as enteral feeds are reintroduced. The specific gravity of the urine is checked to ensure normal renal function. Blood glucose levels are checked as appropriate.

COMMON DRUGS USED IN CARDIAC MANAGEMENT

Chapter 16, on neonatal pharmacy, covers points on general administration, absorption and transport of drugs. Condition-specific drugs are considered here.

Adrenaline

This is a hormone normally produced by the adrenal gland as part of the fight/flight response. Adrenaline is a catecholamine, which produces an adrenergic effect. It is a powerful vasoconstrictor, prescribed for hypotension and bradycardia, and is effectively used during resuscitation. The drug will increase mean arterial and diastolic pressure.

Administration can be by bolus endotracheal, IV and, occasionally, intra-cardiac injection. Side-effects include tachycardia, vasoconstriction, and impaired renal and mesenteric perfusion and, if given via an intravenous infusion, supportive vasodilator therapy should be considered. To maintain infant's safety, dosage should be checked against local protocols and policies. In an emergency an IV bolus of 0.1–0.3 mls/kg of a 1:10 000 solution may be given quickly. A high dose given via endotracheal tube (1 ml/kg) may be tried. An infusion of 0.05–0.15 microgrammes/kg/min could be considered within a therapeutic range.

Atropine

Atropine is an anticholinergic agent that inhibits the action of acetylcholine, a chemical transmitter found in the parasympathetic nervous system. Administration in an arrest situation is intended to free the heart from the inhibitory effects of the vagus nerve, so increasing heart rate and strength. It is often used in conjunction with adrenaline, particularly if bradycardia was thought to have occurred as a result of vagal stimulation. It may be given by bolus intravenous injection and occasionally by endotracheal instillation. To maintain infant's safety, dosage should be checked against local protocols and policies; 0.01–0.02 milligrammes/kg could be a therapeutic dose. This drug is frequently prescribed in microgrammes so extra attention to the detail on the drug chart is essential.

Adenosine

Adenosine slows conduction of the atrio-ventricular node and inhibits re-entry pathways. It is used for supra-ventricular tachycardia. It has a swift action within 10–20 seconds of rapidly given bolus intravenous administration. Its short half-life of 10–15 seconds reduces the chances of side-effects. To maintain infant's safety, the dosage should be checked against local protocols and policies; an initial dose of 0.05 milligrammes/kg could be tried; the dose range is 0.05–0.3 milligrammes/kg, increasing the dose carefully by 0.05 milligrammes/kg.

Caffeine

Full understanding of exactly how caffeine works has not yet been achieved. It may enhance contractility of the diaphragm and/or stimulate the respiratory centre. It certainly increases the heart rate and may cause tachycardia. It may be given orally or intravenously. It is given frequently to pre-term infants to prevent bradycardia of prematurity. For it to be most effective the infant needs to be 'loaded'. To maintain infant's safety, dosage should be checked against local protocols and policies. Locally, we use a loading dose of 10 milligrammes/kg and a maintenance dose of 2.5 milligrammes/kg. Some units like to do caffeine levels to check any toxicity.

Digoxin

This cardiac glycoside has mainly an inotropic action. It is prescribed to improve the contractility of the myocardium in heart failure and to control ventricular arrhythmias. It slows and strengthens the heart rate and function. Its use in the pre-term infant is controversial, as it can be rapidly toxic. If it is decided to commence the infant on digoxin the infant has to be 'loaded' and needs to be fully monitored, until blood levels are taken and the correct maintenance dose established for maximum stability. Digoxin may be given orally or intravenously. It may take up to 6 hours to work and may precipitate ventricular fibrillation and increased blood pressure. Nurses should refer to local practice, policy and protocols for dosage. Range varies widely between digitalisation and maintenance, and between pre-term and term neonate (see Table 9.4).

Table 9.4   Digoxin dosage range for pre-term and term infants

	Loading (microgrammes/kg)	Maintenance daily dose (microgrammes/kg/day)
Pre-term	10–20	5
Term	30–40	5–10

Dopamine

This is a precursor of noradrenaline and has sympathomimetic properties. It is prescribed in the treatment of shock and hypotension associated with cardiovascular surgery, sepsis and severe asphyxia. It is given by continuous IV infusion because of its short half-life and should not be infused with alkali as this will cause inactivation. It has a useful therapeutic effect, increasing stroke volume and cardiac output, raising the mean arterial pressure and improving urine volume depending on the dose regime (Keeley and Bohn, 1988). Dopamine causes blanching of the skin overlying the vein so central access is preferred. To maintain infant's safety, dosage should be checked against local protocols and policies. The dose range is 1–5 microgrammes/kg/min.

Dobutamine

This increases the contractility and output of the heart and systemically vasodilates, so improving tissue perfusion. The drug has a dose-dependent benefit and has a short half-life necessitating a continuous IV infusion (Keeley and Bohn, 1988). Tachycardia has been reported as a side-effect requiring discontinuation. To maintain infant's safety, dosage should be checked against local protocols and policies. The dose range is 2–20 microgrammes/kg/min.

Frusemide

This is a powerful diuretic, which acts by preventing the reabsorption of sodium and thus eliminating excess water in the loop of henle, proximal and distal tubules in the kidneys. It may be given intravenously or a larger dose may be given orally. To maintain infant's safety, dosage should be checked against local protocols and policies. The ranges are 1–2 mg/kg/dose (IV), 1–4 milligrammes/kg/dose (oral).

Indomethacin

This is a prostaglandin synthetase inhibitor and is sometimes used to close the ductus arteriosus. Although the pharmacokinetics are not fully known, the drug is thought to block the action of naturally occurring prostaglandin, which has a role in maintaining this unwanted channel. Monitoring of the infant's fluid balance is vital during administration as indomethacin reduces renal blood flow and fluids are often restricted to try to reduce the circulating volume to help close the duct. The drug may be given orally or intravenously during a course of three to six bolus doses 8–12 hours apart. To maintain infant's safety, dosage should be checked against local protocols and policies. The dosage is 200 microgrammes/kg/dose.

Lignocaine

This is an anti-arrhythmia agent used for serious ventricular arrhythmia. It is given as an initial intravenous bolus followed by a continuous intravenous infusion. To be effective high serum concentrations are needed and the drug has been reported as causing seizure activity. To maintain infant's safety, dosage should be checked against local protocols and policies. Given as a bolus, the range is 1–2 mg/kg/dose; the dosage of an infusion may range between 10 and 20 microgrammes/kg/min.

Prostaglandin E

This is used to maintain the patency of the ductus arteriosus in cyanotic malformation – for example, pulmonary atresia, tetralogy of Fallot and tricuspid atresia – until corrective surgery can be performed. It is given intravenously. To maintain infant's safety, the dosage should be checked against local protocols and policies. The initial bolus dose may be 0.1 milligramme/kg, diluted carefully. Infusion protocols may range from 0.025–0.1 microgrammes/kg/min. The line should not be flushed.

Prostaglandin E has many side-effects, such as apnoea, pyrexia, increased bronchial secretions and jitteriness, and the infant should be carefully monitored during administration. The drug may be prescribed in nanogrammes so careful checking of the detail on the prescription chart is required.

In the case of all drugs listed the infant should be on a cardiac monitor and have regular blood pressure readings as clinically appropriate. Any bradycardia or tachycardia should be reported and if necessary the drug or drugs should not be given until medical advice is sought.

CONCLUSION: THE PRESENT AND THE FUTURE

Many current and effective methods of management started off as experimental treatment options. Cardiac surgeons have always been regarded as pioneers, but there has been much public scrutiny over some surgical techniques and success rates (DoH, 2001). Public expectations have risen, yet many people are reluctant to donate organs or to allow research into growing alternatives. This attitude makes the job of the entire cardiac team much more difficult. Medical colleagues need to remain confident and feel positive that their team will support them, particularly as they trial new techniques or work with increasingly smaller and sicker infants, with higher risk.

There have been some technical improvements in the mechanical devices that assist the left ventricle, and some progress may be made in neonatal cardiac care with these. However, for the foreseeable future, even when they are sufficiently refined these will only be able to act as holding devices for the few. The definitive repair or replacement will still be the answer to a near-normal life. Research into cardiac anomalies is ongoing, old remedies are being questioned and new treatments are developing all the time (Westaby *et al.*, 1999). Pre-natal prevention of the development of lesions is desirable where possible, and health promotion encouraging sensible drinking and an awareness of the link between some drugs and defects, aims to reduce the incidence. Ultrasound scanning is now used routinely to check the development of the heart in utero.

Many young women planning a family who have a CHD themselves have survived thanks to modern medicine, but they need counselling, rigorous antenatal screening and pre-conception advice. Counselling should also be offered to parents with a family history of cardiac anomalies, and those who feel that they may be at risk, perhaps from environmental factors such as industrial pollution.

To give infants with cardiac abnormalities the best chance of survival, and a good quality of life, it is important to pick up any defects early and to diagnose them correctly in the neonatal period (Ainsworth *et al.*, 1999; Wren *et al.*, 1999). A blue infant gives a dramatic clue to all observers that something is seriously amiss. In general, if the infant is displaying respiratory distress (gasping, grunting or indrawing), although cardiac pathology cannot be ruled out, the infant needs respiratory support. If the infant is settled, comfortable but blue, then a cardiac condition is suspected.

SAMPLE EXAMINATION QUESTIONS

Question 1
Draw and label the normal anatomy of the human heart. (*30 marks*)
Describe the flow of blood through the heart. (*30 marks*)
What are the structural and functional differences between the foetal heart and the mature anatomy? (*40 marks*)

Question 2
What pre-procedural observations would the nurse make on a 3-day-old infant prior to transfer to the cardiac catheterisation suite? (*50 marks*)
What post-procedural observations would be made? (*50 marks*)

Question 3
Winston is a 3-week-old term infant who has not gained weight since birth and looks lethargic, puffy and breathless. His GP has suspected a heart murmur and has arranged admission to the cardiac ward for observations and investigations.
What are some of the more common investigations and how would you explain them to Winston's parents? (*50 marks*)
What can the nurse do to reassure Winston's parents and ensure that their stay is as comfortable as possible? (*50 marks*)

REFERENCES

Ainsworth, S., Wyllie, J. and Wren, C. (1999) Prevalence and clinical significance of cardiac murmurs in neonates, *Archives of Disease in Childhood* 80(1), 43–5

Children's Heart Federation (2000) website: www.childrens-heart-fed.org.uk/ E-mail: chf@dircon.co.uk

Department of Health (2001) *Learning from Bristol: A Report of the Public Inquiry into Children's Heart Surgery at the Bristol Royal Infirmary 1984–95*, Department of Health, London

Furdon, S. (1997) Recognising congestive heart failure in the neonatal period, *Neonatal Network* 16(7), 5–13

Harris, M., Valmorida, J., Carey, B. and Trotter, C. (1997) Neonates with congenital heart disease, Part III. Congenital cardiac defects with decreased pulmonary blood flow, *Neonatal Network* **16**(2), 59–63

Hazinski, M. (2000) Cardiovascular Disorders (Chapter 5). In: Hazinski, M. (ed.) *Manual of Paediatric Critical Care*, Mosby, St Louis, IL

Jones, E. and Steer, B. (2000) Care and management of infants and children requiring cardiac surgery (Chapter 9). In: Williams, C. and Asquith, J. (eds), *Paediatric Intensive Care*, Churchill Livingstone, Edinburgh

Keeley, S. and Bohn, D. (1988) The use of inotrophic and afterload reducing agents in neonates, *Clinics in Perinatology* **15**(3), 467–84

Klassen, L. (1999) Complete congenital heart block: a review and case study, *Neonatal Network* **18**(3), 33–42

MacGregor, J. (2000) *Introduction to the Anatomy and Physiology of Children* (Chapter 4), Routledge, London

Massin, M., Maeyns, K., Withofs, N. *et al.* (2000) Circadian rhythm of heart rate and heart rate variability, *Archives of Disease in Childhood* **83**(8) 179–82

Moniaci, V. and Kraus, M. (1997) Determining the relationship between non-invasive and noninvasive blood pressure values, *Neonatal Network* **16**(1), 51–6

Page, J. and Hosking, M. (1997) An approach to the neonate with sudden dysrhythmia: diagnosis, mechanisms and management, *Neonatal Network* **16**(6), 7–18

Paul, K. (1995) Recognition, stabilisation and early management of infants with critical congenital heart disease, presenting in the first days of life, *Neonatal Network* **14**(5), 13–20

Quan, R., Yang, C., Rubinstein, S., Lewiston, N. *et al.* (1994) The effect of nutritional additives on anti-infective factors in human milk, *Clinical Pediatrics* **33**(6), 325–8

Rikard, D. (1993) Nursing care of neonates receiving prostaglandin E therapy, *Neonatal Network* **12**(4), 17–22

Ruth-Sanchez, V. (1998) Cardiac anomalies restricting blood flow to the left atrium, *Neonatal Network* **17**(6), 7–17

Sansoucie, D. and Cavaliere, T. (1997) Transition from fetal to extrauterine circulation, *Neonatal Network* **16**(2), 5–12

Schindler, M. (1999) Cardiovascular system (Chapter 3). In: Macnab, A., Macrae, D. and Henning, R. (eds) *Care of the Critically Ill Child*, Churchill Livingstone, Edinburgh

Stork, E., Carlo, W. and Kleigman, R. (1984) Hypertension redefined for critically ill neonates, *Paediatric Research* **18**(1), 32

Spilman, L. and Furdon, S. (1998) Recognition, understanding and current management of cardiac lesions with decreased pulmonary blood flow, *Neonatal Network* **17**(4), 7–18

Sreeram, N. and Wren, C. (1990) Supraventricular tachycardia in infants; response to initial treatment, *Archives of Disease in Childhood* **65**(1), 127–9

Tibby, S., Hatherill, M. and Murdock, I. (1999) Capillary refill and core-peripheral temperature gap as indicators of haemodynamic status in paediatric intensive care patients, *Archives of Disease in Childhood* **80**(2), 163–6

Turner, S., Hunter, S. and Wyllie, J. (1999) The natural history of ventricular septal defects, *Archives of Disease in Childhood* **81**(11), 413–16

Verklan, T. (1997a) Diagnostic techniques in cardiac disorders, *Neonatal Network* **16**(4), 9–15

Verklan, T. (1997b) Diagnostic techniques in cardiac disorders, *Neonatal Network* **16**(5), 7–13

Vrijheid, M., Dolk, H., Stone, D., Abramsky, L., Alberman, E. and Scott, J. (2000) Socio-economic inequalities in risk of congenital anomaly, *Archives Disease in Childhood* **82**(5), 349–52

Westaby, S., Franklin, O. and Burch, M. (1999) New developments in the treatment of cardiac failure, *Archives of Disease in Childhood* **81**(9), 276–7

Witt, C. (1997) Cardiac embryology, *Neonatal Network* **16**(1), 43–9

Witt, C. (1998) Cyanotic heart lesions with increased pulmonary blood flow, *Neonatal Network* **17**(7), 7–16

Wood, M. (1997) Acyanotic lesions with increased pulmonary blood flow, *Neonatal Network* **16**(3), 17–25

Wood, M. (1998) Acyanotic cardiac lesions with normal pulmonary blood flow, *Neonatal Network* **17**(3), 5–11

Wren, C., Richmond, S. and Donaldson, L. (1999) Presentation of congenital heart disease in infancy: implications for the routine examination, *Archives of Disease in Childhood* **80**(1), 49–53

FURTHER READING

Boxwell, G. (2000) *Neonatal Intensive Care Nursing*, Routledge, London

Hazinski, M. (1999) *Manual of Pediatric Critical Care*, Mosby, St Louis, IL

MacGregor, J. (2000) *Introduction to the Anatomy and Physiology of Children*, Routledge, London

Macnab, A., Macrae, D. and Henning, R. (1999) *Care of the Critically Ill Child*, Churchill Livingstone, Edinburgh

Royal College of Paediatrics and Child Health (1999) *Medicines for Children*, RCPCH, London

Williams, C. and Asquith, J. (2000) *Paediatric Intensive Care Nursing*, Churchill Livingstone, Edinburgh

Yeo, H. (1998) *Nursing the Neonate*, Blackwell Science, Oxford

10 CARE OF INFANTS WITH RENAL DISORDERS

Eileen Brennan

Aims of the chapter

This chapter introduces the normal processes of renal development and function during the embryonic and neonatal period. This provides a framework for understanding the factors that may affect the neonate in renal failure. The concept of homeostasis and electrolyte balance is reviewed and the nursing care of infants with some of the more common renal conditions is considered.

INTRODUCTION

Over the past decade, improvements in dialysis technology and surgical procedures have meant that the success rate of treatment for infants in renal failure has dramatically improved. However, there is still no consensus of advisability for initiating peritoneal dialysis (PD) in the very young infant with chronic renal failure (Geary, 1998). The data collected by Ledermann and colleagues supports the vision that PD, in conjunction with an intensive nutritional programme and optimal management, can provide a favourable outcome (Ledermann *et al.*, 2000). It is well recognised that infants with other co-morbid conditions have a higher rate of morbidity and mortality (Ellis *et al.*, 1995). This should be taken into consideration when counselling parents who wish to start long-term treatment for their infant in chronic renal failure.

Management of the neonate with renal failure is best done in specialist units although impaired renal function can co-exist with and complicate other pathology. Low-birthweight and pre-term infants with renal obstruction will need to have surgical treatment quickly for best outcome, even though they require other forms of management for other reasons. Renal function at birth is limited and sick neonates have a high risk of renal impairment in the first few weeks of life. The condition of these neonates may change rapidly and they can deteriorate quickly without specific management. To maintain adequate homeostasis, the renal structure must develop quickly and function effectively during foetal life. Following birth, the renal system must adapt rapidly.

EMBRYOLOGICAL DEVELOPMENT OF THE KIDNEY

An adequate knowledge of embryological development is vital in understanding renal disorders. Abnormalities in the first trimester may result in agenesis or hypoplasia. Renal obstruction can cause cystic kidney disease. Renal development begins in the first week after conception and progresses through three stages: pronephros, mesonephros and metanephros.

Between the 3rd and 5th weeks of gestation, the pronephros and mesonephros appear. These then further divide to form a solid nephrogenic cord. Subsequently, this develops a lumen, giving rise to a nephric duct that opens into the cloaca of the embryo. At 5 weeks, a ureteric bud grows from the mesonephric duct, giving rise to the pelvis, calyces and collecting tubules of the kidney. The metanephrogenic cap surrounding the bud forms in the eleventh week. Vesicles extend to form nephrogenic tubules, one end fusing with the collecting tubules and the other forming the glomerulus. At this stage, small amounts of urine are being produced. Disordered embryogenesis during this period may result in renal agenesis (Chevalier, 1994). Branching continues until 32–34 weeks gestation, at which time nephrogenesis is complete.

Functional maturity continues into infancy and performance is largely dependent on gestational age (Levene et al., 2000). The glomerular filtration rate (GFR) transiently falls in the first few hours following birth, then slowly increases throughout infancy to reach adult values by 12–18 months (Wolfish and Mongeau, 1983). Urine production (determined by ultrasonography) has been found to rise from 12 ml/h at 32 weeks gestation to 28 ml/h at term (Chevalier, 1994). Failure to pass urine within the first 24 hours is associated with abnormalities of perfusion-filtration or obstruction. Ninety per cent of all infants are expected to pass urine within the first 24 hours of life and 98% within 48 hours (Levene et al., 2000). Failure to do so is associated with renal failure. Approximately 0.1% of all deliveries require peritoneal dialysis for acute renal failure (Haycock, 1993).

RENAL FUNCTION

Concentration and dilution

During the first few hours of life a low urine output is expected in all infants who weigh less than 1.5 kg, however, a urine output of <1 ml/kg/hour is cause for concern. Even though a neonate's ability to dilute urine is regarded as adequate at about 32 weeks, their ability to concentrate urine is limited (Levene et al., 2000). Mechanisms for prevention of hypovolaemia are limited. Fluid replacement should be administered with caution at 10–20 mls/kg plus urine output. Patent ductus arteriosus, bronchopulmonary dysplasia and necrotising enterocolitis are known complications of over-expanding the infant's extracellular volume (Roberton, 1997). Neonates and low-birthweight infants become dehydrated easily due to the greater surface area proportional to weight, higher metabolic rate, greater proportion of total body water in the extracellular space and a reduced ability to concentrate the urine (Levine et al., 1997).

A pre-term infant is born with a very low GFR, controlled by a delicate balance of intrarenal vasoconstrictor and vasodilator forces. If these are disturbed, forcing the already low GFR down, acute renal failure may follow (Toth-Heyn and Drukker Guignard, 2000).

CHEMICAL EQUILIBRIUM AND ELECTROLYTE DISTURBANCES

Sodium

While term infants are capable of sodium conservation, pre-term infants have difficulty reabsorbing sodium due to the immaturity of the proximal and distal tubules; rapid maturity of the proximal tubule cells occurs between 32 and 35 weeks (Jones and Smith, 1999). For this reason some neonates require a higher sodium intake (greater than the customary 3 mmols/kg/day) (Roberton, 1997). In the sick infant, many factors are present that can severely disrupt sodium homeostasis.

Hypernatraemia can occur if water losses exceed sodium losses. This may occur as a result of an inadequate fluid intake, renal failure, dehydration due to overhead heaters, phototherapy, excessive amounts of intravenous 10% dextrose, diarrhoea or excessive salt supplements.

Clinical presentation may include hypertension with a high risk of central nervous system damage due to the changes in intracerebral fluid distribution. Careful rehydration will be necessary. Sometimes an infant may appear to have a low sodium level and this may be as a result of dilution owing to fluid overload.

Low sodium may be seen in acute renal failure and nephrotic syndrome and, with diuretics or dialysis, the sodium level may return to within normal limits. Giving salt supplements in this situation can be detrimental to the infant, causing retention of more water, making the infant hypertensive and overloaded.

With true hyponatraemia, infants become listless, may develop an ileus, and can be hypotensive. In addition, fitting may be evident. Children in chronic renal failure are often salt losers but are usually polyuric with no sign of hypervolaemia. It is crucial to be able to differentiate between the two types in order to prescribe the correct treatment. This would involve either removal of water or replacement of salt, depending on the reason for hyponatraemia. If the infant is passing urine, a specimen should be taken to see how much salt is being passed in the urine. This may help in deciding treatment.

Potassium

The kidney has limited powers of potassium conservation in term and pre-term infants. Potassium levels are determined by intake, extent of muscle breakdown, aldosterone levels, sodium intake and intracellular hydrogen ion concentration (Gower, 1991).

Hyperkalaemia is the most dangerous of all the electrolyte disturbances. The insidious onset and lack of clinical signs can lead to cardiac arrest, so prompt action is essential. Causes of hyperkalaemia include acute and chronic renal failure, potassium supplements, blood transfusions, acidosis and low renin hypoaldosteronism. Haemolysis of the blood sample may also give an inaccurately high potassium result. Signs and symptoms in the older infant would include muscle weakness and abdominal pain. The neonate may experience vomiting, arrhythmias and diarrhoea. Changes that may be seen on ECG include peaked T waves, reduced R wave, increased PR interval and QRS blends with T waves (Gower, 1991).

Treatment of hyperkalaemia

- 6-hourly calcium resonium enemas of 0.5g/kg – this exchange agent exchanges potassium for calcium ions. It is a very effective short-term treatment but care must be taken with it, as the resin can cause constipation and obstruction, making careful monitoring of bowel function necessary.
- Sodium bicarbonate infusion may be administered to correct acidosis, which reduces the amount of potassium in the blood. It also reduces the level of serum calcium, so an awareness of ionised calcium levels is necessary.
- 10% calcium gluconate 2 ml/kg by slow infusion has a direct antagonist effect on the action of potassium.
- Glucose and insulin infusion in a ratio of 1 unit of insulin per 3 g of dextrose.
- A solution of 0.5 g dextrose as concentrated as possible will encourage the body to produce its own insulin.
- Salbutamol via nebulisers or intravenous infusion may be given at a rate of 4 microgrammes/kg over 20 minutes.

The last three treatments all cause potassium ions to cross the cell membrane and move into the intracellular compartment away from the extracellular space. It is important to monitor blood sugar levels throughout the treatment because hyper/hypoglycaemic episodes may occur. These treatments can be very effective in reducing the potassium level, either until the renal failure resolves or dialysis is commenced (Daugirdas, 1994; Roberton, 1997).

Hypokalaemia

This most commonly occurs due to excessive diarrhoea and vomiting, but may be due to diuretic therapy or over-zealous dialysis. Signs and symptoms are muscle weakness, ileus and arrhythmias. The treatment is simply to manage the underlying cause and give potassium supplements.

Calcium and phosphate

Calcium has an important role in clotting, neurotransmitter release, muscle contraction and the normal heartbeat. Following delivery, calcium values are generally elevated due to the active transfer of calcium from the mother to the foetus in utero. This in turn induces hypoparathyroidism, which raises the infant's phosphate level. In the sick infant with renal insufficiency, calcium disturbances are common. It is important to check the serum albumin, and allowances must be made for co-existent hypoalbuminaemia. On average, the serum calcium can fall by 0.1 mmol/l for each 4 g decrease of serum albumin

(Roberton, 1997). Levels below 1.5mmol/l will begin to cause problems and need to be corrected.

Hypocalcaemia can be induced by giving sodium bicarbonate to correct acidosis. Hypocalcaemia is often seen in acute renal failure. Signs and symptoms to observe are tetany and a positive Chvostek's sign, with ECG changes of prolonged QT interval (with subsequent risk of cardiac arrest). Hypocalcaemia can occur as a result of vitamin D deficiency, hypoparathyroidism and as a side-effect from bicarbonate infusions to correct acidosis. Calcium chloride or gluconate must be given intravenously, with great care, as there is a high risk of causing calcium burns. It is very important during this acute stage to monitor the ionised serum and give calcium gluconate to maintain normal levels.

Hypercalcaemia is rare but can occur as a result of over-zealous treatment of phosphate binders, causing hyperparathyroidism. Symptoms may not be obvious but there may be vomiting, and ECG changes with shortened QRT interval and prolonged P-R interval. Infants in renal failure on calcium carbonate and vitamin D therapy are at risk as well as infants with hyperthyroidism or hyperparathyroidism. Treatment aims to suppress the production of parathyroid hormone (PTH) by correcting phosphate levels and also involves a reduction of any calcium supplements in the form of diet and medication.

Those in renal failure usually require phosphate binders and treatment with vitamin D to maintain calcium levels. An infant in renal failure is unable to excrete phosphate, and this causes a reduction in hydroxylation of vitamin D, which decreases intestinal calcium absorption. This results in the elevation in serum PTH resulting in Ca mobilisation from bone, causing osteodystrophy and an elevation in serum phosphate (see Figure 10.1). This cycle needs to be controlled by giving phosphate binders with each feed and vitamin D supplements.

ACID BASE BALANCE

Acid base balance is about maintaining the constancy of the pH of body fluids. This scale measures the concentration of free hydrogen ions in fluid. As the pH reduces, the hydrogen ion concentration increases. Normal pH is between 7.35 and 7.45 (Wharton, 1998). Acids and bases that work together to minimise changes in pH are called buffers and the most important of these is the bicarbonate buffering system.

The carbonic acid–bicarbonate system plays a primary role in the regulation of bicarbonate concentration through tubular secretion. Bicarbonate ions are freely filtered by the glomerulus. When the plasma bicarbonate is normal, all the filtrate bicarbonate will be reabsorbed. However, if it is higher than normal, the excess is excreted in the urine (Wharton, 1998). Plasma bicarbonate concentration should be around 18 μmols/l at birth increasing to 20 μmols/l by 3 weeks. They will then slowly increase to adult levels (Chevalier, 1994). Acute and chronic renal failure or proximal and distal tubular dysfunctioning causes renal losses of bicarbonate. Treatment by supplements of sodium bicarbonate will help maintain an adequate level until the cause is resolved or dialysis is commenced.

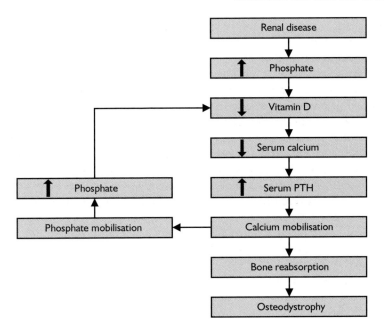

Figure 10.1 Cycle of phosphate excretion in an infant in renal failure

IDENTIFICATION OF DISORDERS

In the first week of life a pre-term infant on established feeds would be expected to lose approximately 1–3% of body weight per day (Roberton, 1997). If weight gain is greater than expected with a raised creatinine, this may indicate overload and renal failure. If weight gain is less, with a rising creatinine, the infant may be dehydrated and require a fluid challenge. Studies have shown that, regardless of gestational age, an infant usually passes urine within the first 24 hours (Chevalier, 1994). Percussion and palpation of the bladder may reveal a distended bladder secondary to urethral obstruction. An infant producing less than 1ml/kg urine per hour after 48 hours would be classed as oliguric (Chevalier, 1994).

One of the first signs of renal failure in the hospitalised infant is raised creatinine in the blood test. An infant with renal disease develops metabolic acidosis through loss of bicarbonate or accumulation of acid (Gower, 1991).

ASSESSMENT AND DIAGNOSIS OF DISORDERS

A pre-natal history of oligohydraminos, with a history of low APGAR score, and perinatal asphyxia indicate a high risk of potential problems, which may result in the development of oliguria (urine flow of less than 1ml/kg/hr) and acute renal failure (ARF). The most common anomalies identified by foetal ultrasound are hydronephrosis, multicystic dysplasia, urinary obstruction and duplications of the collecting systems (Gloor *et al.*, 1995).

Early signs would include an increase of weight greater than expected, oedema and hypertension. If a urine sample can be obtained, haematuria may be present, along with a decreasing osmolarity and creatinine. Culture is necessary to eliminate the possibility of a urinary tract infection and the blood chemistry within the first 24 hours of life may be indicative of fluid retention.

Acute tubular necrosis may be suspected if there is evidence of a raised creatinine, phosphate and urea, hyponatraemia, hyperkalaemia, with a falling albumin, bicarbonate and calcium. However, if the renal failure is due to a metabolic reason, the sodium and chloride may increase (Haycock, 1993).

An abdominal ultrasound of the kidneys and bladder may help to differentiate between an acute or chronic cause for the renal failure.

Urinary infection and congenital malformation of the urinary tract

Haematuria is not uncommon in sick infants; most often it is microscopic. A urine sample should be taken for microscopy and culture but renal vein thrombosis (RVT) may be suspected. Potential urological abnormality should be considered at this stage. Urinary culture must be first undertaken for every sick infant in whom illness or fever persists for more than 24 hours.

Urinary tract infection (UTI)

Diagnosis of urinary tract infection (UTI) in the neonatal period can be overlooked, as symptoms of urinary tract infections of this age group may not be obvious. However, 1.2% of boys and 1.1% of girls have symptomatic bacteraemia during the first year of life (Jones and Smith, 1999). UTI in boys is more often secondary to congenital obstruction, which usually presents within the first few weeks of life. After the first year of life, UTIs are more common in girls (about 3%) than in boys (0.1%). About 5–10% of children will develop renal scarring and about 1% of those become hypertensive in later life.

The newborn infant usually presents with sepsis, fever vomiting and persistent jaundice (Jones and Smith, 1999). Vesicoureteral reflux is the most frequent abnormality found in infants. This can be successfully treated with a course of antibiotics and prophylactic dose should be started. If all the tests prove to be normal, these may be discontinued. However, if dilation and hydronephrosis are present, surgery may be necessary to bypass the obstruction.

There is still no consensus as to the best imaging method for infants who present with urinary abnormalities but most current thinking is to use ultrasound to exclude obstruction, then a micturating cystography to illustrate urinary tract dilation. At about 2 months of age a MAG3 scan may be used; it gives useful information on degree of obstruction, relative renal function and renal artery stenosis and is also referred to as a dynamic renography. DMSA, referred to as static scan, is used mainly in children to identify scarring (Harvey and Bromley, 1999).

Posterior urethral valve (PUV)

This is the most common and severe cause of lower urinary tract abnormalities in male infants, and one of the principal causes of renal failure in newborn infants (Atwell, 1983). A poor urinary stream may be the only symptom present, however, many infants would have been diagnosed pre-natally with ultrasound. If the diagnosis is missed, chronic renal failure may follow in later life.

A variety of obstructive disorders occurs in association with kidney disease, with hydronephrosis, posterior urethral valves, ureteric reflux and mega ureters being among the most common. Obstruction causes a retrograde increase in hydrostatic pressure and dilation, resulting in impaired renal structure and function (Brion *et al.*, 1997). The initial obstruction needs to be surgically relieved by a stent, nephrostomy vesocostomy or supra-pubic catheter. Twenty-five per cent of infants with PUV end up with chronic renal failure (Hounsely and Harrison, 1998).

Hypertension

Hypertension is defined as a blood pressure that consistently exceeds the 95th percentile (Dillon, 1994). Hypertension can be described as transient or persistent high blood pressure. Sixty to seventy per cent of hypertension in infants is caused by renal abnormalities with reflux nephropathy, with obstructive uropathy being the most common (Goonasekera and Dillon, 2000).

The most common persistent causes of neonatal hypertension are vascular anomalies and intrinsic renal disease, followed by coarctation. However, common causes of transient hypertension are often seen; these would include excess administration of fluids, plasma or blood. Hypertension may also occur as a result of side-effects of drugs, pain, urinary obstruction, CNS disorders, bronchodysplasia, pneumothorax, infection and salt supplements.

Pre-renal/renal causes of hypertension account for approximately 60–70% of hypertensive children. These causes include the following:

- renal dysplasia/hypoplasia;
- polycystic kidney disease;
- renal failure;
- obstructive uropathy;
- reflux nephropathy;
- pyelonephritis;
- glomerulonephritis;
- tumour.

A much smaller percentage (10%) are caused by vascular abnormalities including the following:

- renal arterial stenosis;
- renal arterial thrombosis;
- coarctation of the aorta;
- hypoplastic abnormal aorta;
- arterial calcification.

Endocrine abnormalities account for the remaining 20%; they include the following:

- adrenogenital syndrome;
- Cushing's disease;
- hypoaldosteronism;
- thyrotoxicosis.

Assessment and diagnosis

Blood tests should be taken for urea and electrolytes, plasma renin, serum aldosterone, catecholamines.

Investigations may include renal ultrasound and Doppler studies, echocardiogram and various scans, to highlight renal scarring and obstruction. Drug treatments should be carefully monitored and controlled as the complications of long-term uncontrolled hypertension are well recognised:

- cardiac decompensation;
- cerebral infarction;
- intracranial haemorrhage;
- encephalopathy;
- facial palsy;
- renal failure.

Treatment of transient hypertension can involve various hypertensive drugs, dialysis or filtration, or surgery for obstruction. However, long-term treatment for severe vascular causes of hypertension can be difficult and dangerous, with a high morbidity and mortality rate (Dillon, 1994).

Renal failure

Most causes of acute renal failure (ARF) are reversible. The incidence of ARF in the NNU has been reported to range from 1.5% to 23% (Brion *et al.*, 1997), with an estimated 1% of admissions requiring peritoneal dialysis. This number is greatly increased in poor and developing countries (Haycock, 1993). Hypoperfusion caused by birth asphyxia, dehydration and sepsis are the most common causes of ARF in the neonate (Stewart and Barrett, 1999). Infants with acute renal failure display a wide spectrum of volume disorders. It is essential to be able to assess the infant's fluid status. This can be achieved by a careful history of the infant's input and output, weight, vital signs, skin turgor, capillary refill and oedema (Siegel *et al.*, 1994).

The causes of renal failure may be divided into the categories of pre-renal, renal and post-renal.

Pre-renal

- Perinatal asphyxia is the most common cause of ARF in the newborn infant (Stewart and Barrett, 1999).

- Vascular abnormalities include cortical-medullary necrosis, arterial or venous thrombosis and intravascular coagulation.
- Ischaemic necrosis may be a result of hypoxia, dehydration, haemorrhage, sepsis or respiratory distress syndrome.

Renal

- Congenital abnormalities include hypoplasia, dysplasia, polycystic kidney disease and nephrotic syndrome.
- Pyelonephritis and congenital infection.
- Nephrotoxic drugs include aminoglycosides, amphotericin, radiocontrast (Toth-Heyn and Drukker Guignard, 2000). Antibacterials are the primary cause of drug-induced kidney failure (Fanos and Cataldi, 1999).

Post-renal

Causes in this category include:

- posterior urethral valves;
- bilateral ureteropelvic junction obstruction;
- urethral stricture;
- megaureter;
- ureterocele;
- neurogenic bladder;
- urethral diverticulum.

Outcome

The reversal of the underlying condition is the most important factor in determining prognosis (Bonilla-Felix *et al.*, 1998). Sometimes it can be impossible to predict the outcome of pre-term infants until they have reached their term age, due to the fact that the GFR gradually increases for many weeks following birth. However, long-term sequelae may include chronic renal failure, decreasing GFR impaired tubular dysfunction, nephrocalcinosis and impaired growth (McCourt, 1997).

RENAL VEIN THROMBOSIS (RVT)

Thrombosis in the neonatal period is becoming less common with advances in medical knowledge and nursing care. In a large study in neonatal units in Canada, 89% of arterial and venous thrombosis were associated with an intravascular catheter (Schmidt and Andrew, 1995). However, the most likely causes of renal vein thrombosis include sepsis, hypoxia and dehydration, followed by venous catheterisation. This would most commonly occur in the first month of life. RVT is reported to range from 0.1–1.0% in newborn infants and to be as high as 10% in low-birthweight infants (Brion *et al.*, 1997; Ahmed and Swedlund, 1998).

Infants with this problem may present with any of the following:

- haematuria/proteinuria;
- oliguria/anuria;

- anaemia;
- thrombocytopenia.

Unilateral or bilateral renal masses are often palpable. Conservative treatment is often enough, with fluid restriction and treatments to keep the potassium within an acceptable range. Peritoneal dialysis is occasionally used in the more severe cases. Once the condition begins to resolve, a careful review of electrolytes and fluids is necessary, as these infants may become polyuric during the recovery stage. Long-term complications may include renal tubular dysfunction and hypertension.

KIDNEY DISORDERS

Routine ante-natal screening can now detect many renal tract anomalies in the foetus. This means that neonates, especially those with cystic dysplastic kidney disorders, are being referred to specialist units earlier.

Potter Syndrome

These babies are born with dysmorphic clinical features and bilateral renal agenesis. This is a rare condition of 2 in 4000 births, with a male predominance (Levene et al., 2000). This condition is usually incompatible with life.

Polycystic kidney disease

Polycystic kidney disease is the commonest inherited renal disease in the UK, with an incidence of about 1 in 10 000 to 1 in 40 000 (Levene et al., 2000). It can be divided into two conditions: autosomal recessive polycystic disease (RPKD), a rare condition seen in infants and children, and autosomal dominant polycystic disease (DPKD), which is usually found in adolescents and adults.

RPKD is a rare condition. The infant is usually observed to be severely hypertensive, and the large abdomen often causes vomiting and failure to thrive. Diagnosis is usually made with ultrasound. Prognosis is relatively good if the infant survives the neonatal period. Early detection of the disease and appropriate management of systemic or portal hypertension is crucial. Severity of the condition is variable. Death usually results from a combination of respiratory and renal failure, however, the outlook for those children surviving to a year is surprisingly good (Roy et al., 1997).

Multicystic dysplastic kidney disease

With a reported incidence of 1 in 4300, multicystic dysplastic kidney disease (Brion et al.,1997) is the most common form of renal cystic disease in infants. This form of kidney disease results in renal failure, requiring conservative management, and renal replacement therapy is usually necessary. In the short term, the mortality and morbidity is low but, during the long term, the complications of treatment make the prognosis uncertain.

Bartters syndrome

Bartters Syndrome is characterised by persistent hypokalaemia, hypochloraemia, alkalosis, hypernatraemia and hyperaldosteronism in the presence of a normal blood pressure (Brodehi, 1994). Most infants present in the first few weeks of life with lethargy, vomiting and failure to thrive and are found on blood sampling to have very low potassium. The aim of treatment, once the diagnosis has been made, is to replace the electrolytes and keep the infant adequately hydrated.

Congenital nephrotic syndrome

Congenital nephrotic syndrome is an inherited autosomal recessive disorder characterised by heavy proteinuria, hypoalbuminaemia and oedema. The differential diagnosis includes Drash syndrome, which consists of the triad of Wilm's tumour, male pseudohermaphroditism and progressive renal failure. Congenital infection with syphilis, toxoplasmosis, cytomegalovirus, or human immunodeficiency virus can also present with congenital nephrotic syndrome (Savage et al., 1999). It is a very rare condition that occurs primarily in families of Finnish origin and presents shortly after birth. The expected outcome is uncertain if symptoms of proteinuria >20 g/l and hypoalbuminaemia <10 g/l (Holmberg, 1995) persist.

These infants become a challenge for most renal units and are at high risk of sepsis due to poor immune system from lack of proteins. Hypothyroidism and thrombotic complications are also features of the syndrome. The aggressive treatment of 20% albumin infusions to control oedema is often necessary. The risk of pulmonary oedema is high as the infant's kidney function deteriorates. A chemical nephrectomy can be induced with indomethacin 4 mg/kg/day and captopril 4.5 mg/kg/day (Heaton and Smales, 1999), if the proteinuria cannot be controlled. Good nutritional support is essential followed by peritoneal dialysis and transplantation. Dietary supplementation is very important for these children with a high calorie intake and adequate protein necessary for growth.

The severity of this disease varies considerably. Some children, once stabilised, remain in chronic renal failure requiring only medication for many years, while others require much more aggressive treatment. Once transplanted, most of these children do very well.

NURSING CARE OF AN INFANT WITH RENAL FAILURE

Blood pressure

The British Hypertensive Society (de Swiet and Dillon, 1989) recommends the use of a mercury sphygmomanometer and stethoscope for taking blood pressure. Despite considerable research, this remains the most reliable indirect method for measuring blood pressure (Goonasekera and Dillon, 2000), but it can be quite a difficult technique to perform on a small infant. de Swiet and colleagues (1992) recommend using an ultrasonic Doppler device instead of a stethoscope for infants under the age of 5. The bladder size should be at least 80% of the circumference of the arm with the centre of the cuff placed over the artery. The cuff should be inflated to 40 mm above the anticipated blood pressure and the valve released at 2–3 mm/s; a resting phase of 1–2 minutes between readings is advisable. The systolic reading is the reading taken by most paediatric nephrologists, due to much controversy as to where the diastolic pressure reading is read. There is difficulty in interpreting the 4th and 5th Korotkoff sound and detection by auscultation is unacceptably inaccurate. The 4th phase (muffling of Korotkoff sound) is widely misinterpreted and phase 5 (disappearance of Korotkoff sound) can often be zero (de Swiet *et al.*, 1989). Developing the correct technique for measuring blood pressure in infants is very important as false readings can lead to unnecessary treatment and investigations.

A four-limb blood pressure measurement will help distinguish between coarctation and renal involvement. Arterial monitoring saves the infant from being disturbed too frequently, however, this is a very invasive form of monitoring and is only advocated for the critically ill infant. The blood pressure of a pre-term infant can be variable; large increases that are observed can be due to discomfort, passing urine or before vomiting. Blood pressure can be a very helpful indicator of fluid status, but hypertension can be misleading and does not necessary indicate fluid overload. If used in conjunction with other vital signs, such as peripheral temperature and weight, blood pressure measurement can be very useful in helping to prescribe treatment.

Temperature

A peripheral and core temperature measurement gap can be the first sign of fluid overload or fluid depletion. The peripheral and the core temperature should be within 2 degrees centigrade of each other. An increasing gap may be an early indication of fluid depletion, oedema or septicaemia. It is important to change the position of the probe daily to avoid pressure area problems.

Respiration

Continuous oxygen saturation monitoring would be advisable. Tachypnoea may indicate acidosis and falling saturation could be a sign of fluid overload and pulmonary oedema. This is especially important when administering albumin infusions to infants with renal impairment or on dialysis, as the potential rapid fluid shift can cause pulmonary oedema.

Fluid balance

If hypovolaemia is suspected, a fluid challenge should be given; if the infant remains oliguric, frusemide (1–5 mg/kg/dose) may be given (Siegel *et al.*, 1994). If urinary output remains low, very careful fluid restriction may be necessary. Fluid requirements should be carefully assessed at regular intervals giving insensible losses plus urine output hourly. An accurate fluid balance chart should be maintained, measuring all input and output. An accurate measurement of output can be achieved by weighing nappies before use and afterwards (including urine and stool as output). However, if the infant is nursed in a high-humidity incubator, or exposed under an overhead heater, these methods may not be accurate. Catheterisation is only necessary if the infant is known to have an obstructive nephropathy. However, once it has been established that the infant has an empty bladder, the catheter has very little use and comes to represent an unnecessary risk of infection.

Weight

Increasing/decreasing body weight can be a reliable indicator of fluid gain or loss. Checking weight twice daily is one of the best ways of calculating fluid requirements. However, this may be difficult with a ventilated infant. Bed scales or slings can be very useful.

Medication

Medications at this stage will depend on the clinical signs but may include an infusion of frusemide, antihypertensives, dietary supplements and antibiotics. Due to the impaired kidney function, the dosage of drugs must be calculated accordingly. The kidney is the main excretory organ for many drugs, therefore it may be necessary to do more blood harvests for drug levels.

Albumin infusions may be required, starting at 1–2 g/kg, in two divided doses, daily until stabilised. In infants with congenital nephrotic syndrome, the dose may need to be increased, but careful monitoring of vital signs is essential. Frusemide at less than 2 mg/kg daily could result in ototoxicity, so care should be taken. Indomethacin and aminoglycoside should be monitored regularly. Numerous drugs have significant effects on the kidney, therefore the undesired side-effects of drugs must be considered when evaluating the management of each individual infant.

The absorption and metabolism of drugs is considered further in Chapter 16.

Most infants in chronic renal failure need a large quantity of medication. Most children on end-stage programmes may require all of the following:

- sodium supplements for growth and to maintain an adequate blood pressure;
- sodium bicarbonate to correct acidosis;
- vitamin D to correct and prevent bone disease;
- calcium carbonate as a phosphate binder;
- erythropoietin and iron supplements to maintain an adequate haemoglobin;
- folic acid and pyridoxine, which is lost in the dialysis fluid;
- thyroxine.

Feeding

An intensive nutrition programme is essential. This provides a challenge for most dieticians due to the limited fluid requirement of most infants in renal failure. Enteral feeding is usually necessary, with a high-calorie feed. Data collected suggests that infants in renal failure require 130–140% of the recommended daily allowance (Bunchman, 2000). The protein intake will be calculated according to the infant's need, however, if peritoneal dialysis is required, 3–4 g of protein per kilogram of body weight is necessary for adequate growth (Ledermann *et al.*, 2000).

Blood sugar levels

Blood sugar levels need to be checked every 4 hours if the infant is on acute peritoneal dialysis. It is common to absorb glucose from dialysate, especially when the concentration increases above 1.36%. Dextrose in the dialysate provides the osmotic gradient to achieve fluid removal, however, dextrose absorption can be significant and the increased production of PCO_2 will worsen respiratory failure.

END-STAGE RENAL FAILURE

The term 'end-stage renal failure' is normally used for infants who require long-term renal replacement therapy. Due to advances in surgical techniques and nursing care, more pre-term infants are being taken on to end-stage programmes. Over the last two decades many valuable lessons have been learned about first-line management of infants requiring peritoneal dialysis. Two types of catheters may be used: an acute stiff catheter and a long-term single-cuff Tenckhoff catheter. After years of struggling with mechanical problems of leakage, poor outflow and infection with acute catheters, a surgically placed single-cuff Tenckhoff catheter is often the catheter of choice. If this is placed before the infant is excessively swollen and overloaded, it is far less likely to leak and the potential for infection is dramatically reduced.

Continuous veno/venous haemofiltration (CVVH) is fast becoming a very useful way to treat infants in acute renal failure, or for chronic infants who are too overloaded to have a peritoneal catheter inserted. This form of treatment requires a team of highly skilled nurses and has been successfully used in infants who weigh less than 1kg. Continuous arteriovenous haemofiltration (CAVH) is also an option but is largely dependent on arterial blood pressure, which, in sick infants, is difficult to sustain. Vital signs should be monitored and, as with all sick infants, particular attention should be paid to falling saturation levels, which may be an early sign of pulmonary oedema, and hypertension, a sign of fluid overload. A peripheral skin probe is a particularly valuable tool for assessment of fluid balance and may give first indications of vasoconstriction. A twice-daily weight check is vital to assess fluid requirements. If the infant has oedema special care must be taken of the skin due to its fragile nature.

PERITONEAL DIALYSIS

Peritoneal dialysis would be the treatment of choice in neonates with renal failure as it is a gentle form of dialysis. However, if it is anticipated that the renal failure will be a transient problem, an acute catheter can be very valuable.

The following are indications for dialysis:

- hyperkalaemia;
- fluid overload/acute renal failure;
- rapidly rising plasma urea and creatinine in the presence of oliguria;
- metabolic acidosis;
- to create space for nutrition;
- to remove specific poisons;
- pulmonary oedema;
- end-stage disease.

Peritoneal dialysis is a particularly useful treatment in neonates due to the highly vascular peritoneum. The large surface area of the semi-permeable membrane makes it particularly efficient in the removal of water and electrolytes.

Planning the dialysis

A skilled renal specialist will give a 'dry weight', which is the optimum weight for an infant with a normal blood pressure. This is the target weight for planning the dialysis session. If the infant's albumin is low or he or she has oedema, 20% albumin may be given to help draw fluid back into the circulation. This is a very risky treatment for infants on dialysis and should only be considered in extreme cases. Increasing the protein in the diet usually prevents the need for such extreme measures.

Once the catheter is inserted, dialysis can be initiated. In most neonatal areas a manual peritoneal dialysis set is used. A bag of dialysis fluid, Dianeal 1.36% concentration, is attached to a burette, a warming coil, a draining burette and a drainage bag. The circuit should be changed every 24 hours or every time the lines need to be broken for any reason, and a new set should be run through. Daily specimens of peritoneal fluid should be taken for culture and sensitivity. The dialysis prescription should be reviewed regularly and varied according to individual assessment, blood results and vital signs. The infant's blood chemistry, including plasma albumin and haemoglobin, is checked. Hypoalbuminaemia makes removal of fluid more difficult because of reduced osmotic pressure in the intravascular space. An increase in the concentration of glucose may help, but it should be considered as a short-term solution.

Very careful monitoring of the infant's blood pressure and peripheral and core temperature gap is helpful in the initial stabilisation of fluid status at this time. The Tenckhoff site is cleaned and a Kaltostat (calcium-sodium alginate fibre) dressing is left in situ and changed if it becomes soiled. Tension strapping should always be placed on the Tenckhoff to prevent movement of the catheter.

Cycle volumes are based on the child's weight, at 30–50 mls/kg (Ledermann et al., 2000).

Depending on the infant's blood status, additives may be needed, for example, bicarbonate or potassium. Heparin is added to the infusate (200–500 units/l), unless contra-indicated, and the concentration of glucose varies according to volume status. Lignocaine is added to the dialysate to alleviate abdominal pain and discomfort caused by stretching the peritoneal membrane, but its effects are questionable. Regular blood tests for electrolytes are essential when first starting dialysis. The acidotic infant on bicarbonate dialysis is at risk of becoming hypo-calcaemic and potassium removal is very efficient; the dialysis regime may need to be reviewed and changed.

Cycles

Hourly cycles are usually started but these may be increased according to the infant's needs. More frequent cycles may be used to draw off more potassium but care must be taken.

The hourly cycles may proceed as follows:

Fill time	5–10 minutes
Dwell	30 minutes
Drain	20 minutes

Smaller volumes – 10–15 mls/kg – are used at the beginning, building up to 30–50 mls/kg. Gentle clearance of salts is important particularly in the presence of uraemia, as this can lead to imbalance, with resulting signs of cerebral oedema and raised intracranial pressure.

Fluid requirements for the infant on dialysis may be based on the following:

- insensible losses;
- the amount of ultrafiltrate;
- urinary output;
- weight;
- blood pressure.

Complications

Problems with draining can be associated with a badly positioned infant or catheter. However, with the introduction of the practice to use the more permanent Tenckhoff catheters, these problems have been dramatically reduced. Reabsorption of fluid can be an indication of dehydration or hypoalbuminaemia; the glucose concentration may need to be increased or the fluid intake reviewed. The glucose concentration may be increased by 1% by adding 20 mls of 50% glucose to the litre bags of Dianeal, achieving a concentration of 2.36%. A 4.8% concentration of glucose can be achieved if necessary but the blood glucose level should be monitored.

Mechanical problems with filling are usually catheter-related or due to consti-pation. Omentum (part of the lining of the peritoneum) may adhere to the catheter. First-line treatment would be to stop using the catheter and use heparin. If this is unsuccessful, alteplase, used down the line, may help dissolve the blockage. If this does not resolve the problem, early intervention is essential.

An abdominal X-ray would be valuable to indicate the position of the catheter and surgical intervention may be necessary before the infant becomes over-loaded. If this problem is not addressed immediately, the peritoneum becomes stretched and the likelihood of leakage and infection is greatly increased.

Dyspnoea may result from fluid overload or splinting of the diaphragm especially in ventilated infants. The former is resolved by increasing the glucose concentration and the latter by reducing the cycle volume. Tilting the cot is also beneficial. Inguinal and umbilical hernias are frequently recognised complications (Ledermann et al., 2000).

Hyperglycaemia is sometimes apparent and usually resolved by reducing the glucose in the dialysate. Electrolyte disturbances are frequently seen, especially if the infant's condition begins to improve. Hypokalaemia may also be observed in acute renal failure once dialysis has begun. It may be necessary to add potassium chloride at 4 mmols/l to the bags. Blood chemistry needs to be checked at least twice daily during the acute phase and then less regularly as the infant becomes stable on dialysis. Increasing the cycle volume slowly by 10 mls/kg will improve solute clearance. This should be done with caution as fills of greater than 30 mls/kg in the initial few weeks of life have a greater risk of leakage and may cause inguinal and umbilical hernias.

Peritonitis

Episodes of peritonitis have been greatly reduced with surgical placement of Tenckhoff catheters. Peritonitis is diagnosed by the presence of cloudy fluid containing large numbers of white blood cells in drained dialysate (Ledermann et al., 2000). Good standards and technique are the keys to the avoidance of peritonitis. Staphylococcus epidermidis and staphylococcus aureus account for the majority of episodes (Wild, 1997). Fungal peritonitis is uncommon but is the more serious type and carries with it a high morbidity and mortality (Forwell et al., 1987).

Leakage of fluid around the catheter is an unwelcome complication and is indicative of an over-stretched abdomen due to fluid overload. This may result in an increased risk of infection due to the exit site always being moist with a sugary substance. Using an absorbent calcium-sodium alginate dressing, which absorbs serous fluid or leakage and helps to keep the area dry, reduces the risk of infection. Glucose dialysate provides an ideal growth medium for bacteria. If leaking persists once the absorbent dressing is in place, it is advisable for a surgeon to review the position of the catheter, which may need to be replaced in a different site. Fluid volumes for dialysis should be reduced to 10 mls/kg and very gradually increased over 1 to 2 weeks. Ideally, the catheters are left unused for 3 weeks but often this is not practical as the need to remove fluids overrides the risk of using the catheter too early.

Blocked catheters

Omentum or fibrin may become wrapped around the catheter. This may be corrected by repositioning, or relieving constipation. Alternatively, heparin may be added to the infusate. Urokinase used to be the drug of choice to manage occluded lines, however, this will shortly be removed from the market and replaced by alteplase, which is a fibrolytic agent. At present, 2–4 mg are dissolved in 5 mls of saline and should be left in the line for 2–4 hours (Garcia, 1999).

Conclusion

Most causes of renal failure in the neonate are reversible with the correct treatment. Knowledge of renal safety of antibacterial agents and the correct approach to therapeutic drug monitoring are useful elements for preventing iatrogenic renal disorders. However, for those infants who have been left with more permanent damage, the long-term outlook is continuously improving. The treatment of end-stage renal disease by peritoneal dialysis in many young infants does continue to present not only an ethical dilemma, but also a very real practical challenge (Geary, 1998). Ledermann and colleagues (2000) suggest that the outcome for the infant is somewhat related to the ability of the health-care team but is mostly related to the quality of care by the family. A good partnership between the family and health-care professionals is paramount for a good outcome.

For children in end-stage renal failure the aim is to provide adequate dialysis, enhanced nutrition and prevent bone complications and anaemia, to allow the child to grow sufficiently to have a renal transplant. The suitable weight for transplantation is around 10kg, however, smaller infants have received kidney transplants when the options for dialysis have become limited. The significant impact on the infant and on the family is well recognised (Bunchman, 1996). A favourable outcome is expected for most children on long-term programmes. However, the long-term outlook with neurological sequelae of chronic renal failure in the neonate is becoming more evident. Most renal units are now in the second decade of treating very small children with renal replacement therapy.

Interest in xenotransplantation stems from the need to overcome the increasingly severe shortage of human organs. The immunological barriers are fast being reduced through genetic engineering and the development of new drug therapies. However, before this becomes a reality, many complex ethical, social and economic issues must be addressed.

Sample examination questions

Question 1
What techniques can be used to monitor the urine output of a sick newborn infant? (*30 marks*)
How does an ion exchange enema work? (*40 marks*)
What complications may occur during this therapy? (*30 marks*)

Question 2

Jacob was born in a very hypoxic condition 3 weeks ago, and he is still critically ill. He is in renal failure and the consultant has suggested perinatal dialysis. How can the nurse explain this procedure to Jacob's parents? (*75 marks*) What are the long-term complications of this therapy? (*25 marks*)

REFERENCES

Ahmed, S.M. and Swedlund, S.K. (1998) Renal and genitourinary disorders (p. 442). In: Deacon, J. and O'Neill, P. (eds) *Core Curriculum for Neonatal Intensive Care Nursing*, 2nd edition, WB Saunders, Philadelphia, PA, p. 442

Atwell, J.D. (1983) Posterior urethral valves in the British Isles: a multicenter BAPS review, *Journal of Pediatric Surgery* 18(1), 70–4

Bunchman, T.E. (1996) The ethics of infant dialysis, *Peritoneal Dialysis International* 16 [supplement], 3–6

Bunchman, T.E. (2000) Infant dialysis: the future is now, *Journal of Paediatrics* 136(1), 1–2

Bonilla-Felix, M., Brannan, P. and Portman, R.J. (1998) In: Deacon, J. and O'Neill, P. (eds) *Core Curriculum for Neonatal Intensive Care Nursing* (2nd edition), WB Saunders, Philadelphia, PA, pp. 442–73

Brion, L.P., Bernstein, J. and Spitzer, A. (1997) In: Deacon, J. and O'Neill, P. (eds) *Core Curriculum for Neonatal Intensive Care Nursing* (2nd edition), WB Saunders, Philadelphia, PA, pp. 442–73

Brodehi, J. (1994) Renal tubular disorders. In: Postlewaite, R.J. (ed.) *Clinical Paediatric Nephrology* (2nd edition), Butterworth-Heinemann, Oxford, pp. 290 –304

Chevalier, R.L. (1994) Renal disease in neonates. In: Postlewaite, R.J. (ed.) *Clinical Paediatric Nephrology* (2nd edition), Butterworth-Heinemann, Oxford, pp. 373–88

Daugirdas (1994) The possible effects of dialyser membrane on morbidity and mortality, *Nephrol. Dial. Transplant* 1994 2, 145–9

De Swiet, M. and Dillon, M.J. (1989) Measurement of blood pressure in children; recommendations of working party of the British Hypertension Society, *BMJ* 299 (6697), 469–70

De Swiet, M., Fayers, P. and Shinebourne, E. (1992) Blood pressure in the first ten years of life (The Brompton Study) *BMJ* 304, 23–6

Dillon, M. (1994) Hypertension. In: Postlewaite, R.J. (ed.) *Clinical Paediatric Nephrology* (2nd edition), Butterworth-Heinemann, Oxford, pp. 175–95

Ellis, E.N., Pearson, D., Champion, B. and Wood, E.G. (1995) Outcomes of infants on chronic peritoneal dialysis, *Adv Perit Dial* 11, 266–9

Fanos, V. and Cataldi, L. (1999) Antibacterial-induced nephrotoxicity in the newborn, *Drug Safety* 20(3), 245–67

Forwell, M.A., Smith, W.G., Tsakiris, D. *et al.* (1987) Morbidity of fungal peritonitis, *Contrib. Nephrology* 57, 110–13

Garcia, M.G. (1999) *Guidelines and Formulary*, GOSH Pharmacy Department, London

Geary, D.F. (1998) Attitudes of paediatric nephrologists to manage end-stage renal disease in infants, *Journal of Paediatrics* 133(1), 154–6

Gloor, J.M., Ogburn, P.L. and Brekle, R.J. (1995) In: Deacan, J. and O'Neill, P., *Core Curriculum for Neonatal Intensive Care Nursing* (2nd edition), WB Saunders, Philadelphia, PA, p. 448

Goonasekera, C.D and Dillon, M.J. (2000) Measurement and interpretation of blood pressure, *Archives of Disease Childhood*, 82(3), 261–5

Goonasekera, C.D.A, Wade, A., Slattery, M., Brennan, E. and Dillon, M.J. (1999) Performance of a new blood pressure monitor in children and young adults, *Blood Pressure* 7, 231–7

Gower, P.E. (1991) *Handbook of Nephrology* (2nd edition), Blackwell Science, Oxford

Harvey, C. and Biomley, M. (1999) Renal imaging, *Medicine* 27(5), 14–21

Haycock, A. (1993) Acute renal failure in the newborn infant, *Care of the Critically Ill* 9(6), 250–4

Heaton, P. and Smales, O. (1999) Congenital nephrotic syndrome responsive to captopril and indomethacin, *Archives of Disease in Childhood*, 81, 74–175

Holmberg, C., Antikainen, M., Ronnholnm, K. *et al.* (1995) Management of congenital nephrotic syndrome of the Finnish type, *Pediatric Nephrology* 9(1), 87–93

Hounsely, H.T. and Harrison, M.R. (1998) In: Deacan, J. and O'Neill, P., *Core Curriculum for Neonatal Intensive Care Nursing* (2nd edition), WB Saunders, Philadelphia, PA, p. 448

Jones, K.V. and Smith, C.G. (1999) Urinary tract infections in childhood, *Medicine* 27(7), 71–5

Ledermann, S.E., Scanes, M.E. *et al.* (2000) Long-term outcome of peritoneal dialysis in infants, *Journal of Paediatrics* 136(1), 24–9

Levine, E., Hartman, D.S. *et al.* (1997) Current concepts and controversies in imaging of renal cystic disease, *Urology Clinicians (North America)* 24(3), 523–43

Levene, M.D., Tudehope, I. and Thearle, M. (2000) In: *Neonatal Medicine* (3rd edition), Blackwell Science, Oxford

McCourt, M. (1997) In: Deacan, J. and O'Neill, P., *Core Curriculum for Neonatal Intensive Care Nursing* (2nd edition), WB Saunders, Philadelphia, PA

Roberton, N.R.C. (1997) *Neonatal Intensive Care* (3rd edition), Edward Arnold, London, pp. 42–3

Roy, S., Dillon, M.J., Trompeter, R. S. and Barrett, T.M. (1997) Autosomal recessive polycystic kidney disease: long-term outcome of neonatal survivors, *Paediatric Nephrology* 11(3), 302–6

Savage, J.M., Jefferson, J.A., Maxwell, A.P. *et al.* (1999) Improving prognosis for congenital nephrotic syndrome of the Finnish type in Irish families, *Archives of Disease in Childhood* 80(5), 466–96

Schmidt, B. and Andrew, M. (1995) Neonatal thrombosis: report of a prospective Canadian and International Registry, *Pediatrics* 96(5), 939–43

Siegel, N.J., Van Why, S.K., Boydstun Devarajan, P. and Gaudio, K.M. (1994) Acute renal failure. In: Holliday, M.A., Barratt, T.M. and Avner, E.D. (eds) *Pediatric Nephrology* (3rd edition), William and Wilkins, Baltimore, MA, pp. 1176–203

Stewart, C.L. and Barrett, R. (1999) In: Deacan, J. and O'Neill, P., *Core Curriculum for Neonatal Intensive Care Nursing* (2nd edition), WB Saunders, Philadelphia, PA, p. 448

Toth-Heyn, P.A. and Drukker Guignard, J. (2000) The stressed neonatal kidney; from pathophysiology to clinical management of neonatal vasomotor nephropathy, *Paediatric Nephrology* 14(3), 227–39

Wharton, S. (1998) Applied anatomy and physiology. In: Smith, T. (ed.) *Renal Nursing*, Baillière Tindall, London, pp. 31–72

Wild, J. (1997) Peritoneal dialysis. In: Smith, T. (ed.) *Renal Nursing*, Baillière Tindall, London, pp. 247–319

Wolfish, N.M. and Mongeau, J.G. (1983) Pediatric nephrology. In: Levine, D.Z. (ed.) *Care of the Renal Patient*, WB Saunders, Philadelphia, PA, pp. 133–4

11 NURSING CARE OF AN INFANT WITH A NEUROLOGICAL DISORDER

Doreen Crawford

Aims of the chapter

This chapter outlines the anatomy and physiology of the developing brain. This developmental overview is related to the conditions most commonly seen on the neonatal unit. The essential nursing care of an infant with a neurological condition is considered, and the implications of altered anatomy and functioning in the individual is discussed.

INTRODUCTION

Although the brain and central nervous system develops in advance of most of the other organs and systems in the body, it is still relatively immature at term (MacGregor, 2000). The brain of the infant born before term is very vulnerable. Because the brain is such a key organ there is the risk that even 'minor' damage can result in catastrophic implications for the individual. The brain is susceptible to malformation and damage during embryonic and foetal life and hazards include viral infection, radiation, drugs, and other toxins such as excessive alcohol. Insult to the neurological tissue can result from foetal hypoxia and malnourishment, from placental insufficiency, as well as severe maternal illness and deprivation.

There are critical periods of development during which these hazards can exert their influence and cause damage, perhaps before the mother is aware of her pregnancy. The earliest recognisable neuro tissue is found approximately 18 days after conception. Dating is approximate, as there is debate about the accuracy of staging in embryology. The embryogenesis of the brain and central nervous tissue is complex, but a basic comprehension of normal development allows appreciation of the structure and function of the central nervous system, and aids understanding of defective development and neuro-pathology.

RELEVANT ANATOMY OF THE CENTRAL NERVOUS SYSTEM

Neurological development continues throughout gestation and is not complete until the end of the first decade of life.

Embryological development is divided into three stages:

- neuralation;
- secondary canalisation;
- retrogressive differentiation.

Neuralation (very early development)

This stage covers post-conceptual age 18–27 days. During this time early neuro tissue appears as an area of thickened embryonic neuroectoderm. This becomes known as the neural plate, which will eventually develop into the brain and spinal cord. The neural plate invaginates (it forms a groove), flanked by the neural folds. As this groove deepens, the top-most edges of the neural folds begin to fuse, at approximately 22–24 days, giving rise to the neural tube. The neural folds do not fuse simultaneously. Initially they fuse near the middle of the neural tube, opposite somites 2–7 (O'Rahilly *et al.*, 1977) and continue in both cephalic (towards the top) and caudal (towards the bottom) directions. The neural tube is formed by the 4th week of pregnancy.

Neural tube defects, such as anencephaly and myelomeningocele (*see below*), are a result of failure of the neural tube to fuse.

Secondary canalisation

This stage covers day 28 to day 51 – a period of explosive development. With neural tube closure, the cephalic end expands and constrictions appear. These constrictions divide this part of the neural tube into three primary brain vesicles called the prosencephalon (the forebrain), the mesencephalon (the midbrain) and the rhombencephalon (the hindbrain).

Further sub-division of the forebrain and hindbrain results in five structures called the secondary brain vesicles. The prosencephalon divides and forms the telencephalon (endbrain) and diencephalon (interbrain). The telencephalon, with further development, eventually results in the cerebral hemispheres. The diencephalon is the posterior part of the forebrain. Three swellings occur on each side of the diencephalon, eventually resulting in the thalamus, epithalamus and the hypothalamus.

The mesencephalon remains undivided.

The rhombencephalon has constricted to form both the metencephalon (afterbrain), which becomes the pons and cerebellum, and the myelencephalon (spinal brain), which becomes the medulla oblongata.

The midbrain and hindbrain structures, with the exception of the cerebellum, eventually become the brain stem.

Retrogressive differentiation

This occurs between 52 and 80 days. Some of the embryonic landmarks are lost, like the tail and structures within it.

During embryogenesis the brain develops its general shape, which is a framework for the sophisticated nervous system. In the period following embryogenesis, there is rapid neuroblast multiplication, when the adult numbers of cells are laid down. Final maturation of these cells with myelination may not occur until the individual is several years old (MacGregor, 2000).

Development of the ventricles

The central cavity of the neural tube remains continuous and becomes enlarged in four areas, resulting in the ventricles. They are lined by ependymal cells and filled with cerebrospinal fluid (CSF). With the convolutions of the brain and spinal cord, owing to the restricted space for development, the lateral ventricles become well-defined C-shaped structures by approximately 12 weeks gestation. Each lateral ventricle communicates with the third ventricle and the third ventricle is continuous with the fourth. Within the fourth ventricle, there are three apertures, which connect with the subarachnoid space and bathe the brain in CSF.

Close to the ventricles is the highly vascular subependymal germinal matrix. Between 10 and 20 weeks gestation this area serves as a main site of cerebral neuroblasts. It is of particular interest to neonatal nurses as it is the area where intraventricular haemorrhage (IVH) most commonly originates. The many thin-walled blood vessels around this area are prone to bleeding, in certain circumstances, if premature delivery has occurred. As the foetus matures, the matrix progressively decreases in size. By 36 weeks it has undergone nearly complete involution (Volpe, 1989).

Development of the cerebral hemispheres

The cerebral hemispheres arise from the telencephalon. Owing to rapid growth and restricted space, they are forced backwards and sideways (posteriorly and laterally), and shroud the diencephalon and midbrain.

At 15 weeks gestation, the cerebral hemispheres are smooth and have no sulci and gyri. Convolution of the cerebral cortex, which gives the cerebral hemispheres their familiar external pattern, facilitates an increase in cortical size without an increase in cranial volume. The number of sulci and gyri increases until, at birth, the surface of the cerebral cortex covers twice the visible area. Because of the rapid growth there are high 'fuel' requirements. Unfortunately the blood supply to these areas is single and fairly tenuous; it is almost a case of the levels of growth outstripping the supply. If delivery occurs between 24 and 28 weeks, and adequate oxygen fails to reach these areas, they are particularly susceptible to ischaemia and will infarct. Clinically these are classed as areas of periventricular leucomalacia and will show up on ultrasound scan as 'flares'. Depending on the size of the infarcted areas they may then become cystic-forming cavities in the brain giving a characteristic appearance on the ultrasound scans. Interconnection of the network of blood vessels to supply the brain becomes more complex from about 30 weeks gestation and the brain becomes less vulnerable to ischaemic injury.

There are many causes of neuropathogenesis, some related to deviation from normal development. Few conditions have such an impact on the individual and their family as malformation or malfunction of the neurological system. The nurse is in a unique position to support and care for all concerned whatever the reason for admission.

Table 11.1 From embryo to foetus: early brain development

Neuralation	18–27 days	Thickened embryonic neuroectoderm; invagination of the neural plate, formation of the neural folds, fusion of the neural folds; formation of the neural tube
Canalisation	28–51 days	Cephalic end of the neural tube expands; constrictions appear on the neural tube to form the forebrain, midbrain and hindbrain; further sub-divisions of forebrain and hindbrain; out-growths of the forebrain develop into eyes; development of the cranial nerves
Retrogressive differentiation	52–80 days	Loss of embryonic structures such as tail; rapid neuroblast multiplication; enlargement of central cavity of neural tube resulting in ventricles
Foetal development	12–20 weeks	Ventricles are well-defined C-shaped structures; rapid growth in restricted space forces the developing cerebral hemispheres to shroud and cover the midbrain; initially cerebral cortex is smooth; rapid convolution of cortex forms sulci and gyri, giving increase in surface area

NEUROLOGICAL CONDITIONS SEEN ON THE NEONATAL UNIT

Neurological conditions seen on the NNU include the following:

- neonatal intracranial haemorrhage;
- hypoxic-ischaemic encephalopathy/birth asphyxia and sequel;
- seizures;
- structural malformations and hydrocephalus;
- meningitis;
- neonatal hypotonia/the floppy infant.

This list is not exhaustive or in any order of priority, and some of the conditions are seen more frequently than others. Some of the most common conditions are discussed below.

Neonatal intracranial haemorrhage

There are several types of intracranial haemorrhage:

- periventricular intracranial haemorrhage;
- subarachnoid haemorrhage;
- cerebellar haemorrhage;
- subdural haemorrhage.

The most common is the periventricular-intraventricular (PVH-IVH) haemor-rhage of the pre-term infant. Although this can be regarded as a complication of prematurity it is also to be found in the term infant. For guidance on the care of a pre-term infant with this condition, *see* below.

The true incidence of subarachnoid haemorrhage in neonates is probably unknown, as minor bleeding could occur during birth and the infants remain stable and well. A few red blood cells or mild xanthochromia (the result of red cell breakdown) in the cerebro-spinal fluid is often a coincidental finding on lumbar puncture or post-mortem in infants not previously suspected of having suffered a haemorrhage. Mercuri *et al.* (1998) found a surprisingly high number of intracranial ultrasound abnormalities in a random selection of well term infants on the post-natal ward. Significant subarachnoid haemorrhage, however, may result in seizures and hydrocephalus. The prognosis is variable.

Cerebellar haemorrhage is infrequent but may be seen as an extension from other bleeds. It may also be seen where the infant has been heparinised for extra-corporeal management or where the infant has a major metabolic error, resulting in bizarre blood pictures and clotting abnormalities.

Subdural haemorrhage is rare but may be seen following traumatic deliveries with a prolonged second stage and excessive moulding. The clinical presentation depends on the extent of the bleed, with severe bleeds being associated with early signs of raised intracranial pressure, unresponsiveness and deterioration in condition. More moderate bleeds may involve a fluctuation in level of consciousness, jaundice and anaemia. Later presentations include subdural haematoma irritability, altered consciousness, poor feeding, vomiting, generally not thriving and an infant who is difficult to soothe and mother (Pellock and Myer, 1993).

Improvements in obstetric management and in neonatal care have significantly improved the morbidity and mortality attributed to periventricular-intraventricular haemorrhages, although it is still one of the most serious and common neurological conditions (Schwartz *et al.*, 1993). Although the exact pathogenesis of periventricular-intraventricular haemorrhage is not understood, several factors are thought to predispose to the rupture of delicate blood vessels. These are: poor condition at birth, respiratory distress syndrome, acidosis and high levels of CO_2. Sudden swings between hypoxia and hyperoxia and infusion of base may also be implicated. Coagulation abnormalities, fluctuation of blood pressure may also contribute, as may sudden stresses such as insensitive handling, physiotherapy and endotracheal suction (Perlman and Volpe, 1983; Wallace, 1998).

The sicker and earlier the infant, the higher the likelihood of intraventricular haemorrhage. As always, prevention is preferred to cure. Nursing interventions to reduce the risk of IVH include consideration of the infant's position – intracranial pressure was found to be lowest when the head was slightly elevated and in the midline (Kling, 1989). Obstruction of venous outflow caused by tight strapping to protect infusion sites or secure endotracheal tubes has been implicated. Whenever possible, strapping should not circumvent the head. The aim of all nursing interventions must be to handle the infant as gently and as little as possible, to prevent sudden swings in pressure, which may affect cerebral blood flow. Other causative factors are beyond medical control and nursing prevention.

Different therapeutic agents have been tried to limit the occurrence and extent of haemorrhage, including vitamin E, fresh frozen plasma and indomethacin. It is difficult accurately to predict the final extent of disability, if any (Andersen, 1989).

Birth asphyxia (hypoxic-ischaemic encephalopathy)

Asphyxia as a term has become less than useful and it has been suggested that the terminology be modified, to decrease the possibility of misunderstanding (Committee on Obstetrical Practice, 1994; Holbrook *et al.*, 1997). The term 'hypoxia' refers to diminished oxygen delivery to tissues despite adequate blood flow. 'Anoxia' refers to the absence of oxygen delivery to tissues despite adequate blood flow. 'Asphyxia' encompasses both terms and in addition involves tissue-damaging acidotic changes in the infant's blood gas picture (Holbrook *et al.*, 1997). The distinction is important, as there is an increasing trend towards litigation as parents seek to provide for a damaged child. Volpe (1987) has suggested that 90% of hypoxic, ischaemic, cerebral injuries occur antepartum or intrapartum.

Regulation of the cerebral blood flow

Under normal circumstances the control of the cerebral blood is tightly regulated with the local blood vessels vasodilating and constricting in response to subtle changes in blood gas. This process is called autoregulation and is independent of normal systemic blood pressure fluctuations. The regulation of this in the pre-term infant is thought to be less precise, creating a more pressure-passive cerebral circulation. Nelle and colleagues (1997) found that even bolus feeds caused significant swings in cerebral blood flow velocity, attributed to the infant digesting their meal. Animal models have suggested that hypoxia before or during birth, even at term, can also stretch the cerebral pressure-compensating mechanisms to the limit, particularly if the insult is prolonged (Gunn *et al.*, 1997; Holbrook *et al.*, 1997).

As obstetric screening procedures become more sophisticated, the number of severely asphyxiated infants and the number subjected to unnecessary obstetric intervention should decline. Hypoxic insult is no respecter of gestation terms; although the pre-term infant is more at risk, the term infant can also be affected.

There are various degrees of severity. Infants with mild hypoxia who respond rapidly to minimal resuscitation, who have good APGAR scores and observant mothers, may not even be admitted to a neonatal unit. Others are less fortunate and need a period of observation. Severely asphyxiated infants, who have been in terminal apnoea, have a variable and not always favourable prognosis. Many of these will require full supportive pulmonary ventilation and some may never be able to self-ventilate.

Following terminal apnoea, spontaneous respiration cannot occur. Prolonged resuscitation can occasionally revive an infant who is profoundly asphyxiated but may result in severe neurological sequel. Initial assessment cannot accurately predict outcome. Levene (1988, 1995) and Zideman and colleagues (1998) concluded that resuscitative measures should be abandoned if an infant has had no cardiac output for 10–15 minutes or has made no effort to breathe spontaneously by 30 minutes after establishment of cardiac output (*see* Chapter 5).

Complications of severe hypoxia

Infants with severe hypoxia are very sick and may have cardiovascular, renal, gastro-intestinal complications, as well as cerebral complications (Perlman, 1989).

Cardiovascular effects of severe hypoxia may result in instability, with hypotension and poor perfusion. The heart, although more resilient than some other organs, can be damaged by ischaemia, resulting in arrhythmia and cardiac failure.

If treatment is to continue, the infant will need skilled medical and nursing care. This may involve the management of several lines, giving infusions of volume expanders such as human albumin, to maintain blood pressure and help correct acidosis, as well as dopamine, to improve vascular tone and raise blood pressure. Such fluid input needs to be balanced with careful monitoring of fluid output as it is vital not to overload these infants.

These infants are prone to cerebral oedema occurring as a result of intracellular and extracellular accumulation of fluid; little can be done for this, except restriction of fluids. Mannitol and frusemide may be used, provided that cardiac and renal perfusion is adequate. Cerebral oedema may give rise to signs of raised intracranial pressure such as increasing blood pressure, decreasing heart rate and irregular respiratory pattern. Regular observation of these vital signs can greatly assist management.

Cerebral oedema and brain injury may result in an irritable and restless infant who can be hyper-responsive to stimulation. The infant should be kept warm and comfortable in a quiet environment with muted light, and should not be over-stressed with too much handling.

Care has focused on the supportive management of a critically unstable infant having suffered hypoxia. In the future, nurses may be actively involved in efforts to protect the infant's brain by using a cooling cap to induce selective hypothermia. This is based on the principle that there may be a therapeutic window of time before the intracellular events that lead to brain cell death begin their catastrophic cascade (Robertson and Edwards, 1998). Animal studies have suggested that rapid death did not result in observable changes to brain tissue, whereas necrotic changes were observed in the survivors (Holbrook *et al.*, 1997).

Impaired renal function is common, even in cases of mild hypoxia. Severe anoxia can result in both tubular and cortical necrosis. Pressure or displacement can cause inappropriate antidiuretic hormone release and subsequent fluid retention. These infants need careful monitoring of fluid balance and all urine needs to be tested for protein and blood. If the damage is minimal, no further intervention is required. Others will require resin ion exchange enemas or dialysis (*see* pages 218–21).

Gastro-intestinal complications, such as necrotising enterocolitis (NEC), may occur from intestinal tissue hypoxia. (For more on NEC, *see* Chapter 5.)

The prognosis for asphyxiated infants is variable. Recovery can occur within hours. On the other hand, if, after a few days, other signs of neurological abnormality occur, the prognosis is bleak. Severe hypoxia may result in profound stupour or convulsions, which may be difficult to control.

Neonatal seizures

The incidence of neonatal seizures varies from 1.5 to 14 per 1000 live births, depending on the sample (Painter and Gaus, 1993). However, for the neonatal nurse, witnessing a seizure is a common event. The seizure activity may be the first manifestation of neurological dysfunction over a variety of insults (Evans and Levene, 1998). Convulsions, fits, seizures, blue do's, funny turns, twitching, and jitteriness are all terms which are frequently heard and understood in the NNU culture and understanding is easy when there is an infant in front of you, displaying the described activity. Brown and Minns (1988) suggested that the term 'seizure' should be used to describe any paroxysmal event, which may or may not be a fit. Evans and Levene (1998) modified a classification of seizure types, which is extremely easy to understand, and have focused on subtle, clonic, myoclonic and tonic activity. Many seizure activities, reported by nurses, are generalised motor disturbances, which may be accompanied by apnoea.

Management of seizure activity is aimed at the underlying cause as well as control. Prescribed medication by bolus or by continuous infusion may include drugs such as phenobarbitone, phenytoin, benzodiazepines such as diazepam and clonazepam as well as paraldehyde.

Causes of seizure activity

Causes of seizure activity may include the following:

- asphyxia/profound hypoxia;
- metabolic disturbance;
- intracranial haemorrhage;
- malformation;
- genetic;
- infection;
- toxicity.

Asphyxia

Asphyxia, resulting in hypoxic ischaemic encephalopathy, is the most common cause of neonatal seizure activity. The seizures may be difficult to control (Levene, 1987; Evans and Levene, 1998). The full range of anticonvulsants may be tried, singly or in combination, until activity is controlled. This may result in high serum drug levels in infants who have ischaemic damage to other organs and such drastic polypharmacy may be hazardous (Mizrahi, 1989). According to Evans and Levene (1998), the positive benefits of seizure control outweigh the deleterious effects of anticonvulsant medication. However, the drugs are often ineffective in controlling all seizures either clinically or electrically.

Clark (1989) suggested that some seizure activity may be the result of excitatory amino acids in the traumatised brain, resulting ultimately in neuronal death. This research suggests it may ultimately be possible to block the activity of such amino acids with a therapeutic agent.

Metabolic seizures
Hypoglycaemia, hypocalcaemia and hyponatraemia all cause seizure activity that responds to correction of the underlying cause. Rare metabolic disturbances are best left to specialist units to diagnose and manage. Unfortunately, the ability to diagnose exceeds the ability to cure. For many of these families, genetic advice is necessary to prevent recurrence.

Intracranial haemorrhage
Seizure activity resulting from intracranial haemorrhage occurs owing to the presence of blood in the meninges or ventricles, brain tissue damage, compression from extensive blood clot or ischaemia from interruption of blood supply.

Malformation
A structurally malformed brain or a rare genetic syndrome may manifest seizure activity, as may cystic areas that are the result of periventricular leucomalacia. Hydrocephalus results in surprisingly few seizures, provided that the intracranial pressure is not elevated. Management of the infant with a hopelessly abnormal brain may result in ethical dilemmas, during which the parents and the family will need all the support that the nurse can give.

Infection
Infants with severe infection and meningitis may display seizure activity, which should be treated by anticonvulsants. The cause of seizure activity from infection varies. It may arise from secondary metabolic disturbance, dehydration or neurotoxins produced by bacteria, as well as meningeal irritation, emboli or thrombosis. Final resolution of this seizure activity depends on the initial cause and success of antibiotic therapy.

Toxicity
Kernicterus is now a rare cause of neonatal seizures although, with increasingly early discharge and a growing interest in home births, it may make a rare comeback in a few cases. Seizures from foetal alcohol syndrome and withdrawal from narcotics in the infants of addicted mothers are rare. Seizure can be caused by toxins produced by infection (*see above*).

The prognosis from neonatal seizure is variable; poorly controlled seizure, with early severe onset has a poor prognosis (Painter and Gaus, 1993). Temple and colleagues (1995) suggested that, with children who survived and were thought to be normal, the long-term follow-up indicated that they tended to have more difficulties with memory, arithmetic and spelling despite 'normal intelligence'.

Structural malformations and hydrocephalus

The main categories of structural malformation are:

- anencephaly;
- encephalocele;
- spina bifida occulta;
- spina bifida cystica.

In anencephaly there is developmental failure resulting in the absence of forebrain. The incidence is about 1 in 1000 (Roberton, 1993) and the defect is incompatible with life. No attempt at resuscitation should be made. Sometimes there are signs of life and the infant may move and occasionally gasp, but the situation remains hopeless. Where possible, the family should be cared for together with sensitive support for the parents. There is some risk of reccurrence and the families involved need counselling. Increasingly, parents of affected infants are asking about donation of their infant's organs.

Encephalocele occurs when there is a failure of midline closure; it is comparatively rare and 80% of these lesions are occipital (Levene, 1987). These defects can be skin-covered. The prognosis can be poor and depends on how much brain tissue is in the sac. Complications during delivery can result in severe damage and full assessment should be made as soon as possible.

Spina bifida occulta is a defect in the spine. In many cases the diagnosis is made by X-ray for unrelated problems or by examination and chance; many cases go undetected. The cord and meninges are normal and no disability need be involved.

Spina bifida cystica can be further divided into meningocele and meningomyelocele. Meningocele is a herniation of the meninges and gathering of cerebrospinal fluid within the defect. It can occur anywhere along the spinal cord and disability need not arise as the cord is structurally normal. Rapid surgical intervention is recommended. In meningomyelocele the defect can be open and much more severe as it can involve the spinal cord. Disabilities resulting from this lesion can be extensive.

These structural malformations are caused by a failure of part of the tube to fuse. This occurs in the first month of pregnancy and many factors have been incriminated, such as genetic, familial, dietetic, toxins and environmental factors; sadly, there is a high risk of recurrence. Research has supported the use of additional folic acid in women who wish to become pregnant and during the first trimester. Folic acid has a role to play in the development of neural tube defects (Czeizel, 1993). This is an example of positive health promotion, but the increased awareness and extensive media coverage may also cause women with affected foetuses to experience guilt in relation to their diet and lifestyle. Improvements in pre-natal diagnosis and the increase in pregnancy terminations has resulted in fewer of these infants coming to the NNU (Seller, 1989).

Much work has been done since Lorber (1971) initially postulated that surgery at all costs was not always in the best interests of the child. The decision to treat actively or conservatively is not made in isolation but involves family, physiotherapists, medical and nursing staff. Prior to active treatment, careful assessment is made and surgery performed as soon as possible, provided that there is adequate skin cover, to prevent ascending infection. Tissue expansion is now possible (Moss, 1992), which can provide extra skin but, if the lesion is so vast that early primary closure is not possible, the resulting neurological, urological and orthopaedic deficit may be equally extensive.

Improved surgical techniques have enhanced the overall prognosis (Noetzel, 1989) of infants with myelomeningocele. For infants with hydrocephalus at birth, simultaneous shunt placement is desirable. Not all NNUs have facilities for neurosurgery and the infant may need to be transferred. Photographs of the child should be taken for the parents whether the child is malformed or not.

Surgeons' preferences and local protocols differ. However the lesion should be kept covered and moist with a non-adherent sterile dressing or saline gauze. In small infants, who have difficulty maintaining their temperature, this may not be ideal. A sterile U drape, as used in transporting exomphalos infants, could be used, as could cling film or other non-adherent materials. None of these are absolutely ideal or universally recommended.

To try and minimise contamination by soiling and limit any further neurological damage, the infant should be kept prone. This method of management usually means that they are nursed exposed in an incubator, to maintain warmth and facilitate observation. This, unfortunately, provides a physical barrier between the parents and their offspring.

There is no reason why the infant cannot be fed milk until approximately 4 hours prior to surgery, when a dextrose infusion should be started, to maintain hydration and blood glucose.

Post-operatively, the infusion is continued until the infant is ready to consume milk. The cannula is maintained for antibiotic therapy, if prescribed. The infant is nursed prone and the dressing and drainage monitored for signs of oozing. Frequent observation of head circumference is vital, to detect hydrocephalus. Nursing observation of bowel and bladder function can be useful to establish the extent of associated urinary and bowel problems and occasionally manual expression of the bladder may be necessary to prevent urinary stasis.

Once the infant has recovered and the lesion has healed sufficiently, intensive limb physiotherapy is commenced. At this stage, the parents can make up for all the cuddles they were perhaps afraid to give pre-operatively.

Hydrocephalus is treated by the insertion of a shunt, which prevents intracranial pressure from building up because of dilated fluid-filled ventricles.

Surprisingly, the procedure disturbs the infant very little unless complications occur. Many return from theatre hungry and ready to feed.

Meningitis

Infection of the meninges (the two delicate membranes covering the brain) may occur before, during or after birth. Intra-uterine infection assumes transplacental crossing of organisms or severe ascending infection following premature rupture of the membranes. Infection during birth and in the neonatal period can come from contamination by hands, instruments, inhalation, ingestion or inoculation. The sicker the infant, the greater the intervention required and therefore the more likely the risk of infection.

The pre-term infant has a less than effective immunity system, with reduced levels of immunoglobulin synthesis, few circulating white cells and complement levels that are about half that of an adult (Davies, 1988).

Prevention of such infection would be ideal and stringent hygiene regulations apply at all times when caring for such vulnerable infants.

Unfortunately, neonatal meningitis is common and a major neonatal emergency. The initial signs are often non-specific. In neonatal unit jargon, infants may present as follows:

- They may go 'off their feeds', meaning not taken their usual amount of feed with the accustomed enthusiasm or not tolerating the feed, and vomiting.
- They may look 'off colour', meaning they are pale, mottled, flushed or jaundiced.
- They may not 'handle well', meaning that they may be irritable, and not settling, not welcoming attention, arching and fussing, tense or hypotonic.

The infant's temperature may fluctuate and there is often a wide gap between the core and peripheral temperature owing to poor perfusion. Blood glucose may be elevated as part of a generalised stress reaction. Vital signs may deviate from the usual baseline. Later signs include seizure activity, tense and bulging fontanelle, posturing such as opisthotonos and increasing head circumference. Neonatal nurses are in a prime position to detect the early signs. If their intuition is to prove useful to the infant, resulting in prompt detection and treatment, nurses need to be specific and make accurate descriptions.

Most units readily perform full infection screens, including lumbar puncture, and some may commence intravenous broad spectrum antibiotic therapy on clinical suspicion, while awaiting the results.

Lumbar puncture is not well tolerated by very small, sick infants, who tend to get cold and stressed. Owing to the extreme back bend required to widen intervertebral spaces, their respiratory function is compromised. The nurse assisting with the procedure should ensure that emergency equipment is close at hand and that the supplementary O_2 is available should the infant change colour and became cyanosed. In infants who are bordering on needing ventilatory assistance, it is often preferable to intubate and secure the airway prior to performing the puncture.

Debate exists about the necessity of lumbar puncture. Research has suggested that, in cases of meningitis, there is concurrent septicaemia and positive microbial results would be obtained from blood culture. Such an invasive procedure should not be routine (MacMahon *et al.*, 1990).

Neurological observations are open to wide interpretation but posture, irritability and rousability are good guides to neurological stability. Meningeal irritation can result in a high-pitched cry. Head circumference should be monitored and vital signs monitored during the acute stage of the illness, to detect raised intracranial pressure or deteriorating condition. To prevent cerebral oedema, fluid restriction may be prescribed and balanced with accurate measurement of output. Some infants will require anticonvulsants and some will develop neurological sequelae.

Infants with meningitis are often very sick and need full intensive care. The care of the family and siblings is very important and these families need a great deal of support.

Neonatal hypotonia

The term 'floppy infant' describes a loss of body tension and tone, which results in an abnormal posture when the infant is handled and delayed developmental motor milestones. It can originate centrally as a result of severe asphyxia or from the neurological sequel of illness and damage. It may also be caused by a genetic defect such as Down's syndrome or a neuromuscular disorder, many of which are very rare. Roland (1989) gives a comprehensive review of causes of neuromuscular disorders. Some disorders are progressive, such as the muscular dystrophy group, which may not be evident in the newborn. These infants, if admitted for any other reason, should be actively treated as they can live to their late teens or early twenties. Their families require diagnostic assessment and genetic counselling, which should be performed on an outpatient basis, with the support of the health visitor.

Infants with spinal muscular atrophy (Werdnig-Hoffman disease) may require admission to the NNU because of respiratory distress, and may initially be ventilated. They pose difficult ethical problems owing to their very bleak prognosis. There is no treatment available and arguably the only kind method of management is nursing care. This would ideally be done at home, although it can be difficult to withdraw ventilator support from an infant with breathing difficulties. Many of these conditions result from consanguineous relationships or genetic abnormalities, and genetic advice is recommended.

INVESTIGATIONS USED TO AID DIAGNOSIS

A lumbar puncture is performed to obtain a specimen of cerebrospinal fluid (CSF) for examination by culture or chemistry. This is one of the most invasive, yet most common, investigations to take place on the NNU. A number of exciting studies suggest that the measurement of levels of certain proteins in the CSF could be used as 'marker' proteins to indicate areas and levels of damage

(Whitelaw *et al.*, 2001). However, the neonatal nurse would be unlikely to welcome repeated CSF sampling, which could compromise the stability of an infant under care. The ventricular tap is a variation on the lumbar puncture, and may be used to aid the diagnosis of haemorrhage.

Ultrasound scans are not invasive but do involve handling of the infant. There is some indication that the results are not always interpreted as accurately as one would wish (Reynolds *et al.*, 2001). The equipment is large and may intimidate parents, so a brief, reassuring explanation is necessary, along with their consent. Increasingly, other methods of imaging are being employed, such as computerised axial tomography (CAT) scans and magnetic resonance scans. *See* Trounce and Levene (1988) for a description of these and discussion of their advantages and disadvantages.

CONCLUSION

The care of neonates with neuropathology is a challenging and expanding one. There are very few certainties involved and it is very difficult to give parents an accurate prognosis. Some infants whose scans are interpreted as normal go on to suffer profound consequences of their neonatal career; others who have clear damage seem to function later apparently normally. The difficulties seem to be compounded as the outcome is so often not only variable but clouded by the occurrence of other factors (Salamon *et al.*, 2000). Sadly some of the treatment strategies used to protect life may have a profound influence on the subsequent quality of life. For example, Shinwell *et al.* (2000) found that dexamethasone-treated infants had a higher incidence of cerebral palsy than those not treated. The parents' perception of the disclosure of the diagnosis of cerebral palsy (Baird *et al.*, 2000) is very important and one area where the neonatal nurse can be of enormous help to the medical team. With good teamwork, vague comments that the infant may have a 'touch of cerebral palsy' (Marlow, 2001) should never be heard.

Socially, parents cope with damaged children in different ways but the coping abilities need to be seen against the social and economic context of parenting (Taylor *et al.*, 2000). There is good argument for extensive and long-term follow-up (and support) of all neonatal graduates, as a surprisingly high proportion of children born pre-term have minor neurological signs and perceptual motor difficulties in the absence of major neurological impairment. These problems may affect the child's ability to function in everyday life (Jongmans *et al.*, 1997). Cerebral palsy comprises a heterogeneous group of movement disorders caused by damage to the brain. In each child there is an individual blend of impaired motor function (including spasticity), muscularskeletal deformations, dyskinesia, dystonia, ataxia, sustained developmental implication and impaired neural control (Forssberg *et al.*, 1999).

A Health Economics Group in 1993 questioned the concept of care for infants weighing less than 500 grams. Other ethical issues concern the donation of organs from infants with anencephaly (Frost, 1989) and the measurement of neonatal brain death (Ashwal, 1989). (For a full discussion of ethical issues, *see* Chapter 2.)

SAMPLE EXAMINATION QUESTIONS

Question 1
What antenatal factors can disrupt the normal formation and functioning of the brain? (*40 marks*)
What help and support networks are available for the parents of a profoundly damaged infant following discharge from hospital? (*60 marks*)

Question 2
What factors may cause seizure activity in the neonate? (*50 marks*)
What are the nursing priorities in caring for an infant during a generalised seizure? (*50 marks*)

Question 3
Baljit suffered prolonged hypoxia during birth. Her parents are keen to take her home. She is not feeding by mouth because of a poor swallow reflex and is profoundly hypotonic. As her primary nurse, what discharge plans are you going to make and what teaching packages are you going to implement? (*100 marks*)

REFERENCES

Andersen, G. (1989) Prediction of outcome in infants born after 24–28 weeks gestation, *Acta-Paediatric Scandinavian Supplement* **360**, 56–61

Ashwal, S. (1989) Brain death in the newborn, *Clinics in Perinatology* **16**(2), 501–18

Baird, G., Conachie, H. and Scrutton, D. (2000) Parents' perceptions of disclosure of the diagnosis of cerebral palsy, *Archives of Disease in Childhood* **83**(12), 475–80

Brown, F. and Minns, R. (1988) Seizure disorders. In: Levene, M., Bennett, M. and Punt, J. (eds) *Foetal and Neonatal Neurology and Neurosurgery*, Churchill Livingstone, Edinburgh, pp. 487–513

Committee on Obstetrical Practice, American College of Obstetricians and Gynaecologists (1994) *Committee Opinion on Fetal Distress and Asphyxia*, No. 137, Committee on Obstetrical Practice/American College of Obstrtricians and Gynaecologists, New York

Clark, G. (1989) Role of excitatory amino acids in brain injury caused by hypoxic ischaemia, status epilepticus and hypoglycaemia, *Clinics in Perinatology* **16**(2), 459–74

Czeizel, A. (1993) Prevention of congenital abnormalities by periconceptual multi-vitamin supplementation, *British Medical Journal* **6893**(306), 1645–48

Davies, P. (1988) Bacterial and fungal infections. In: Levene, M., Bennett, M. and Punt, J. (eds) *Foetal and Neonatal Neurology and Neurosurgery*, Churchill Livingstone, Edinburgh, pp. 427–49

Evans, D. and Levene, M. (1998) Neonatal seizure, *Archives of Disease in Childhood* **78**(1), 70–5

Forssberg, H., Eliasson, A., Zouitenn, C., Mercuri, E. and Dubowitz, L. (1999) Impaired grip-lift synergy in children with unilateral brain lesions, *Brain* **122**(6), 1157–68

Frost, N. (1989) Removing organs from anencephalic infants – ethical and legal considerations, *Clinics in Perinatology* **16**(2), 331–7

Gunn, A., De Haan, H. and Gluckman, P. (1997) Experimental models of perinatal brain injury (Chapter 4). In: Stevenson, D. and Sunshine, P. (eds.) *Fetal and Neonatal Brain Injury; Mechanisms, Management and the Risks of Practice*, Oxford Medical Publications, Oxford

Holbrook, H., Gibson, R., El Sayeed, Y. and Seidman, D. (1997) Chapter 5. In: Stevenson, D. and Sunshine, P. (eds) *Fetal and Neonatal Brain Injury; Mechanisms, Management and the Risks of Practice*, Oxford Medical Publications, Oxford

Jongmans, M., Mercuri, E., de Vries, L., Dubowitz, L. and Henderson, S. (1997) Minor neurological signs and perceptual motor difficulties in prematurely born children, *Archives of Disease in Childhood* 76(1), 9–14

Kling, P. (1989) Nursing interventions to decrease the risk of periventricular haemorrhage, *Journal of Obstetrics, Gynaecology and Neonatal Nursing* 18(6), 457–64

Levene, M. (1987) *Neonatal Neurology; Current Reviews in Paediatrics*, Churchill Livingstone, Edinburgh

Levene, M. (1988) Management and outcome of birth asphyxia (Chapter 34). In: Levene, M., Bennett, M. and Punt, J. (eds) *Foetal and Neonatal Neurology and Neurosurgery*, Churchill Livingstone, Edinburgh

Levene, M. (1995) Management and outcome of birth asphyxia. In: Levene, M. and Lilford, R. (eds.) *Fetal and Neonatal Neurology and Neurosurgery*, Churchill Livingstone, Edinburgh

Lorber, J. (1971) Results of treatment of myelomeningocele; an analysis of 524 unselected cases with special reference to possible selection for treatment, *Developmental Medicine and Child Neurology* 13, 279–303

MacGregor, J. (2000) *Introduction to the Anatomy and Physiology of Children* (Chapter 3), Routledge, London

MacMahon, P., Jewes, L. and de Louvois, J. (1990) Routine lumbar punctures in the newborn, are they justified? *European Journal of Pediatrics* 149(11), 797–9

Marlow, N. (2001) A touch of cerebral palsy, *Archives of Disease in Childhood* 84(1), 4–5

Mercuri, E., Dubowitz, L., Paterson-Brown, S. and Cowan, F. (1998) Incidence of cranial ultrasound abnormalities in apparently well neonates on a postnatal ward, *Archives of Disease in Childhood* 79(11), 185–9

Mizrahi, E. (1989) Consensus and controversy in the clinical management of neonatal seizures, *Clinics in Perinatology* 16(2), 485–500

Moss, A. (1992) Plastic surgeons' notebook: the technique of tissue expansion, *Professional Care of Mother and Child* 2(10), 330

Nelle, M., Hocker, C. and Linderkamp, O. (1997) Effects of bolus tube feeding on the cerebral blood flow velocity in neonates, *Archives of Disease in Childhood* 76(1), 54–6

Noetzel, M. (1989) Myelomeningocele; current concepts of management, *Clinics in Perinatology* 16(2), 311–29

O'Rahilly, R. *et al.* (1977) The developmental anatomy of the human central nervous system. In: Vinken, R. and Bruyn, G. (eds) *Handbook of Clinical Neurology; Congenital Malformations of the Brain and Skull*, Myrianthopoulos, Amsterdam XX, pp. 15–40

Painter, M. and Gaus, L. (1993) Neonatal seizure (Chapter 2). In: Pellock, J. and Myer, E. (eds) *Neurologic Emergencies in Infancy and Childhood* (2nd edition), Butterworth-Heinemann, Oxford

Pellock, J. and Myer, E. (eds) (1993) *Neurologic Emergencies in Infancy and Childhood* (2nd edition), Butterworth-Heinemann, Oxford

Perlman, J. (1989) Systemic abnormalities in term infants following perinatal asphyxia; relevance to long-term neurologic outcome, *Clinics in Perinatology* 16(2), 475–84

Perlman, J. and Volpe, J. (1983) Suctioning in the pre-term infant; effects on cerebral blood flow velocity, intracranial pressure and arterial blood pressure, *Pediatrics* 72(3), 329–34

Reynolds, P., Dale, R. and Cowan, F. (2001) Neonatal cranial ultrasound: a clinical audit, *Archives of Disease in Childhood* 84(3), 92–5

Roland, E. (1989) Neuromuscular disorders in the newborn, *Clinics in Perinatology* 16(2), 519–47

Roberton, N.R.C. (1993) *A Manual of Neonatal Intensive Care* (3rd edition), Edward Arnold, London

Robertson, N. and Edwards, A. (1998) Recent advances in developing strategies for perinatal asphyxia, *Current Opinions in Pediatrics* 10(6), 575–80

Salamon, M., Gerner, E., Jonsson, B. and Lagercrantz, H. (2000) Early motor and mental development in the very pre-term infants with chronic lung disease, *Archives of Disease in Childhood* 83(7), 1–6

Schwartz, J., Ahmann, P., Dykes, F. and Brann, A. (1993) Neonatal intracranial haemorrhage and hypoxia (Chapter 1). In: Pellock, J. and Myer, E. (eds) *Neurologic Emergencies in Infancy and Childhood* (2nd edition), Butterworth-Heinemann, Oxford

Seller, M. (1989) Perinatal diagnosis of neural tube defects, *Midwife, Health Visitor and Community Nurse* 25(11), 458–62

Shinwell, E., Karplus, M., Reich, D., Weintraub, Z. *et al.* (2000) Early post-natal dexamethasone treatment and increased incidence of cerebral palsy, *Archives of Disease in Childhood* 83(11), 177–81

Taylor, J., Spencer, N. and Baldwin, N. (2000) Social economic and political context of parenting, *Archives of Disease in Childhood* 82(2), 113–20

Temple, C., Dennis, J., Carney, R. and Sharich, J. (1995) Neonatal seizures: long-term outcome and cognitive development among normal survivors, *Dev Med Child Neurol* 37, 109–18

Trounce, F. and Levene, M. (1988) Ultrasound imaging of the neonatal brain. In: Levene, M. and Lilford, R. (eds) *Fetal and Neonatal Neurology and Neurosurgery*, Churchill Livingstone, Edinburgh, pp. 139–48

Volpe, J. (1987) *Neurology of the Newborn*, WB Saunders, Philadelphia, PA

Volpe, J. (1989) Intraventricular haemorrhage and brain injury in the premature infant: neuropathology and pathogenesis, *Clinics in Perinatology* 16(2), 361–86

Wallace, J. (1998) Suctioning – a two-edged sword, *Journal of Neonatal Nursing* 4(6), 12–17

Whitelaw, A., Rosengren, L. and Blennow M. (2001) Brain-specific proteins in posthaemorrhagic ventricular dilatation, *Archives of Disease in Childhood* 84(3), 90–2

Zideman, D., Bingham, R., Bettie, T. *et al.* (1998) Recommendations on resuscitation of babies at birth, *Resuscitation* 37, 103–10

PART THREE

TREATMENT AND CARE STRATEGIES

12 NURSING CARE OF THE INFANT IN PAIN AND DISCOMFORT

Margaret Sparshott

Aims of the chapter

This chapter considers the effects of pain and discomfort on newborn infants. It reviews the infant's responses to pain on both physiological and behavioural levels. To help the neonatal nurse care for infants in pain, assessment tools are reviewed and some nursing strategies are provided.

INTRODUCTION

It is the duty of a nurse to act as the patient's advocate. This is especially the case for the neonatal nurse, whose charges cannot speak of their sufferings and cannot protect themselves either by flight or fight. (For more on advocacy, *see* Chapter 2.) This inability had led many people to doubt that newborn infants could feel pain at all. If nurses are obliged to inflict pain for the good of others, maybe the task is made easier if they are able to pretend that it is not felt. In this way, they can absolve themselves of all guilt and proceed without worrying about the distress that is being caused. However, research has shown that infants who are given analgesia during heart surgery tend to be less distressed, both during and after the operation, than those who have had to do without (Anand and Hickey, 1987).

EFFECTS OF PAIN AND DISCOMFORT ON NEWBORN INFANTS

The elements involved in the pain pathway are in place from an early gestational age. Recent research has suggested that infants are neurologically capable of feeling pain from 20 weeks gestation, and probably before (Glover and Fisk, 1999). Foetal development can be affected by life events, stress in the mother and, since this is a time of rapid increase in cortical brain cell structure, an adverse experience may affect the balance of neurological development of the cerebral cortex (Connolly and Cullen, 1983; Anand and Hickey, 1987; Grunau, 1999). The question of pain and its effects on the newborn is therefore of vital importance when future quality of life is considered.

Newborn infants have no subjective experience of pain. They have, as yet, no knowledge of their environment – they absorb this from day to day. Infants develop and grow through their relationship with the encompassing world and the people it contains. It is mainly through this relationship that personality comes into being. For this development, a gradual awareness of pain and discomfort is essential, as the surroundings will aid an infant to pass from complete dependence to independence. Both positive and negative experiences are necessary for the growth of the individual, but this must come about gradually. Winnicott (1965) referred to the process as 'graduated failure', meaning that no mother is perfect, and that this is one of the things that every infant must learn.

It is potentially harmful if the environment impinges too soon, too sharply or too persistently. Infants will not be able to cope with the adaptation necessary to withstand it. They are forced into a knowledge that is totally inappropriate at this stage, and to defend themselves they may regress and withdraw (Huteau, 1988). This regression can be beneficial if it is only temporary and, once the cause is removed, it can be reversed. Psychoanalysts have attributed feelings of persecution in adulthood to traumatic, prolonged experiences in infancy (Balint, 1968). A syndrome of 'needing' pain has been identified in some small children who have undergone traumatic experiences in infancy (Herzog, 1983).

The environment of a neonatal unit, in which fragile infants are maintained, is inappropriate at best and frequently appears to offer nothing but discomfort. To keep such infants alive, it may be necessary to inflict many traumatic procedures upon them. Having to do this knowingly can only add to the stresses of the caregiver. It is a serious dilemma faced daily by those caring for sick newborns.

INFANT RESPONSES TO PAIN AND DISCOMFORT

In order to improve the care of sick and pre-term infants in hospital, neonatal nurses must first understand how those infants communicate their feelings, as they are unable to use words to express how they feel. The response that each infant makes will depend on its gestational age, physical condition and state of consciousness.

The 'states of consciousness' or 'sleeping/waking states' are a cycle of states in which healthy newborn infants pass their daily life. They progress from deep sleep to light sleep (rapid eye movement, or REM, sleep), then through drowsiness to a quietly awake and alert state, and from wakefulness with considerable motor activity and some fussy crying, to crying, as they become hungry. Once hunger is satisfied, they retreat into a deep sleep and the cycle begins again (Brazelton and Nugent, 1995).

The internal 'state' of infants will affect their ability to receive stimuli from and respond to their environment. It is at the time of quiet wakefulness that infants are most attentive to what is going on around them and this is the time when they need stimulation from their care-givers. Their attention span is short, however, and a well term infant is able to retreat into a state of sleep, shutting off unwanted external stimuli (Wolff, 1966). A sick or pre-term infant may be incapable of this response and will consequently be at the mercy of environmental pressure. It is important that infants exhibiting 'shut out' signs are handled as little as possible (Als, 1986).

Infants 'speak' through their actions and reactions and are incapable of telling a lie. If infants show signs of stress, something is wrong. They may be complaining of the onset of pain, or simply of a soiled nappy. It is the degree of behavioural and physiological expression, combined with the care-giver's own knowledge and understanding of the infant, that will guide the carer to the root of the problem.

A newborn infant can experience three types of pain, with symptoms that can be distinguished from each other:

- acute;
- extreme;
- chronic or long-lasting pain.

Acute pain

This is usually highly localised, sharp and transitory. This is the type of pain that may be experienced by an infant during the performance of a traumatic procedure. It may occur when an infant is handled post-operatively, for example, or spontaneously in conditions such as colic.

Extreme pain

Extreme pain may be experienced in illnesses such as necrotising enterocolitis, meningitis or glaucoma.

Chronic (or long-lasting) pain

This type of pain is intractable and persists over a period of time. It is usually associated with illnesses such as cancer, but the symptoms may also be seen in infants who, due to their precarious state, are repeatedly subjected to traumatic procedures (Sparshott, 1989, 1997).

BEHAVIOURAL RESPONSES TO ACUTE PAIN

Vocalisation

Infants may indicate that they are distressed by the way they cry. Interpretation of sound spectography of infants' crying suggests that cries differ not so much in their origin (resulting from hunger or pain, for example) as in their intensity, pitch and duration (Michelsson et al., 1983). Hunger is probably not distinguishable from pain to an infant and the fussy crying of a hungry infant will eventually lead, if not satisfied, to the cry of pain. This 'pain cry' has been described as 'a sudden long and strong initial cry ... followed by a long period of absolute silence, due to apnoea, ultimately this gives way to short gasping inhalations alternated with expiratory coughs' (Bowlby, 1969). If there is no response to this cry, it will develop into the loud, braying cry of anger or tantrum, which is very difficult to appease.

Sound spectography also shows that sick, light for gestational age, pre-term infants or infants who have suffered from birth trauma have a particularly high-pitched, shrill, penetrating cry, which is hard to ignore and demands a response

(Michelsson *et al.*, 1983). Very low-birthweight infants undergoing ventilation may be seen to gape round the endotracheal tube (Figure 12.1). This is known as the 'silent cry' (Wolke, 1987; Sparshott, 1989, 1997).

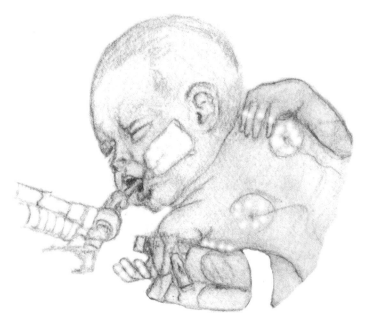

Figure 12.1 The 'silent cry'

Facial expression

The Neonatal Facial Coding System (NFCS) was devised by Grunau and Craig in 1987, using adult facial coding systems and an infant's response to a painful stimulus (heel prick blood sampling). These specific facial changes – eye-squeeze, brow contraction, nasolabial furrow, taut/cupped tongue and open mouth (Figure 12.2) – were quite different from facial responses to other stimuli, such as rubbing the heel. For practical purposes, this pattern of reaction may be termed a 'pain expression'.

Grunau and Craig discovered that healthy term infants disturbed for heel prick during deep sleep would, provided they were not over-handled, react less violently than infants disturbed during the quiet alert state (Figure 12.3). Infants also react differently to different technicians, suggesting that it is to the infant's advantage if they are handled by someone who has a good technique (Grunau and Craig, 1987; Craig *et al.*, 1993).

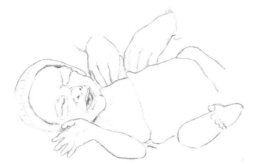

Figure 12.2 A 'pain expression'

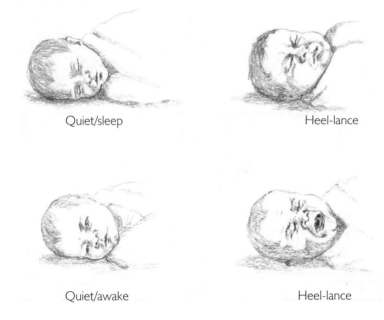

Quiet/sleep

Heel-lance

Quiet/awake

Heel-lance

Figure 12.3 Facial behaviour of the newborn

Body movements

The Infant Body Coding System (IBCS) showed the many complex ways that infants might react to pain by movements of the body (Craig *et al.*, 1993). There is frequently a violent thrashing or extension of all extremities and sometimes a withdrawal of the affected limb from the site of the injury. A well term infant may even sideswipe with the unaffected limb, showing considerable motor coordination at this stage (Dale, 1986). The Moro reflex may be present, but it is less specifically associated with pain and its origin may rather be a fear of falling.

PHYSIOLOGICAL CHANGES IN ACUTE PAIN

Cardiovascular

Increases as well as decreases in heart rate have been observed during procedures in healthy term infants, but bradycardia is more frequent in fragile infants (Williamson and Williamson, 1983; Anand and Hickey, 1987; Brown, 1987). Increases in blood pressure have been noted during traumatic procedures. Increases in cerebral blood flow and increases in intracranial pressure can occur during endotracheal suctioning (Perlman and Volpe, 1983; Brown, 1987).

Respiratory

Hyperventilation can follow prolonged crying in term infants, but a decrease in respiratory rate and apnoea is more likely to occur in fragile infants (Brown, 1987; Wolke, 1987). Increase in $TcPO_2$ may occur, owing to crying, but a decrease will be more common (Williamson and Williamson, 1983; Brown, 1987; Wolke, 1987). Over-handling and suctioning can cause $TcPO_2$ to fall (Long et al., 1980). Oxygen saturation will be affected in the same way.

Temperature regulation

Increase in central/peripheral temperature differential is an indication of stress response in sick or pre-term infants, although the stress may be caused by factors other than pain. Temperature differential is significant, however, in a context where pain or distress are suspected (Mok et al., 1991).

Emotional sweating

Sweating from the palm of the hand and the sole of the foot is determined by emotional factors. It is increased by fear, anxiety and concentration, and decreased by contentment, relaxation, and sleep. Palmar sweating increases during painful procedures in infants from at least 37 weeks gestation (Harpin and Rutter, 1982).

Endocrine

Changes in the endocrine system have been observed following ventilation, chest physiotherapy, endotracheal suctioning and circumcision with minimal anaesthetic, a response which was measurably decreased in sedated infants (Anand and Hickey, 1987). Over-handling can also lead to a release of plasma catecholamines; raised levels of these hormones are associated with stress (Lagercrantz et al., 1986).

Palmar sweating and the endocrine response are of no practical value to nurses assessing infants in their care. The other physiological changes mentioned are alarm signals and, when they are observed, every possible source of stress should be investigated. Physiological changes are the only means open to very pre-term infants to indicate stress from whatever cause, since these infants are too immature to coordinate behavioural responses.

Responses to extreme pain

Since crying cannot indicate the intensity of pain felt, it is sometimes difficult to assess when an infant is in extreme pain. There are certain abnormal positions of the limbs, an axial stiffness with head extension and an antalgic position of the body at rest, which may indicate intense suffering (see Figure 12.4) (Gauvain-Piquard, 1989a; Sparshott, 1996, 1997). The antalgic position is a defensive attitude adopted by the body against pain. Infants in extreme pain may stop crying for a short while when picked up and cuddled but, since the pain persists, they will begin again as soon as they are returned to their cot.

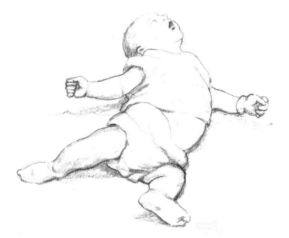

Figure 12.4 Abnormal position of an infant in extreme pain (adapted from Gauvain-Piquard, 1989b)

Responses to chronic or long-lasting pain

Lasting pain has a very different symptomatology. It may endure for several hours, days or weeks, and is not easy to diagnose, as the symptoms are more discreet. If infants suffer for a long time without relief, they will cease to struggle or cry, since this wastes valuable energy. They will withdraw into themselves (as already described) and, the younger the infant and the greater the intensity of the pain, the quicker they will cease to make responses. It is hard to recognise the fact that such infants are suffering. The signs are negative: no crying, reduced motor activity, diminished communication with the outside world, diminished alertness and sometimes even an expression of hostility. The infant appears listless, apathetic, and unresponsive to the care-giver (Gauvain-Piquard, 1989a; Sparshott, 1997).

PAIN SCORING SYSTEMS

Johnston and Strada (1986) offered a multidimensional description of acute pain response in infants. Gauvain-Piquard described reactions of the non-verbal child to extreme and long-lasting pain in 1989. Some of these reactions were adapted for the newborn and used by Sparshott (1989) in a nursing care plan for the management of pain in the special care unit (Table 12.1). This care plan also included a chart showing an individual infant's reaction to pain, and what nursing actions could be used to return the infant to stability (Table 12.2).

Table 12.1 Nursing care plan for the management of pain in the special care unit

Problem	Goal	Nursing intervention	Nursing evaluation
Pain from:			
Traumatic procedures	Prevention of unnecessary suffering Maintenance of a safe environment: Restoration to a state of equilibrium	1 Observe: a) state of consciousness; b) physiological signs prior to procedure.	Goal is achieved when infant is restored to state of equilibrium; the shorter the time, the greater the success of the nursing intervention
		2 Perform or assist with procedure: a) cause as little disturbance to baby as possible; b) maintain safe environment by keeping infant warm and in most comfortable position; c) suggest administration of local anaesthetic if appropriate.	
		3 Note time taken over procedure.	
		4 Note immediate behavioural and physiological response.	
		5 Comfort and console infant until calm once procedure is completed.	
		6 Suggest administration of analgesia if necessary.	
		7 Observe state of infant and physiological changes.	
		8 Note time taken and methods used to restore baby to a state of equilibrium.	
Post-surgery	As above	1 Anticipate that pain will be experienced.	
		2 Ensure that appropriate analgesia has been prescribed.	
		3 Observe for signs of pain.	
		4 Take appropriate action by: a) alleviating symptoms; b) administering analgesia.	
		5 Observe state of infant and physiological changes.	
		6 Note time taken and methods used to restore baby to equilibrium.	As above
Illness (extreme and lasting pain)	As above	As in post-surgery.	As above

Note: Observations of state, maintenance of safe environment and attempts to comfort and console should be made in all cases.

Table 12.2 Chart showing infant's reaction to pain and nursing actions required to return the infant to stability

Date and time									
STATE (before procedure)									
Asleep									
Awake									
Crying									
Heart rate									
Respiration									
Blood pressure									
TcPO$_2$ (or O$_2$ sat)									
PROCEDURE									
time taken (minutes)									
REACTION									
NURSING ACTION									
Voice									
Stroking									
Massage									
Cuddle									
Rocking									
Swaddle									
Non-nutritive sucking									
Breast-/bottle-feed									
Analgesia									
RESULT									
Asleep									
Awake									
Crying									
Heart rate									
Respiration									
Blood pressure									
TcPO$_2$ (or O$_2$ sat)									
ACHIEVED									
1–3 minutes									
3–5 minutes									
5–10 minutes									
CODE									

Lawrence *et al.* (1993) published a description of the Neonatal Infant Pain Score (NIPS), a tool devised to assess the behavioural reactions of pre-term and full-term infants to the painful stimulus of needle puncture. Operational definitions described changes in facial expression, cry, breathing patterns, the movements of arms and legs, and state of arousal. More recently, the Premature Infant Pain Profile (PIPP) has proved useful in assessing pain by means of observation of facial expression, heart rate, oxygen saturation, and behavioural state, in the context of gestational age (Stevens *et al.*, 1996). PIPP is used to evaluate procedural pain in pre-term infants of more than 28 weeks gestational age, and more recently has been validated for evaluating post-operative pain in neonates. (These and other pain scores have been discussed in detail by Stevens *et al.*, 1999.)

Table 12.3 Distress Scale for Ventilated Newborn Infants (DSVNI) showing examples of facial expression and body movement

Behavioural score	0	1
Facial expression	**Relaxed**	**Anxious**
	Smooth muscled, unlined, relaxed expression	Anxious expression, frown; REM; wandering gaze; eyes narrowed; lips parted; lips pursed
	Deep sleep state	Eyes tightly closed, pursed lips
	Quiet alert state	Eyes narrowed/wandering gaze; lips pursed; slightly parted
Body movement	**Relaxed**	**Restless**
	Relaxed trunk and limbs; body in tucked position; hands in cupped position or willing to grasp a finger	Moro reflex, startles; jerky or uncoordinated movement of limbs; flexion extension of limbs; attempt to withdraw limb from site of injury
	Relaxed trunk and limbs Tucked position	Limb withdrawal
Colour	Normal skin colour (depending on skin type)	Redness; congestion

(Continued)

Table 12.3 Continued

Behavioural score	2	3
Facial expression	**Anguished**	**Inert**
	Anguished expression/crumpled face; brow bulge; eye-squeeze; nasolabial furrow pronounced; square-stretched mouth; cupped tongue; 'silent cry'	(Only during or immediately following traumatic procedure); no response to trauma; no crying; rigidity; gaze avoidance; fixed/staring gaze; apathy, diminished alertness
	Silent cry	Gaze avoidance
	Cupped tongue	Fixed/staring gaze
Body movement	**Exaggerated**	**Inert**
	Abnormal position of limbs; limb/neck extension; splaying of fingers and or toes; flailing or thrashing of limbs; arching back; sideswiping/guarding site of injury	(Only during or immediately following traumatic procedure); no response to trauma, inertia; limpness/rigidity; immobility
	Exaggerated neck extension, flailing arching back Exaggerated limb extension, finger/toe splay	Rigidity
Colour	Pallor, mottling, grey	Baseline colour, pallor, mottling, grey

From Sparshott (1996)

Distress Scale for Ventilated Newborn Infants

The Distress Scale for Ventilated Newborn Infants (DSVNI) was devised to assess the physiological and behavioural responses of the ventilated newborn infant to trauma (Sparshott, 1996, 1997). The scale includes the reactions of infants who have been subjected to repeated traumatic procedures, as well as immediate reactions to acute pain. Behavioural responses include degrees of facial expression, body movement, and colour. Except for the 'silent cry', differences in cry have not been included in the scale, as this response is not available to the ventilated infant. Examples of facial expression and body movement are accompanied by illustrations (Table 12.3). Physiological changes include changes in heart rate, blood pressure, oxygenation, and temperature differential (Table 12.4).

Table 12.4   Physiological changes during stress

Physiological changes are not scored, but read directly from the monitors. Changes indicative of stress, read from baseline, are:

Heart rate	Increase; decrease; bradycardia frequent in fragile infants
Blood pressure	Increase
Oxygenation	Commonly a decrease; occasionally increases due to crying and consequent increased intracranial pressure
Temperature differential	Widening gap between core and peripheral temperature; decrease in peripheral temperature

Lability of skin colour is an indication of physiological instability. For the caregiver performing or assisting with a traumatic procedure, colour changes are easily discernible; therefore, as fluctuations in colour are associated with stress, colour is included in the DSVNI. A score sheet shows recordings at baseline, during procedure, after procedure, and time taken to return to baseline (Table 12.5).

The DSVNI is based on the following validated scoring systems:

- Neonatal Behavioural Assessment Scale (NBAS) (Brazelton and Nugent, 1995) (state of consciousness, colour);
- Assessment of Pre-term Infant Behaviour (APIB) (Als *et al.*, 1982) (facial expression, body movement, colour);
- Neonatal Facial Coding System (NFCS) (Grunau and Craig, 1987) (facial expression);
- Infant Body Coding System (IBCS) (Craig *et al.*, 1993) (body movement);
- Gustave-Roussy Child Pain Scale (Gauvain-Piquard, 1989a; Sparshott, 1989) (extreme and long-lasting pain).

The behavioural scale is assessed on a score of 0 to 8 (Table 12.6), but caregivers should be aware that infants differ widely in their behavioural reactions to stress. The nurse's knowledge of the individual infant, their gestational age, and

Table 12.5 Score sheet for Distress Scale for Ventilated Newborn Infants (DSVNI)

DSVNI score sheet

Name:	Date:	Time:	Hospital number:
Gestation:	Age:	Birth weight:	

Main diagnosis:

Type of ventilation:	Duration of ventilation:

Analgesia or local anaesthetic:	Dose:
Bolus/infusion:	Time since last given:

Traumatic procedure: No. of attempts:
Duration of procedure:

Score	Baseline	During procedure	After procedure		Time taken to return to baseline
			At 3 mins	At 1 hr	
Facial expression					
Body movement					
Colour					
Heart rate					
Blood pressure					
Oxygen saturation					
Temperature – skin					
– toe					
Total					

Codes for invasive procedures:

CD	Chest drain insertion	LP	Lumbar puncture
INT	Intubation	VP	Venepuncture
ETS	Endotracheal suctioning	AS	Arterial stab
OPS	Oropharangeal suctioning	HL	Heel-lance
CPAP	Continuous positive airways pressure	Other	

Note: To avoid more disturbance to the baby, these observations need only be made if monitoring equipment is already in place.

From Sparshott (1996)

the context and the cause of the pain, should guide any response (Sparshott, 1997).

Although the DSVNI is principally designed to assess reaction to invasive procedures, care-givers may well observe the same distress signals demonstrated by a fragile infant subjected to over-stimulation – handling that is too rough or too brusque for the rapidly developing nervous system to maintain.

Table 12.6 Assessment of behavioural score

0	Relaxed – infant comfortable, not distressed
1–2	Some transitory distress caused; returns immediately to 'relaxed'
3–4	Transitory distress, likely to respond to consolation
5	Infant experiences pain; if no response to consolation, may require analgesia
6	'Anguished' and 'exaggerated' – infant experiencing acute pain; unlikely to respond to consolation, will probably benefit from analgesia
6–8	'Inert' – (no response to traumatic procedure); infant is habituated to pain, will not respond to consolation; systematic pain control by analgesia should be considered

CATEGORIES OF ENVIRONMENTAL DISTURBANCE

Once the nurse has interpreted the infant's cues and believes that the infant is in pain, he or she needs to decide what action to take. This will depend on the type of pain suffered and the individual infant's response to treatment. A chart showing the main sources of pain, discomfort and disturbance likely to be encountered in the NNU, balanced by the corresponding ways in which they may be treated, should help the nurse to identify the problem and choose the most acceptable way of providing comfort (Table 12.7). Since the infant has, as yet, no subjective experience, the items of these categories are interchangeable. For example, a heel prick may be hardly disturbing to the term infant who is in deep sleep but will be painful to the fragile infant who is unable to 'shut off' unwanted experience. It is for the nurse, who knows the infant, to determine which method of consolation is best (Sparshott, 1991a).

Disturbance and cherishment

Disturbance can be prevented by attention to light and sound levels. Permanent lighting, providing no difference between night and day, may contribute to the absence of circadian rhythm, which is present in intra-uterine life (Dreyfus-Brisac, 1983). Dimmer switches can be used in special care nurseries. In intensive care, individual lamps reduce the light intensity, as does the partial covering of the incubator, allowing observation but protection from direct light (Sparshott, 1997).

Sound levels in excess of 60 dB(A) are potentially harmful to the newborn infant. British and American safety standards require that this level should not be exceeded within an incubator (Wolke, 1987). Noise can be reduced by avoiding the slamming of incubator doors or the placing of solid objects on the top of incubators, and by being aware of the disturbance caused by such extraneous sounds as the radio, loud voices and laughter. It is the behaviour of care-givers that is responsible for most of the raised sound levels. Infants do respond well to the sound of a gentle human voice and parents should be helped to understand that speaking lovingly to their child should contribute to the child's well-being (Sparshott, 1995). Music has also been used to good effect as a source of calm and comfort (Kirby, 2000).

Table 12.7 Categories of environmental disturbance and their treatment

Pain	Discomfort	Disturbance
• Intubation	• Monitoring	• Light
• Chest drain insertion	• Physical examination	• Noise
• Venepuncture	• Extubation	• Cold
• Heel prick	• Range finding, due to insecurity	• Heat
• Suctioning	• Chest physiotherapy	• Nappy change
• IM injection	• Electrode removal	• Position change
• Wound cleansing	• Rectal temperature	• Nakedness
• CPAP	• Passage of NG or OP tube	• Weighing
• Lumbar puncture	• IV medication	• Over-handling
• Arterial or supra-pubic stab	• Splinting	• Feeding by NG or OP tube
• Surgery	• Physical restraint	• Bottle-feeding when too weak
• Illness, ie: meningitis, necrotising enterocolitis	• Phototherapy	• Isolation
	• Urine bag removal	• Separation
	• Adhesive tape removal	• Lack of stimulation if well
	• Hunger	• Noxious taste/odour
Therapy	**Consolation**	**Cherishment**
Prevent pain by:	• Music and sound	• Day and night lighting
• technique	• Provision of boundaries	• Noise reduction
• preparation beforehand	• Containment	• Minimal handling or
• choice of equipment	• Stroking and massage	stimulation
Abstention	• Swaddling	• Clothing and coverings
Grouping care	• Rocking	• Parental presence
Treat pain by:	• Non-nutritive sucking	• Soft toys
• analgesia	• Breast-feeding	• Musical toys and cassettes
• local anaesthetic	• Encouragement of self-	• Pictures
• anaesthetic cream	consolation (hand-to-mouth	• Mirrors
Treat intractable pain by:	movement)	• Mobiles
• relief of symptoms	• Encasement	• Baby carriers
• containment	• Correct positioning	• Baby chairs
• narcotic analgesia		• Skin-to-skin contact
		• Pleasant taste/odour

Strict observance of 'minimal handling' will allow periods of rest for the fragile infant. Ways to accomplish this are by the introduction of 'quiet hours', when sound and light are reduced, and nursing and medical procedures are kept to a minimum, and for care-givers to group the infants' care. Neonatal nurses should help parents to see for themselves when it is best not to disturb their infant and when to offer suitable stimulation. A booklet designed for the parents of a pre-term infant, explaining how the infant is likely to behave and what actions can be taken to maintain a state of well-being, will help to make them to feel involved (Sparshott, 1990).

Discomfort and consolation

The integrity of the skin as the surface of the body is of vital importance to the newborn infant, both physiologically and psychologically (Sparshott, 1991b, 1991c). Attention should be paid to the siting of electrodes and the use of adhesives and strapping. The positioning of splints is also important, to ensure that the limbs are maintained in as natural a position as possible.

Infants do not like to feel exposed and will waste energy 'range finding'. Suitable clothing, swaddling, comfortable support for the body and limbs and the provision of barriers against which they can rest will promote a sense of security (Sparshott, 1997).

Following a traumatic procedure, the care-giver should offer consolation in the way that is best suited to the individual infant (*see* Table 12.6). This will be observed over a period of time by trial and error, and parents should be encouraged to play the role of comforter. The isolation of the newborn infant in an incubator is one of the most unnatural features of neonatal intensive care, and parents should be encouraged to participate in the care of their child as soon as they feel confident to do so. Parents who constantly watch their newborn soon become sensitive to their needs and quickly learn what form of stroking and caressing suits them best.

For the fragile infant for whom even the gentle stimulation of stroking is too much, the technique of 'containment' may be beneficial (Als, 1986; Sparshott, 1997). The care-giver places one hand gently over the top of the infant's head and the other hand gently over the trunk, thus containing the body in the warmth of human contact, without demanding any response in return.

Pain and therapy

Unfortunately, many of the traumatic experiences that infants undergo in the NNU are unavoidable if they are to survive with a good quality of life. It is the task of the care-giver to alleviate this suffering as much as possible.

Some pain and unnecessary suffering can be prevented by attention to such details as choice of equipment, preparation of the infant beforehand, planning, grouping and sharing periods of handling. For example, the use of mechanical lancets for the taking of blood samples has been shown to cause the least damage, whereas over-zealous squeezing of the heel adds to the trauma (Harpin and Rutter, 1983). Studies of infants undergoing circumcision without local anaesthetic have shown that as much distress was caused by the immobilisation on a cold slab and drenching with cold antiseptic solution, as by the incision itself (Williamson and Williamson, 1983). Doctors and nurses co-operating with each other to arrange for the care and treatment of the infant to coincide will allow longer periods for rest and sleep.

The practice of good techniques is also essential to avoid inflicting unnecessary suffering. Nurses and doctors are more likely to become skilled at such procedures as heel-prick blood sampling and the siting of intravenous infusions with experience, and this is enhanced by the establishment of permanent qualified staff in NNUs.

Intractable pain can be alleviated by as far as possible relieving the symptoms, and by the use of narcotic analgesia. Consolation techniques are unlikely to benefit the infant in extreme or long-lasting pain.

PHARMACOLOGICAL AND NON-PHARMACOLOGICAL PAIN TREATMENT

A wide spectrum of analgesics have been used in systemic analgesic therapy in the treatment of pain from different sources (Anand et al., 1999). Morphine is the opioid analgesic most commonly used in the treatment of both acute and chronic pain. It is usually administered intravenously, either by bolus or, preferably, by continuous infusion (Gauntlett, 1987; Anand et al., 1993). Morphine syrup is more useful in the treatment of long-lasting pain, such as the mature infant with BPD who can be fed orally. Close monitoring and strict observation are necessary in view of the possible side-effect of depression of respiration, and facilities for ventilation should be at hand (Koren et al., 1985). Fentanyl and alfentanyl have also been used in the anaesthesia of newborn infants with good effect (Anand et al., 1997), but withdrawal symptoms (though rare) appear to be more common with fentanyl than with morphine (Levene and Quinn, 1992). Of the non-opioid analgesics, paracetamol is the most widely used, particularly in the treatment of peripheral pain. Its preparation for infants is in the form of an elixir or rectal suppositories.

Lignocaine is the most widely used nerve block and is effective as a local skin anaesthetic, as it works rapidly. For example, it can be used in the elective insertion of a chest drain. Its disadvantages are that it is not suitable for use in an emergency and that, since it is administered by subcutaneous injection, it is in itself painful. Epidural local anaesthesia can also be administered, most commonly using the caudal approach (Sethna and Koh, 1999). EMLA cream is a local anaesthetic used topically to anaesthetise the skin, but it needs to be applied at least 1 hour before the performance of a traumatic procedure. EMLA cream is used in some units for the term infant, but as yet it is not recommended by the manufacturers for use with pre-term infants of below 37 weeks gestation (EMLA Monograph, 2000).

Some non-pharmacological pain treatments have been tried, such as massage of the affected part, reflexology, therapeutic touch (Sparshott, 1997), and auricular acupuncture (Yuan-Chi Lin, 2000). The most successful and the most widely used is the oral administration of sucrose combined with non-nutritive sucking (Johnston et al., 1999).

PAIN MANAGEMENT

The belief that infants are incapable of the pain experience is a protective mechanism against the stress of being obliged to inflict pain on a being that is helpless. To see an infant in pain is shocking; to be forced to inflict pain, even in the infant's interests, makes it even less supportable. But pain does exist and denying it will not make it go away.

The nurse, acting as the advocate, should be able to demonstrate the infant's reactions to painful stimuli. Accusing the doctor of hurting an infant will only lead to antagonism, since traumatic procedures must be performed for ultimate well-being. However, if the nurse can show that the infant is suffering, or is maybe even compromised by the pain felt, the doctor is more likely to avoid inflicting pain, by the use of analgesia or other means.

The most reliable way to maintain adequate sedation for the newborn is for the medical staff to establish a 'pain protocol', such as that proposed by Andrews and Wills (1992). For neonatal nurses, the care plan for the pain management of the newborn infant (*see* Tables 12.1 and 12.2) can be used to show the individual infant's reactions to the traumatic procedure, and can demonstrate which method of consolation or analgesia proved to be the most effective (Sparshott, 1989).

CONCLUSION

An understanding of infant behaviour is of vital importance to neonatal nurses. Not only will this enable them to identify the signs of pain and discomfort in their patients, it will also allow them to see when they are comfortable and at rest. Individual infants have their own needs and what pleases one will not always satisfy another. It is by means of behavioural responses and physiological changes that they communicate pain and pleasure. Once these are understood, all the actions listed in Table 12.7 (and many more) are available for the nurse to try; and if they fail, an alternative can be chosen. The infant will soon let the nurse know when the right choice has been made.

SAMPLE EXAMINATION QUESTIONS

Question 1
What are the common physiological responses to pain and discomfort?
(*50 marks*)
What combined medical and nursing strategies can be adopted to ensure the comfort of these infants? (*50 marks*)

Question 2
Anna is currently ventilated following repair of a tracheo-oesophageal fistula. What nursing assessments and actions are going to be undertaken to ensure that she remains comfortable during the first 48 hours? (*100 marks*)

REFERENCES

Als, H. (1986) A synactive model of neonatal behavioural organisation: framework for the assessment of neurobehavioral development in the premature infant and for the support of infants and parents in the neonatal intensive care environment. In: Sweeney, J. (ed.) *The High Risk Neonate*, Haworth Press, London, pp. 3–53

Als, H. *et al.* (1982) Manual for the assessment of pre-term infant behaviour (APIB). In: Fitzgerald, E., Lester, B.M. and Yogman, M.H. (eds) *Theory and Research in Behavioural Pediatrics*, Vol I, Plenum Press, New York

Anand, K.J.S. and Hickey, P.R. (1987) Pain and its effects in the newborn neonate and fetus, *The New England Journal of Medicine* 317(21), 1321–9

Anand, K.J.S., Shapiro, B.S.and Berde, C.B. (1993) Pharmacotherapy and systemic analgesics. In: Anand, K.J.S. and McGrath, P.J. (eds) Pain in neonates, *Pain Research and Clinical Management*, Vol 5, Elsevier, Amsterdam

Anand, K.J.S., Menon, G., Narsinghani, U. and McIntosh, N. (1997) Long-term effects of pain in neonates and infants. In: Jense, T.S., Turner, J.A. and Wiesenfeld-Hallin, Z. (eds) *Progress in Pain Research and Management*, Vol 8, IASP Press, Seattle, pp. 881–92

Anand, K.J.S. *et al.* (1999) Systemic analgesic therapy. In: Anand, K.J.S., Stevens, B.J. and McGrath, P.J. (eds) *Pain in Neonates* (2nd edition), Elsevier, Amsterdam, pp. 159–88

Andrews, K. and Wills, B. (1992) A systematic approach can reduce side-effects: a protocol for pain relief in neonates, *Professional Nurse* 7(8), 528–32

Balint, M. (1968) *The Basic Fault*, Tavistock Press, London

Bowlby, J. (1969) *Attachment*, The Hogarth Press and the Institute of Psycho-Analysis, London

Brazelton, T.B. and Nugent, J.K. (1995) *Neonatal Behavioral Assessment Scale* (3rd edition), Mac Keith Press, London

Brown, L. (1987) Physiological responses to cutaneous pain in neonates, *Neonatal Network* 6, 18-22

Connolly, J.A. and Cullen, J.H. (1983) Maternal stress and the origins of health status. In: Call, J.D., Galenson, E. and Tyson, R.L. (eds) *Frontiers of Infant Psychiatry*, Basic Books, New York

Craig, K.D., Whitfield, M.F., Grunau, R.V.E., Linton, J. and Hadjistavropoulos, H.D. (1993) Pain and the pre-term neonate: behavioral and physiological indices, *Pain* 52, 287–99

Dale, J.C. (1986) A multidimensional study of infants' responses to painful stimuli, *Pediatric Nursing* 12(1), 27–31

Dreyfus-Brisac, C. (1983) Organisation of sleep in prematures: implications for care giving. In: Call, J.D., Galenson, E. and Tyson, R.L. (eds.) *Frontiers of Infant Psychiatry*, Basic Books, New York

Emla Monograph: Emla Cream and Emla Patch (2000) Astra Zeneca Pharmaceuticals

Gauntlett, I.S. (1987) Analgesia and the neonate, *British Journal of Hospital Medicine*, June, 518–19

Gauvain-Piquard, A. (1989a) *Douleur Enfant Gustave-Roussy (DEGR)* (Gustave-Roussy Child Pain Scale), Unite de psychiatric et d'oncologie, Institut Gustave-Roussy, Villejuif, Paris

Gauvain-Piquard, A. (1989b) Le douleur d'un enfant, *Revue de l'Infirmière* 15

Glover, V. and Fisk, N.M. (1999) Fetal pain: implications for research and practice, *British Journal of Obstetrics and Gynaecology*, 106, 881–6

Grunau, R.V.E. (1999) Long-term consequences of pain in human neonates. In: Anand, K.J.S., Stevens, B.J. and McGrath, P.J. (eds) *Pain in Neonates* (2nd edition), Elsevier, Amsterdam, pp. 55–76

Grunau, R.V.E. and Craig, K.D. (1987) Pain expression in neonates: facial action and cry, *Pain* 28, 395–410

Harpin, V.A.H. and Rutter, N. (1982) Development of emotional sweating in the newborn infant, *Archives of Disease in Childhood* 57, 395–410

Harpin, V.A.H. and Rutter, N. (1983) Making heel pricks less painful, *Archives of Disease in Childhood* 58(3), 226–8

Herzog, J. (1983) A neonatal intensive care syndrome: a pain complex involving neuroplasticity and psychic trauma. In: Call, J.D., Galenson, E. and Tyson, R.L. (eds) *Frontiers of Infant Psychiatry*, Basic Books, New York

Huteau, M. (1988) Travail de recherche sur les sons et les prematures, *Soins Gyn-Obs-Puer-Ped* 84, 11–20

Johnston, C.C. and Strada, M.E. (1986) Acute pain response in infants. A multidimensional description, *Pain* 24, 373–82

Johnston, C.C., Stremler, R., Horton, L. and Friedman, A. (1999) The effect of repeated doses of oral sucrose for decreasing pain from heelstick in pre-term neonates, *Biol Neonate*, 75, 160–6

Kirby, H. (2000) Reverie pour enfant malade: The therapeutic power of music, *Journal of Neonatal Nursing* 6(2), 56–8

Koren, G., Butt, W., Chinyanga, H. *et al.* (1985) Post-operative morphine infusion in newborn infants: assessment of deposition characteristics and safety, *Journal of Pediatrics* 107(6), 963–7

Lagercrantz, H., Nillson, E., Redham, I. and Hjemdahl, P. (1986) Plasma catecholamines following nursing procedures in a neonatal ward, *Early Human Development* 14, 61–5

Lawrence, J., Alcock, D., McGrath, P. *et al.* (1993) The development of a tool to assess neonatal pain, *Neonatal Network* 12(6), 59–66

Levene, M.I. and Quinn, M.W. (1992) Use of sedative and muscle relaxants in newborn babies receiving mechanical ventilation, *Archives of Disease in Childhood* 67(7), 870–3

Long, J.G., Philip, A.G.S. and Lucey, J.F. (1980) Excessive handling as a cause of hypoxaemia, *Paediatrics* 65, 203–7

Michelsson, A-L., Jarvenpaa, A-L. and Rinne, A. (1983) Sound spectrographic analysis of pain cry in pre-term infants, *Early Human Development* 8, 141–9

Mok, Q., Bass, C.A., Ducker, D.A. and McIntosh, N. (1991) Temperature instability during nursing procedures in pre-term neonates, *Archives of Disease in Childhood* 66(7), 783–6

Perlman, J.M. and Volpe, J.J. (1983) Suctioning in the pre-term infant: effects on cerebral blood flow velocity, intracranial pressure, and arterial blood pressure, *Pediatrics* 72, 329–34

Sethna, N.F. and Koh, J.L. (1999) Regional anaesthesia and analgesia. In: Anand, K.J.S., Stevens, B.J. and McGrath, P.J. (eds) *Pain in Neonates* (2nd edition), Elsevier, Amsterdam, pp. 189–201

Sparshott, M.M. (1989) Pain and the special care baby unit, *Nursing Times* 85(41) 61-4

Sparshott, M.M. (1990) *This is Your Baby* (booklet for parents of pre-term babies), available from NICU/Derriford Hospital, Plymouth P16 8DH

Sparshott, M.M. (1991a) Creating a home for babies in hospital, *Paediatric Nursing* 3(8), 20–2

Sparshott, M.M. (1991b) Maintaining skin integrity, *Paediatric Nursing* 3(2), 12–13

Sparshott, M.M. (1991c) Psychological function of the skin, *Paediatric Nursing* 3(3), 22–3

Sparshott, M.M. (1995) The 'sound' of neonatal nursing care, *Journal of Neonatal Nursing* 1(2), 7–9

Sparshott, M.M. (1996) The development of a clinical distress scale for ventilated newborn infants: identification of pain and distress based on validated behavioural scores, *Journal of Neonatal Nursing* 2(2), 5–11

Sparshott, M.M. (1997) *Pain, Distress and the Newborn Baby*, Blackwell Science, Oxford

Stevens, B., Johnston, C., Petryshen, P. and Taddio, A. (1996) Premature infant pain profile; development and initial validation, *Clinical Journal of Pain* 12, 13–22

Stevens, B., Johnston, C., and Gibbins, S. (1999) Pain assessment in neonates. In: Anand, K.J.S., Stevens, B.J. and McGrath, P.J. (eds) *Pain in Neonates* (2nd edition), Elsevier, Amsterdam, pp. 101–34

Williamson, P.S. and Williamson, M.L. (1983) Physiological stress reduction by a local anaesthetic during newborn circumcision, *Paediatrics* 71(1), 360–400

Winnicott, D. (1965) The theory of parent–infant relationship. In: Winnicott, D. (ed.) *The Maturational Process and the Facilitating Environment*, Hogarth Press, London

Wolff, P.H. (1966) *The Causes, Controls and Organization of Behaviour in the Neonate*, International University Press, New York

Wolke, D. (1987) Environmental and developmental neonatology, *Journal of Reproductive and Infant Psychiatry* 5, 17–42

Yuan-Chi Lin (2000) *Complementary treatments for painful neonatal procedures.* Workshop at ISPP 2000, 5th International Symposium on Paediatric Pain, June, London

13 TRANSPORT OF INFANTS

Alison Gibbs and Andrew Leslie

Aims of the chapter

This chapter introduces the reader to the complexities of transporting infants, some of whom will be critically ill. It considers the transfer process, and reviews the needs of the infant in transit and the qualities required in the transport team. It emphasises the importance of communication between hospitals, individuals and the infant's parents. Guidance is given on the extra requirements of transporting infants with specific conditions.

INTRODUCTION

The ideal for an infant is to receive post-natal care at the hospital of delivery. This is not always possible, due to the often unexpected nature of neonatal problems, and the lack of availability of specialist equipment or expertise. If a planned *in utero* transfer is not possible, a neonate may require post-natal transfer.

The first reports of modern neonatal transport (Wallace *et al.*, 1952) date from the period following the Second World War, at a time when neonatal intensive care was being developed. Neonatal transport in the UK has developed as the neonatal speciality has become established. The Report of the expert group on special care for babies (Department of Health and Social Security, 1971) recommended that neonatal intensive care be centralised and that the tertiary units maintain a transport facility for infants. The degree of central planning and regionalisation has fluctuated since that time, but the safety concerns, as highlighted in the TINA Report (Medical Devices Agency, 1995), coupled with broader issues of resource allocation and clinical effectiveness, have tended to encourage centralisation of transport facilities in recent years. These developments look as if they will continue.

Today, sick and premature infants still need to be transferred between hospitals and the basic necessities of warmth and oxygen must be provided, along with a range of other intensive care modalities. The success of a transfer depends upon the people who do the transfer, and their operation within a service that is properly trained and where quality is monitored and improved. There is substantial evidence that transport may be hazardous for infants (Harding and Morton, 1993; Leslie and Stephenson, 1994) and further work strongly suggests that these hazards are minimised by using staff who are trained in transport and whose skills are used frequently (Chance *et al.*, 1978; Leslie and Stephenson, 1997).

This chapter outlines an approach to transport that recognises the additional hazards outlined in Table 13.1 and makes attending to these a routine part of transport practice. A quality service is best provided when proper and balanced attention is given to all aspects, including training of staff, equipment and quality monitoring with improvement.

Table 13.1   Hazards of neonatal transport

Infants are vulnerable to:	• Temperature instability • Handling
Staff are remote from:	• Familiar environment • Advice and help • Replacements for failing equipment
The transport environment has:	• Extremes of temperature • Vibration • Poor light • Limited supplies of power and gases
The transport equipment is:	• Unfamiliar

THE TRANSFER PROCESS

Infants may be transferred for many different reasons. This section takes retrieval as an example situation, where a team from a tertiary unit goes to another hospital to stabilise and transfer a sick infant. The general principles may be applied to most transfer situations.

Referral

The process begins when the referring hospital has made the decision that transport is necessary. This decision should always be made carefully, with consideration given to alternative possibilities, for example, if an extra member of staff coming in might allow the infant to stay. Transport is a potentially risky process, and should never be considered the easy option in a cot crisis.

The transporting unit needs information in order to make important decisions about personnel, clinical supplies, equipment and speed of journey. To facilitate this it may be best to utilise a standard proforma that prompts staff to ask about significant issues (*see* Figure 13.1). The referral acceptance form allows the team to enquire into the condition of the infant in order to enable them to prepare appropriately. This preparation may include the incorporation of additional equipment, such as nitric oxide, which is not routinely carried. Present management may be discussed and an estimated time of arrival offered. The information given at this stage will help the team decide on mode and speed of transfer, depending on the condition and stability of the infant.

Nottingham Transport Referral
Acceptance Form

Date: [　　　　　]   Referring unit: [　　　　　　　　　　]

Time: [　　　　　]   Transport nurse: [　　　　　　　　　　]

Transport required
to / from: [　　　　　　　　　　　　　　　]

Baby name: [　　　　　　　　　　　　　　　]

Gestation: [　　　　]   (Birth) Wt: [　　　　]   D.O.B: [　　　　]

Diagnosis / reason for referral: [　　　　　　　　　　]

SUPPORT

PIP / PEEP: [　　/　　]   BPM: [　　　　]   FiO$_2$: [　　　　]

I.V. Fluids and infusions: [　　　　　　　　　　]

Is an I.A. line in situ? [Yes / No]   Searle? [Yes / No]

CURRENT STATUS
Recent blood gas:

Time: [　　　　]   Cap. / Art? [　　　　]

pH: [　　　　]   pO$_2$: [　　　　]   pCO$_2$: [　　　　]

Base Ex: [　　　　]   Bicarb: [　　　　]

Temp: [　　　　]   B.P: [　　　　]   Blood sugar: [　　　　]

Please add any other relevant details on the reverse, including summary of any advice given.

Figure 13.1   Transport referral proforma

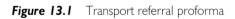

Outward journey

Safety is the most important feature of all ambulance journeys. The safety of the team members, ambulance crew, infant, observers or other road users should be paramount, and no unnecessary risk should be taken. To minimise hazards the following steps should be attended to, both in planning for transport and in the conduct of the day-to-day activity.

- Securing the transport system: effective systems must be in place to secure transport incubator systems in vehicles, and all the staff involved in transport must know how to use these properly.
- Securing other equipment: all other items carried, including monitors, infusion pumps, gas cylinders and bags of clinical supplies, must be secured in the vehicle so that they do not become missiles in the event of a crash.
- Speed of journey: the only indication for using extraordinary measures to move through traffic is that the infant will be placed at unacceptable additional risk by not doing so. Transfer with blue lights/sirens undoubtedly places the team and other road users at additional risk (Auerbach *et al.*, 1987) and there is some evidence that, particularly in urban settings, it may not make a clinically important difference to the journey time (Hunt *et al.*, 1995).

At the referring hospital

The initial step is to obtain a thorough handover, following which an initial assessment can be made. *See* Table 13.2 for the major areas to which the attention of the transport team should be directed in order for the infant to be properly prepared for transfer. There is good evidence (Chance *et al.*, 1978; Hood *et al.*, 1983; Leslie and Stephenson, 1997) that time spent thoroughly attending to stabilisation – a so-called 'stay and play' approach – yields better transport outcomes and results in fewer adverse events during the journey.

Even after extensive stabilisation, some infants may still be too sick to move. This situation always needs input from senior staff, and it may be necessary to seek advice from the base unit. It may be beneficial to return 24 hours later, once the infant is more stable and fit for transfer. A balanced decision needs to account for those infants where the treatment they need is at the other end of the journey and the risk of the journey is outweighed by the benefits of a treatment such as ECMO at the receiving hospital. Transfer should not be attempted when the situation is hopeless, and transport teams may be required to play a part in end-of-life decisions.

The stabilisation period is a time when both the transport team and the resident team need to be aware of, and show consideration towards, each other's views and sensitivities. Anecdotally, some transport teams behave with unacceptable rudeness and insensitivity while on other units, and some units are unhelpful to the transport team. The retrieval team can do much to influence this issue, by showing consideration and respect to the resident team, and by offering a rationale for their activities. For example, changing the endotracheal

Table 13.2 Key activities for stabilising infants for transfer

Objective	Action/rationale
A = Airway	**B = Breathing**
Reliable airway	Should the infant be intubated prior to transfer? Threshold for intubation is lower than on the NNU, to minimise potential for needing to intervene in transit. In an infant >30 weeks gestation if the vital signs (pulse, blood pressure, respiratory rate, temperature) have been consistently stable in oxygen <50% and if the pCO_2 is normal it may be acceptable to move the infant without intubation. However, if the infant is unstable; has a rising oxygen requirement >50%; has a rising pCO_2; has recurrent apnoea; or is < 30 weeks gestation, then intubation and respiratory support are highly likely to be required, at least for the duration of the journey.
Confirm ETT size, X-ray position and ensure well secured	If already intubated, the tube must be correctly positioned and secure. ETTs must be secured to a high standard to avoid dislodgement and need for subsequent intubation during transfer.
Confirm ETT is patent	This is to avoid increased airway impedence due to secretions. All ETTs should be suctioned prior to transfer.
Sufficient respiratory rate	Ventilate infants for apnoea/poor respiratory drive. It is important to avoid the need for intubation in the ambulance. All ventilated transported infants should receive sedation. An infant with an asynchronous respiration may need muscle relaxation, though this is not routinely indicated for transport.
Adequate surface area for gaseous exchange	Appropriate ventilatory pressure. Use surfactant – take your own if necessary. Drain pneumothoraces before the journey, as an undrained small pneumothorax can become larger (especially if flying) and a tension pneumothorax can occur.
Appropriate gaseous exchange has occurred	Monitor oxygenation and CO_2 levels. An arterial blood gas measurement is a necessity for decision-making and for calibration of the transcutaneous monitor.
C = Circulation	
Normal heart rate and blood pressure	Measure the blood pressure, preferably via arterial access. The use of core/toe gap monitoring of temperature may also be helpful (gap >1.5°C and worsening may indicate poor/deteriorating perfusion). Management of hypotension may require inotropes or colloid.
D = Drips/drugs	
Glucose maintenance	The brain makes a constant demand for glucose that a neonate may be unable to meet due to inadequate stores or an inability to utilise those stores. This will vary from infant to infant, so a constant supply of glucose will be needed, by intravenous infusion, and monitoring of blood glucose continued.
Hydration	A supply of water must also be provided. Neonates requiring strict monitoring of input and output may need to be catheterised.
Venous access	Before leaving a referral site ensure that all cannulas are patent and well fixed. If a cannula is required for more than one infusion mixture, another should be inserted before leaving.

(Continued)

Table 13.2 Continued

Prevent aspiration	Best avoided by not feeding in transit, and draining the stomach of any large feed volumes. A nasogastric tube left on free drainage will also help to decompress the stomach when flying and avoid compression of the diaphragm.

E = Exposure

Normothermia	There is evidence that hypothermia significantly worsens the risk of death for transported premature infants (Leslie & Stephenson, 1994). Attention to achieving and maintaining a normal temperature should be a priority. It may be necessary to run the transport incubator at its top setting (39–40°C) as heat is lost much more rapidly to the environment on a transfer than in a well-heated NICU.
Reduction of heat loss	For those infants (less than 29 weeks gestation) at risk of heat loss by evaporation, incubator humidity should be provided if possible. Infants experiencing difficulty in maintenance of temperature may benefit from a chemically activated warming mattress. Transfer from isolette to transport incubator should take no longer than 15 seconds from start to finish. Further heat loss can be minimised by adding a heat and moisture exchanger to the ventilation circuit. Continuous monitoring of temperature is obligatory, with the sensor placed in a core position – for example, under the infant or fixed with a spot plaster in the axilla.

F = Family

Parental contact	Tell parents the important things first – what's wrong, what is being done about it, and how they can visit – and repeat them if necessary. Provide leaflets, videos, maps, etc., to back up the essential information. This time may be very important in the care of the infant where the prognosis may be poor. Photographs, bravery awards or mementoes may be helpful for some parents. The opportunity must be made for the mother to view her infant before transfer, even though this may involve a journey via the labour suite in the transport incubator before boarding the ambulance.
Unit liaison	Keep your own team updated regarding changes and expected departure time for the return journey, so that they can commence any preparations required.

tube may be necessary, if it is too long, too short, blocking or not secure, but this can be interpreted by the resident team as criticism of the work they had done prior to arrival of the transport team. The transport team needs to represent such activities as part of the necessary preparation for transport (Leslie and Middleton, 1995).

Preparation for the return journey should include restocking of any of the unit's equipment used, having a pre-prepared ETT in case a sick infant should extubate, and gathering together items necessary for transfer, such as maternal blood, X-rays and documentation. Thorough stabilisation and preparation for transfer before leaving the referring unit includes ensuring that all the necessary monitoring is in place and working properly.

Return journey

The same considerations regarding the use of blue lights and sirens apply to the return journey as the outward journey. On most transfers, provided the activities of the stabilising period have been properly attended to, it should be possible to complete the return journey without opening the incubator doors, to reduce the heat loss via the portholes to the cooler ambulance environment. Adverse events are minimised by this preparation of the infant and team. However, should they occur, they need to be dealt with promptly and efficiently. The back of the ambulance is an unsuitable site for major resuscitative procedures. There is limited space and pairs of hands, and infants soon become cold. A skilled team will have the knowledge and confidence to consider all the factors and options available should a major adverse event, such as pneumothorax or extubation, occur. It may be best to consider performing a limited procedure in the ambulance, for example, needle aspiration of pneumothorax, and then diversion to another hospital, to allow definitive treatment. Whatever is required, the confines of an ambulance create a difficult work situation and consideration needs to be given to this prior to departure and while on the journey.

Continuous monitoring of vital signs should be documented every 15 minutes, as well as any adverse event. Unfortunately, it is not unknown for in-transit care to be legally challenged, and so it is essential that the team are able to demonstrate, perhaps many years later, that the infant was properly monitored and cared for in transit in order to defend litigation.

Completion

The transfer is complete when the infant is in an incubator on the receiving unit and a comprehensive handover has been given. The equipment must then be prepared for the next call. It is polite to telephone the referring unit to inform them of the infant's safe arrival and also to contact the parents to give them an update. Routine monitoring should include the recording of important parameters, such as temperature and pH, on completion of the transfer to facilitate a quality improvement programme (Hermansen *et al.*, 1988).

The back transfer

Preparation for back transfer should start as soon as an infant is transferred or admitted to a unit that is not the most local for the family. At that time, and throughout the subsequent period of specialist care, it should be made clear to families that their infant will be returned to the sending unit as soon as the condition allows. It is highly counterproductive in this respect for the specialist centre to imply that it provides 'better' care than the sending unit, as this will tend to make the family reluctant to return. An approach that recognises that different units offer different facilities, but that all provide good care, is far superior.

Specialist units need to prepare parents for a change in the technological environment and there should be regular feedback of information between the original referring hospital and the parents. The referring hospital needs to welcome the parents and help them with settling back in, offering a pre-return visit and supplying local information, perhaps in the form of photographs or videos of the unit, to the retrieval hospital for the parents to utilise.

The transport team

The modern transport process and the composition of the team have evolved since the 1950s and there have been a number of studies of the optimal team configuration (Chance *et al.*, 1978; Hood *et al.*, 1983; Leslie and Stephenson, 1997). These data do not achieve a consensus view, but a number of clear principles emerge. First, whatever the professional background of the attending staff, they should be thoroughly trained in the supervision of transfers. It appears that the transport process is sufficiently different from work on neonatal units to mitigate against transport being reliably led by staff who are good at unit work, but who are without transport training and experience.

Second, staff attending transfers should be able to adapt a full range of neonatal interventions to the constraints of the transport setting. There are data suggesting that teams who do not have the traditional doctor/nurse configuration may be equally good at this. In the USA, neonatal nurses, trained for the role, are widely used and appear to be equally effective when compared to traditional teams (Cook and Kattwinkel, 1983). In the UK, the development of the advanced neonatal nurse practitioner (ANNP) role has led to increasing numbers of transfers being led by this group, but their role has yet to be properly evaluated (Leslie and Bose, 1999).

As the numbers of registrars and the hours they work continue to contract, it may be that an approach that ensures a trained, experienced interested neonatal transport nurse is present on every transfer, as the cornerstone of good practice, is best (Leslie and Stephenson, 1997). The team leader can be an ANNP or specialist registrar as required, recognising that their training and expertise may be variable.

A transport programme of education needs to incorporate a number of pertinent issues (*see* Table 13.3). The training programme should start with a period of induction, including supervised clinical practice supported with theoretical perspectives. It is important during this initial period that protected, supervised exposure to real transfers is available, and that education is focused on key principles that will equip the new team member with skills and knowledge that are transferable between situations. An assessment strategy is necessary, to ensure satisfactory completion of training (Budd and Donlen, 1984), and this should be constructed to be congruent with established transport policies and procedures. This initial foundation needs to be followed by ongoing education of the team. This is of critical importance in transport work, as the key practice of team members happens away from the scrutiny of their peers, unlike work on the NNU.

Appointment of a team member responsible for induction and education of transport team members may be a helpful part of developing a rounded, comprehensive transport programme.

Team-member selection is a key issue for the effective running of the team. Some of the key qualities for transport team nurses are the following:

- good intensive care experience (at least 1-year post-ENB Course 405);
- evidence of a teaching interest;

- the ability to work independently, especially in a crisis; and
- commitment to co-operative teamworking.

Table 13.3 Education of transport personnel

Induction	Assessment strategy
• Management of potentially life-threatening situations	• Reflective practice diary
• Transport equipment, including trouble-shooting	• Summative assessment
• Clinical transfer issues, eg, stabilisation of airway	• Demonstration of practice
• Communication	• Demonstration of practice
• Documentation	• Demonstration of practice
Ongoing	
• Audit and subsequent care management	• Monitoring tool/audit form
• Critical incident analysis/workshop analysis (past or potential)	
• Review of recent transport research	
• Revision of pathophysiology	
• Equipment updates	
• Clinical supervision	

Some authors advocate key personality traits, such as diplomacy and assertiveness, for transport team members. However, for team growth, development and stability, these issues seem less important than selecting people who are interested and enthusiastic, and who meet the basic criteria.

EQUIPMENT

Equipment needs to meet the needs of critically ill infants and offer a high standard of intensive care during the journey. A number of conflicting constraints influence the design and construction of equipment for neonatal transport.

Characteristics of transport equipment

Reliability
Vibration is bad for electrical equipment. In general it is preferable to use equipment that has been engineered specifically to deal with the more hostile transport environment. Replacement equipment is not available during transfer.

Simplicity
Transport equipment will often be different from that used on the NNU. For it to be used effectively by staff who may not attend transfers very often, it should be as simple and intuitive to use as possible. Complex equipment in general has more to go wrong. It is preferable to use a simple and reliable gas-driven ventilator rather than one with complex electronic monitoring and control facilities, as these are unlikely to be sufficiently robust for transport.

Flexibility (in terms of power/gas supplies)

As far as possible, electronic equipment should be able to run from a mains supply as well as internal batteries and the ambulance power supply. Gas supply may be from cylinders on the system, external sources or from a compressor. For both batteries and gases it is prudent to plan for providing independent supplies based on double the longest routine journey undertaken.

Weight

For transport equipment to be effectively secured in the vehicle, the weight has to minimised. It is likely that the European Standards Organisation will impose a maximum weight of 150kg for transport systems, as well as other restrictions.

Securing equipment

Effective securing devices need to be provided in vehicles as a result of planning with the local ambulance service, and the devices must be used properly by the staff attending each transfer. Cargo straps provide a simple and effective solution to securing most items. It is the responsibility of the neonatal team to ensure that all the equipment on the system is properly secured. Bags of clinical supplies, for example, must be secured properly. The transport team should avoid carrying any other items of equipment that cannot be secured in the vehicle.

Items included in a typical transport system

A typical transport system configured for emergency transfers may comprise the following items. Operational characteristics are also outlined. The European Standards Organisation may make it obligatory for clinicians to purchase fully configured, off-the-shelf equipment, but at present no such equipment exists.

Trolley

The trolley needs to be compatible both with ambulance service fittings and with the equipment to be mounted on it. A trolley that can be raised to a reasonable working height is helpful, and it needs to have space for incubator, monitors and other components according to local needs.

Incubator

A thermo-neutral environment is the starting point for the transfer of neonates. The incubator should readily heat to 39–40^{0}C, with a humidification facility for the most immature infants. It should run from battery, ambulance power and mains electricity. Double incubator walls help minimise heat loss. A light is helpful.

Gas supply

Oxygen and air are needed, in flexible configurations. Cylinders must be properly secured.

Ventilator

A ventilator for neonates needs to provide facilities for pressure-limited, time-cycled ventilation, as well as CPAP. A full range of FiO_2 should be available, from 0.21–1.0. It should be able to draw gas from the hospital wall supply, from the ambulance oxygen during transfer, and from the system cylinders. Other ventilation modes, such as patient-triggered ventilation and high-frequency oscillation are not necessary as part of the routine transport equipment, although they may be utilised by specialist units. Disconnect alarms and a device for monitoring FiO_2 are essential. Humidity may be provided by a disposable heat and moisture exchanger in the ventilator circuit. Electric water-bath humidifiers, like those used on the NNU, are likely to have large power consumption and be unreliable, with substantial motion moving the water around.

Monitors

A number of transport monitors are available that will provide monitoring of heart rate, respiratory rate, oxygen saturation, invasive and non-invasive blood pressure and two temperatures, all in a single relatively small box with good battery and power characteristics. In adults, blood pressure monitored via the arterial line is more reliable than a cuff recording when in transport (Runcie *et al.*, 1990), and can provide a more reliable heart rate than chest leads, which are susceptible to motion artefacts. A transcutaneous monitor has been shown to produce better transport outcomes by providing information on ventilation and enabling ventilator adjustments in transit (O'Connor and Grueber, 1998).

Infusion devices

A variety of infusion devices are available but the quality of the battery facilities is variable and the ease and security of mounting to the transport system must also be considered. Once they have been purchased, their battery life can be further maximised by restricting their use to transport.

Nitric oxide

Nitric oxide can also be introduced, as small cylinders and portable monitors are available. This should, in general, be restricted to centres that can give proper attention to the exceptional health and safety considerations.

Supporting items

A number of supporting items are needed to facilitate a safe neonatal transfer. These may include equipment for the following:

- airway control;
- resuscitation, basic and advanced;
- drugs administration;
- fluid maintenance;
- monitoring;

- essential infant care equipment;
- staff care, eg, travel sickness tablets, cold drinks.

These should be configured according to local practice and carried in transport packs. All items of equipment must be properly secured in the vehicle.

COMMUNICATIONS

The greater part of a nurse's work involves communications: across the multidisciplinary team and with the parents and families. Transportation only allows a very short time frame in which to achieve effective communication. This time needs to be used constructively in order to ensure that all the necessary communication takes place.

Communication with parents

Shellabarger and Thompson (1993) remind the nurse that the NICU experience on its own is fraught with anxiety and recommend ways to address the needs for parental communication. Cross *et al.* (1995) researched the content of the communications strategies adopted on transport in Nottingham, and found that using a portable video to support other information was well accepted.

Mehrabin (1971) observed that only 7% of communication is verbal, the remaining being comprised of tone, pitch and intonation. Proper understanding of important information is further hindered by the use of medical language (Ley and Spelman, 1967) and a third of the information given will not be retained. Jupp (1992) recommends that when giving bad news to parents the information is given based upon just five questions; these can be further reduced to three questions for the transportation process:

1   What are your child's needs?
2   What will happen to your child?
3   What do you need to do to help, or be with your child?

These three questions must address the most important factors first, and may require repetition. In practice this can be complemented by the use of video and information booklets. Photographs and bravery certificates help to mark the significance of the event and provide lasting memories.

Multidisciplinary communication

It is essential that the relations between units be based on mutual trust and respect for each other's experience. The retrieval team and the referring hospital must work effectively together, using the skills of the retrieval team and the local knowledge of the referring hospital with mutual respect and courtesy. The need for referral must never be regarded as in any way a failure of the referring staff. The responsibility of each unit is indicated on the graph in Figure 13.2. The key points to draw from this conceptual graph are that, while the transport team assumes the majority of the responsibility for the infant after receiving handover (the point where the lines cross), the transport team has some responsibility before then, and the referring team retains some responsibility after then (Brimhall, 1994).

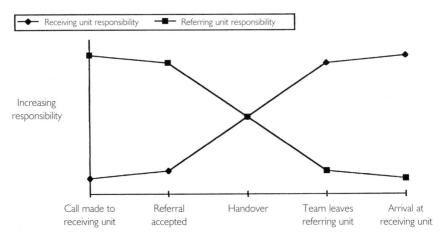

Figure 13.2   Responsibility of each unit

The transport team should listen to everything that the referring team has to say, remembering that they are there at the request of the referring team. Those referring should be willing to assist the retrieval team with any further stabilisation measures necessary. Leslie and Middleton (1995) described three specific areas for communication breakdown:

- the transport team 'barging in and taking over';
- critical comments on the quality of care given;
- arbitrary changes in management.

Recognising these issues encourages good working relations to be built up, which can lead to forums for discussion and better management across all types of NNU.

Written communications

An accurate written record of the infant's story is essential, in the form of written communications (medical notes). Although it is not a legal requirement, the nursing documentation could be used as supportive evidence in a court of law, in the event of litigation, when any errors or omissions could become matters of first importance. The details of specific cases may become confused in the memory over time with a host of similar situations, so it is vital to adopt the habit of producing good written records. Even after a relatively short time, the documents may represent the only record that is able to demonstrate decisions and management. Ongoing management can be demonstrated using observation and fluid management charts (*see* Figures 13.3 and 13.4). These records can also be used for audit purposes and to ensure subsequent clinical effectiveness.

NOTTINGHAM NEONATAL SERVICE TRANSPORT RECORD (1)   DATE   A GIBBS 01/00

NAME

DATE OF BIRTH	NAME BANDS	E.T.T. SIZE
REFERRAL HOSPITAL	TIME OF BIRTH	CUT AT
REFERRAL HOSPITAL NO.	AGE	LAST TUBE CHANGE DATE
MOTHERS TRANSFER PLAN	CONTACT NO.	GUTHRIE / TSH

Time																								
P.I.P.																								
P.E.E.P. / C.P.A.P.																								
Ti. Time																								
Ventilator rate																								
Respiratory rate																								
FiO$_2$																								
Saturation																								
TcPO$_2$																								
TcPCO$_2$																								
E.T.T.Washout/suction																								
Heart rate																								
Bp mean																								
Systolic/diastolic																								
Baby temperature																								
Incubator temperature																								
Comments/actions Location																								

| NAME | SIGNATURE |

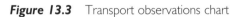

Figure 13.3 Transport observations chart

NOTTINGHAM NEONATAL SERVICE TRANSPORT RECORD (2)   DATE   A.GIBBS.01/00

NAME   D.O.B.   HOSP. NO.   DRUGS

BIRTH WT.   PRESENT WT.   Vit K. O/I.M.

Time	fluids mls/kg	ml/hr	Total	site	ml/hr	Total	site	ml/hr	Total	site	ml/hr	Total	site	ml/hr	Total	site	ml/hr	Total	site	blood sugar	NG ASP		Urine	Bowels	

HISTORY

STABILISATION

IN TRANSIT

NAME	SIGNATURE

Figure 13.4   Transport of fluids chart

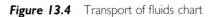

SPECIAL CONSIDERATIONS

Very immature/low birthweight

Infants in this group are particularly vulnerable to cold and this has been shown to be associated with poor outcomes (Leslie and Stephenson, 1994). These infants represent a unique transport challenge, and every effort must be made to promote normothermia. The transport incubator should be double-walled and thoroughly pre-warmed to 39–40°C, with humidity if possible. A chemically activated gel mattress will provide an additional source of heat when placed under the infant. Time spent in handling, or in transfer from the hospital isolette to the transport incubator, will exacerbate heat loss due to time spent in contact with cooler air. A '15-second rule' may help to reinforce the importance of limiting exposure to room air – the nurse should complete the transfer of the infant into (or out of) the transport incubator within 15 seconds, including opening and closing incubator doors. Further optimisation will also occur if the back of the ambulance is heated.

Gastroschisis

Infants with this condition can quickly run into difficulties with hypoglycaemia, hypotension and hypothermia if not actively managed. The infant should be placed up to their armpits into a drawstring type bag, to cover the defect and provide a clean environment for the exposed bowel. Positioning should ensure that the exposed bowel is supported. The bag should be emptied of fluid regularly, to avoid the infant lying in a pool of cold fluid. Fluid losses of 40–60 mls/kg should be anticipated and replaced with human albumin solution. Fluid losses may be estimated by measuring the serous fluid collected from the bag, by measuring BP and tracking the trend of the toe/core temperature gap. The temptation to allow the parents to cuddle their infant should be resisted, as further handling of the gut causes it to become bruised and oedematous, placing the defect at greater compromise.

Oesophageal atresia/tracheo-oesophageal fistula

A double lumen (Replogle) type of nasogastric tube, allowing for frequent suction and wash-out of the secretions collecting within the oesophageal pouch, is needed for infants with oesophageal atresia. Infants should be positioned with the head slightly up, to allow secretions to pool in the oesophageal pouch, from where they can be suctioned. Suction in transit is achieved by turning on the aspirator for a few seconds every 5–15 minutes. Infants with oesophageal atresia and a distal tracheo-oesophageal fistula who have been intubated and ventilated represent a significant surgical emergency and need prompt transfer. Ventilation gas is forced into the gut via the fistula, but cannot escape upwards, due to the oesophageal atresia. This may lead to gross gaseous distension of the abdomen and difficulty with ventilation due to pressure on the chest cavity.

Congenital diaphragmatic hernia

All infants with this condition should be ventilated for transfer. Pharmacological muscle relaxation to reduce swallowing of air, as well as sedation, should be routine. Most infants will have increasing respiratory distress, worsening with bag and mask ventilation. This deterioration with bag and mask ventilation needs to be anticipated before transfer and an ETT prepared to allow for immediate reintubation. A nasogastric tube on free drainage will need to be in situ to deflate the stomach of air and allow for maximum lung expansion.

Acute gastro-intestinal obstruction and/or perforation (including necrotising enterocolitis)

These infants will often be extremely sick and may require full intensive care support for the transfer. Where surgery may be life-saving, the team may have to balance the time spent stabilising against the need for transfer for definitive treatment. These infants may benefit from a continuous plasma infusion as well as glucose intravenously. They will need to be nil orally, with a nasogastric tube on free drainage.

Cardiac lesions

The care of neonates with cardiac lesions during transfer is a continuation of the care given on the NNU. Management for transfer should be guided by discussion with the receiving cardiac centre. Infants with lesions that depend on a patent arterial duct should not be given oxygen supplementation, as this may promote closure of the duct. Such infants will need to be bagged in air, should the situation arise, rather than use the oxygen found in an ambulance cylinder. Infants with cardiac disease may have saturations in the 70s to the 80s and correction should be attempted with prostaglandin therapy rather than oxygen. Infants starting prostaglandin therapy should have a dedicated intravenous line for the infusion, so reducing the risk of inadvertent stoppages or bolus of the drug.

The side-effects of prostaglandin therapy are numerous; most noticeably, apnoea and seizures can occur. It is a wise precaution to allow a few minutes following the commencement of the drug to allow any side-effects to show before departing into the confined space of an ambulance. Some infants will need ventilating to protect their airway. Time spent in stabilisation is valuable and essential but needs to be balanced against the knowledge that definitive treatment commences when the journey concludes at a cardiac centre.

AIRBORNE TRANSFERS

Airborne transfer, by helicopter or fixed-wing aircraft, is useful when long-distance transfer is necessary. It is widely used in parts of the world where the distances between centres are substantial, such as USA and Australia. (American Academy of Pediatrics, 1999; Job et al., 1999). There are significant limitations on where and when aircraft can take off and land, and so it is likely that time will only be saved when the journey time by ground exceeds 1.5–2 hours. Airborne transfer has a number of significant problems, beyond the expense. The working environment, particularly in terms of space and noise, may be significantly worse than that experienced on ground transfer. Altitude has significant effects, particularly reducing the oxygen available in the atmosphere. Another important consideration is that, as atmospheric pressure decreases, trapped gas will expand, tending to worsen pneumothoraces and other air leaks.

Most centres in the UK will not have a routine need to transfer by air, and airborne transport should not be undertaken on an ad hoc basis.

SAMPLE EXAMINATION QUESTION

Question 1
What are the transport team's priorities following their arrival on a unit to collect a sick infant for retrieval? (*70 marks*)
What actions can the nurse take to ensure that the parents have some memories and can maintain contact with their infant? (*30 marks*)

REFERENCES

American Academy of Pediatrics (1999) *Guidelines for Air and Ground Transport of Neonatal and Pediatric Patients* (2nd edition), AAP

Auerbach, P.S., Morris, J.A., Phillips, J.B., Redlinger, S.R. and Vaughn, W.K. (1987) An analysis of ambulance accidents in Tennessee, *JAMA* 258(11), 487–90

Brimhall, D. (1994) Legal aspects of transport. In: Stone Trautman, M. (ed.) *Current Concepts in Transport* (6th edition), University of Utah, Utah

Budd, R.A. and Donlen, J.M. (1984) Clinical evaluation of the neonatal transport team, *Critical Care Nurse*, Sept/Oct, 24–8

Chance, G.W. *et al.* (1978) Neonatal transport: a controlled study of skilled assistance, *Journal of Pediatrics* 93(4), 662–6

Cook, L. and Kattwinkel, J. (1983) A prospective study of nurse-supervised versus physician-supervised neonatal transports, *Journal of Obstetric, Gynecologic and Neonatal Nursing* 12(6), 371–6

Cross, J., Townsend, S. and Leslie, A. (1995) Communication from a distance, *Journal of Neonatal Nursing* 1(4), 32–5

Department of Health and Social Security (1971) *Report of the Expert Group on Special Care for Babies*, Reports on Public Health and Medical Subjects No. 127, HMSO, London

Harding, J.E. and Morton, S.M. (1993) Adverse effects of neonatal transport between Level III centres, *Journal of Paediatrics and Child Health* 29, 146–9

Hermansen, M.C., Hasan, S., Hoppin, J. and Cunningham, M.D. (1988) A validation of a scoring system to evaluate the condition of transported very low-birthweight neonates, *American Journal of Perinatology* 5, 74–8

Hood, J.L. *et al.* (1983) Effectiveness of the neonatal transport team, *Critical Care Medicine* 11(6), 419–23

Hunt, R.C. *et al.* (1995) Is ambulance transport time with lights and siren faster than that without? *Annals of Emergency Medicine* **25**(4), 507–11

Job, L., Deming, D.D., Hopper, A.O. and Peverini, R.L. (1999) Air transport in neonatal medicine, *Seminars in Neonatology* **4**(4), 273–9

Jupp, S. (1992) *Making the Right Start – A Practical Manual to Help Break the News to Families When Their Baby has Been Born with a Disability*, Opened Eye Publications, Cheshire, England

Leslie, A. and Bose, C. (1999) Nurse-led neonatal transport, *Seminars in Neonatology* **4**(4), 265–71

Leslie, A. and Middleton, D. (1995) Give and take in neonatal transport – communication hazards in handover, *Journal of Neonatal Nursing* **1**(5), 27–31

Leslie, A.J. and Stephenson, T.J. (1994) Audit of neonatal intensive care transport, *Archive of Diseases in Childhood* **71**, 61–6

Leslie, A. and Stephenson, T.J. (1997) Audit of neonatal intensive care transport – closing the loop, *Acta Paediatrica* **86**, 1253–6

Ley, P. and Spelman, M. (1967) *Communication with the Patient*, Warren H Green, St Louis, IL

Medical Devices Agency (1995) *Transport of Neonates in Ambulances (TINA)*, Department of Health, London

Mehrabin, A. (1971) *Silent Messages*, Wandsworth, Belmont, LA

O'Connor, T. and Grueber, R. (1998) Transcutaneous measurement of carbon dioxide tension during long-distance transport of neonates receiving mechanical ventilation, *Journal of Perinatology* **18**(3), 189–92

Runcie, C., Reeve, J., Reidy, J. and Dougall, J. (1990) Blood pressure measurement during transport, *Anaesthesia* **45**, 659–65

Shellabarger, S. and Thompson, T. (1993) The critical times: meeting parental communication needs throughout the NICU experience, *Neonatal Network* **12**(2), 39–44

Wallace, H.M., Losty, M.A. and Baumgartner, L. (1952) Report of two years experience in the transportation of premature infants in New York City, *Pediatrics* **22**, 439

14 Neonatal infection

Ann and Daniel Dooley

Aims of the chapter

This chapter introduces the neonatal nurse to some of the factors that contribute to the high incidence of infection on the unit. It aims to inform and guide practice during the collection of specimens, goes on to review specific organisms and describes management. Where appropriate, the disease process has also been considered.

INTRODUCTION

The infant in the neonatal unit is in a uniquely vulnerable situation with regard to infection. Several factors contribute to the high incidence of infection:

- poor immune response in pre-term infants;
- artificially warm, moist, enclosed environment in incubators;
- use of invasive procedures such as ventilation, cannulation and drains;
- exposure to multiple carers and handling.

The rates for neonatal septicaemia give an indication of the increased risk of infection, with pre-term infants experiencing a 5–8 times higher incidence than term infants (Fanaroff *et al.*, 1998).

The newborn infant is unable to communicate verbally the distress caused by infection, and will often lack the classical signs of infection, which would be found in the more mature infant and adult. Careful monitoring of the infant, coupled with appropriate use of infection screen procedures, is vital if any infection is to be diagnosed in its early stages. An understanding of the relevant issues will allow nursing staff to have a greater awareness of the needs of the newborn and to optimise the nursing care provided.

Some neonatal infections can be attributed to the infant having already being infected at time of admission to the NNU, but nursing staff must be aware that nosocomial (hospital-acquired) infection rates in NNUs can be as high as 25% (Donowitz, 1989). Infection control measures must, therefore, be carefully devised and implemented to protect the neonate from further risk of infection. Close collaboration with infection control departments, clinical microbiologists and occupational health departments is a necessity if cross-infection risks are to be reduced as far as is practicable. In addition to the risk of cross-infection between infants, the risk to hospital staff from infectious agents must always be considered. Where particular risks are present these have been discussed within this chapter, as have the risks associated with hospital staff as a potential source of infection.

THE NEONATE'S IMMUNE RESPONSE TO INFECTION

The newborn infant's immune system will offer some degree of protection against infection by certain micro-organisms but the extent of this protection will vary greatly according to the gestational age at delivery. At term, the infant will have high levels of maternal immunoglobulin G. This is the only immunoglobulin class to cross the placenta and will offer protection against the range of pathogens to which the mother has been exposed – streptococci, pneumococci and meningococci. However, in pre-term infants, this level of maternal immunoglobulin G will be reduced, making them particularly vulnerable to infection by these pathogens.

Immunoglobulin M is the immunoglobulin class responsible for combating Gram negative infections but, due to its large molecular size, it does not cross the placenta. Since immunoglobulin M levels in pre-term infants are reduced (even in term infants, they are found at only 20% of adult levels), this predisposes them to Gram-negative infections by organisms such as E. coli. This accounts for the high pathogenicity of these organisms at this stage in life.

The other major class of immunoglobulin is immunoglobulin A. This does not cross the placenta but can be of great significance in the newborn infant's response to infection because it is present, in very high concentrations, in colostrum and breast milk. Also present in breast milk is a protein called lactoferrin, which has a synergistic role with the immunoglobulin A in preventing gastroenteritis caused by pathogenic strains of E. coli. These enteropathogenic E. coli have a high metabolic requirement for iron, to allow replication and growth. However, lactoferrin has a high affinity for free iron, thereby depriving the E. coli of this essential metabolic component and making them susceptible to attack by immunoglobulin A.

SPECIFIC RISK FACTORS FOR INFECTION

Pre-term neonates, born as a result of a labour complicated by prolonged rupture of membranes (PROM), are at a greater risk of infection than those born by non-PROM labours (Levine, 1991). This risk is further increased (twofold) if the duration of PROM was greater than 48 hours. Subsequent delivery by caesarean section is also a risk factor. These neonates may, therefore, require closer observation for any sign of early-onset infection and, according to local policy, may need to be considered for active antimicrobial prophylaxis.

Other researchers have shown that low birthweight and prematurity are, in themselves, specific risk factors, as are abnormal vaginal presentation and antepartum foetal tachycardia (Spaans et al., 1990). Following delivery, other factors associated with increased likelihood of infection have been identified, including the presence of intravenous cannulae (Mullett *et al.*, 1998) and assisted ventilation (Slagle *et al.*, 1989).

ANTIMICROBIAL CHEMOTHERAPY

The administration of antibiotics to neonates occurs as a response to three distinct situations:

1   If the infant meets criteria for prophylactic antibiotics as a result of obstetric risk factors for infection. Examples of this include previous history of group B streptococcus sepsis or prolonged rupture of membranes. Reference should always be made to current local policies and risk assessment algorhythms.

2   If the infant shows clinical signs of infection, but no confirmed microbiological results are yet available, treatment must be started using an empirical regimen directed towards the most likely pathogens. An example of this process would be the choice of gentamicin and benzyl penicillin in cases of suspected early-onset neonatal sepsis, where Group B Strep. is the most common cause. This is in contrast to suspected late-onset sepsis, where a combination of flucloxacillin and gentamicin would be favoured, due to the prevalence of staphylococcal infection in these circumstances.

3   In the case of an infant with confirmed microbiological results demonstrating neonatal infection. Preliminary results will usually only be available 24–48 hours after a specimen is sent to the laboratory, with antibiotic sensitivities requiring a further 24 hours. In many such cases the infant will already have commenced empirical antibiotic therapy, however, prompt response to any culture results must be a priority to ensure the most effective treatment can be given.

DETECTION/DIAGNOSIS OF INFECTION

Specimen taking

Compliance with laboratory requirements, when taking specimens for the detection/diagnosis of neonatal infection, is one aspect of nursing care that is often overlooked. This is, generally, not as a result of failure to follow guidelines, but due to ignorance and lack of communication between laboratory and nursing staff. For example, the type of specimen container and the type of swab used will determine the acceptable delay allowed before processing the specimen in the laboratory. Examples of this are the use of sterile universal containers for urine instead of a urine container with boric acid, and the use of normal transport swabs instead of charcoal swabs when attempting to culture *Neisseria gonorrhoeae* from suspected ophthalmia neonatorum.

In general, swabs, secretions, endotracheal tube tips and intravenous line tips should arrive at the laboratory within 4 hours of being taken. If this is not possible, certain specimens may be placed in a refrigerator overnight, without significant detriment to the culture results. Notable exceptions to this are specimens looking for delicate organisms such as *Neisseria gonorrhoeae*, blood culture bottles and certain virological studies such as *Chlamydia trachomatis* isolation. In these cases, the transport of the specimen, direct to the laboratory specimen reception, should be arranged and, if outside normal working hours, consideration must be given to contacting the laboratory to arrange for urgent processing or appropriate storage upon receipt in the laboratory.

Microbiology/virology request forms

The details provided by medical and nursing staff on microbiology/virology request forms are of great importance in determining the extent of investigation undertaken and the significance placed on any findings in the laboratory. Date of onset of symptoms, duration of illness, other predisposing medical conditions, all recent and current antimicrobial therapy, as well as a full description of specimen site and patient's details, will all influence the final laboratory report and should therefore be included, wherever possible.

The Gram stain

The Gram stain is a laboratory technique that allows visualisation of certain micro-organisms and human cells. When performed directly on specimens, this stain can give an indication of the cellular response to infection (the presence of leucocytes) as well as the type of bacteria/fungi present.

The Gram stain also has a use in the preliminary identification of bacteria according to their Gram reaction. Examples of Gram stain reactions, for commonly encountered pathogens, are given in Table 14.1 (these are also included under the sections dealing with the specific pathogen). The morphology of bacteria is also included in a Gram stain result to aid any presumptive diagnosis of infection.

Table 14.1   Gram stain reaction and bacterial morphology of certain bacterial pathogens encountered in neonatal infections

Gram reaction and morphology	Common neonatal pathogens
Gram-positive cocci	*Staphylococcus aureus*
	Beta haemolytic streptococci
Gram-positive bacilli	*Listeria monocytogenes*
	Clostridium species
Gram-negative bacilli	*Escherichia coli*
	Pseudomonas aeruginosa
Gram-negative cocci	*Neisseria gonnorheae*
Gram-negative cocco-bacilli	*Haemophilus influenzae*

Non-microbiological tests

As well as the bacterial and virology specimens, which will be taken when infection is suspected, other tests will be carried out to aid the diagnosis. These may include:

- haematology requests, such as full blood counts;
- chemical analysis, such as blood gases and electrolyte levels;
- radiography, if respiratory infection or necrotising enterocolitis is suspected.

BACTERIAL AND FUNGAL INFECTION

Beta haemolytic streptococci (BHS)

Beta haemolytic streptococci are a group of Gram-positive cocci, which produce a wide range of toxic factors responsible for their pathogenesis. These include blood-destroying haemolysins, which can be tested for in the laboratory, and are responsible for their name. The BHS are grouped serologically (Lancefield groups), with groups A, B, C, D and G being of most significance in neonatal infection.

Group B streptococci are the major cause of neonatal meningitis at present (Schuchat, 1999). The infection is usually perinatally acquired following prolonged rupture of membranes or during traumatic delivery. Following perinatal exposure, *Group B streptococci* are often isolated from eye, ear and gastric aspirate cultures, hence the value of full infection screens for infants, following a long labour or traumatic birth. Locally we have commenced a rigorous programme of aggressive post-natal prophylaxis for infants of mothers with positive high vaginal swabs.

Group A streptococci are the classical *Pyogenic streptococci*, responsible for scarlet fever, glomerulonephritis and wound infections. They are often responsible, along with *Groups C and G streptococci*, for infected umbilical stumps as well as eye, ear and respiratory infections.

Group D streptococci (faecal streptococci/Enterococcus faecalis) are less pathogenic members of this group but occasionally found in urinary tract infections and septicaemia.

Coliform bacilli

The *coliform bacilli* are a group of Gram negative bacilli, commonly associated with faecal/intestinal origin, but also found in the general environment. Included in this group is *Escherichia coli*. Colonisation of the intestinal tract occurs in the first week of life and superficial skin contamination soon thereafter. Unlike healthy infants, newborns resident in NNUs are initially colonised with the Gram-negative bacterial flora found in the unit, and not from bacteria acquired from the mother perinatally. This may have serious consequences if the unit contains endemic strains of virulent or multiple drug-resistant coliforms. These newly colonised infants represent a reservoir for continued infection within the unit. Examples of this effect have been documented, with particular strains of *Serratia marcescens* causing infection over a long period of time (Jones et al., 2000).

Coliform bacilli do not produce the wide range of toxins found in other pathogens and therefore physical damage to infected areas is less severe. However, prompt treatment of any infected site is essential to reduce the risk of infection spreading, since coliform bacilli are a major cause of neonatal meningitis and septicaemia.

Candida albicans (thrush)

Candida albicans is a commensal of the vaginal tract, found in low numbers in 10–30% of healthy women. During vaginal delivery, the infant is exposed to this opportunistic pathogen and may be at risk from infection. The main sites of candidal infection are the mouth and groin. In the case of oral candidiasis, the mucous membranes develop white spots or coating, which resist gentle scraping. The condition responds rapidly to regular mouth care with anti-fungal gel or drops. Candidiasis of moist skin folds, particularly the groin region, is recognisable by the characteristic reddening of the affected area, often with satellite lesions occurring in close proximity and is treated topically with the same anti-fungal which is used in the mouth. In cases of candidiasis affecting the groin region, there is a risk of subsequent urinary tract infection. If there is any suspicion of this, a specimen of urine should be submitted for culture, specifically requesting candida culture.

Listeria monocytogenes

Listeria monocytogenes is a Gram-positive bacillus, responsible for meningitis and septicaemia in immuno-compromised individuals, pregnant women and newborn infants. The main source of maternal infection is by consumption of contaminated foods, although dietary advice, which is now widely available, appears to be reducing the incidence of adult infections. Maternal infection results in abortion in 90% of cases in pregnant women, whilst an infection at time of delivery places the infant at high risk of developing neonatal meningitis.

Neisseria gonorrhoeae

Neisseria gonorrhoeae (gonococcus) is a Gram-negative diplococcus, and is responsible for the sexually transmitted disease, gonorrhoea. Its main significance, in neonates, is as the cause of the purulent neonatal conjunctivitis (*Ophthalmia neonatorum*), although disseminated infection, involving sites such as the vagina and rectum, can occur if the maternal infection is acute at time of delivery. *Ophthalmia neonatorum* usually presents following undiagnosed gonococcal infection in the mother, resulting in perinatal infection during vaginal delivery, with the characteristic purulent conjunctivitis appearing within 48 hours of birth.

In cases of purulent conjunctivitis, treatment must be started immediately following the taking of swabs for culture, and not delayed until microbiological culture results are available. Any swabs for suspected *Ophthalmia neonatorum* must be taken to the microbiology laboratory without delay if *Neisseria gonorrhoeae* is to be cultured successfully, since these bacteria are very fragile and die off quickly in transport.

Although neonatal gonococcal infection is relatively rare in the UK, recent data shows that the number of newly diagnosed cases of gonorrhoea has risen steadily over the past five years (DHSS and PS, 2000). Of particular concern is the annual rise of 25% in new cases among teenage girls, who are already associated with additional obstetric and neonatal complications.

Haemophilus influenzae

Haemophilus influenzae is a Gram-negative cocco-bacillus that is predominantly a pathogen of the respiratory tract, eyes and ears in neonates. Contrary to common misconception, the bacteria Haemophilus influenzae is not responsible for the illness influenza ('flu'), which is caused by the influenza viruses. In neonates, Haemophilus influenzae is a rare cause of meningitis and septicaemia. Historically, this organism became of increasing importance in older infants and children, being one of the major causes of paediatric meningitis. However, the highly successful HIB vaccination programme has greatly reduced the occurrence of invasive Haemophilus influenzae infection (Slack et al., 1998).

Mycobacterium tuberculosis

Mycobacterium tuberculosis is a bacterium that does not respond to the Gram stain reaction and therefore requires specialised stains for its identification. The most common stain is the Zeihl Nilson stain (ZN stain), which involves treatment with acid and alcohol, giving rise to the terminology acid alcohol fast bacilli (AFB or AAFB). The incidence of neonatal tuberculosis infection in Europe had become very low, but it is now on the increase. This is the result of a combination of factors, including the emergence of drug-resistant strains, an increased reservoir of infection in AIDS patients, and a reduced uptake of vaccination, and there is an accompanying increase in the risk of neonatal tuberculosis.

Intra-uterine tuberculosis is rare and inevitably results in abortion or stillbirth, with perinatal infection from the mother being the main source of infection. If neonatal infection is suspected, as well as investigating the infant, the mother must undergo examination for tuberculosis, since the demonstration of tubercle bacilli in infected neonates is unreliable. Treatment is often started in the absence of proven neonatal tuberculosis due to the devastating consequences of this disease, and consists of long-term multiple antibiotic therapy.

Infected infants and mothers should be nursed in isolation if 'open' tuberculosis is diagnosed. Staff should be screened for tuberculosis when starting work, due to the high infectivity of the disease in neonates and because, in its early stages, tuberculosis may be asymptomatic, yet infectious.

Pseudomonas aeruginosa

Pseudomonas aeruginosa is a Gram-negative bacillus. Its main pathogenesis, in neonates, is in conjunctivitis, skin infections and complications as a result of heavy colonisation of endotracheal tubes. The latter occurs due to the very favourable conditions for the growth of Pseudomonas aeruginosa in the warm, humidified environment and results in greatly increased secretions in heavily colonised infants.

One characteristic of *Pseudomonas aeruginosa* is the production of green pigments, which, when visible in infected secretions and discharges and accompanied by the typical rancid smell of heavy pseudomonal infection, may assist diagnosis before laboratory reports are available.

Staphylococcus aureus

Staphylococcus aureus is a Gram-positive coccus that is responsible for a wide range of infections in neonates. Since the organism is ubiquitously distributed in the hospital environment, colonisation of the infant's nose and skin occurs within 5 days in up to 90% of cases. The most common manifestations of staphylococcus infection are conjunctivitis, omphalitis and skin infections, although abscesses, septicaemia, osteomyelitis and respiratory tract infections also occur. Infections usually respond to flucloxacillin, although certain strains of methicillin-resistant *Staphylococcus aureus* (MRSA) are not responsive and must be treated alternatively.

Other species of staphylococci such as *Staphylococcus epidermidis* (also called *Staphylococcus albus* and *Coagulase negative staph*.) also cause infections in neonates, usually bacteraemia. High-risk factors in this case are the presence of central lines and umbilical catheters, which tend to be colonised from the skin, then giving rise to infection.

Syphilis

Syphilis is caused by the spirochaete organism *Treponema pallidum*. Congenital syphilis has been largely eradicated in developed countries, due to screening in antenatal programmes. Non-attendance for full antenatal care, a primary infection occurring late in the third trimester and failure of treatment in diagnosed cases account for approximately 5–10 cases annually in the UK.

Intra-uterine infection results in very poor prognosis with intra-uterine growth retardation and hydrops foetalis. Pre-term labour is common, if abortion does not occur. Approximately 60% of cases of congenital syphilis have no clinical symptoms apparent at birth, but go on to develop long-term sequelae of ocular and aural impairment, bone lesions and neurological involvement. On the clinically symptomatic infants, the main feature is a macropapular rash, particularly on the back, thighs, palms of hands and soles of feet. Treatment of congenital syphilis is by penicillin, with long-term serological and developmental follow-up.

Chlamydia trachomatis

Chlamydia trachomatis is taxonomically linked to bacteria but diagnosis is made by virological laboratory techniques due to its failure to grow outside human cells. In neonates the main clinical manifestations of infection are conjunctivitis and pneumonia. The increase of sexually transmitted infection in women during the last decade (1600 new cases in 1989 rising to 29 283 new cases in 1999) (DHSS and PS, 2000), is making this organism a pathogen of increasing importance in neonates. Perinatal infection occurs in around 60–70% of cases of maternal infection. Treatment is by erythromycin, either orally or intravenously, since topical treatment of chlamydial conjunctivitis will not prevent any subsequent chlamydial pneumonia.

SITES OF INFECTION

Conjunctivitis

The most common causes of neonatal conjunctivitis are staphylococci and Gram-negative organisms such as *E. coli* and *Pseudomonas aeruginosa*. These generally present as non-purulent conjunctivitis with inflammation of the conjunctiva and eyelids. In more severe cases of purulent conjunctivitis, infection with *Neisseria gonorrhoea* must be considered and aggressive antimicrobial treatment commenced immediately (following the taking of a swab for microbiological confirmation). Another cause of purulent conjunctivitis is perinatal infection with *Chlamydia trachomatis*, so chlamydial cultures should be taken to exclude this.

Meningitis

Neonatal meningitis is one of the most serious bacterial infections encountered in the newborn. Mortality is high, even with early antibiotic treatment, and long-term sequelae are common in survivors (Holt *et al.*, 2001). The classic symptoms of headache, neck stiffness and photophobia cannot be communicated by the infant to their carers, and irritability and poor feeding are often the only visible signs of meningitis. The main causes of neonatal meningitis are *Group B streptococci* and coliforms, although other organisms are occasionally implicated.

In suspected neonatal meningitis, a full infection screen should be performed, including lumbar puncture. The cerebrospinal fluid of a neonate differs in two respects from that of an adult. It contains a higher number of white blood cells (mainly polymorphs) and has a higher protein content. Since both these factors play a role in the diagnosis of meningitis, these differences make the preliminary laboratory results less useful than in adults, due to the overlap with normal ranges found in children and adults. Conclusive evidence of bacterial infection will be available only after 18–24 hours, when cultures have grown, since Gram staining of the CSF will not always show bacteria, if they are present in low numbers. More sensitive tests, such as latex agglutination tests, to confirm the presence of pathogens in CSF are progressively being developed. These are enabling earlier presumptive diagnosis of the causative agents of meningitis to be made, although antibiotic sensitivities must still wait for culture results to be available.

Septicaemia/bacteraemia

The routine inclusion of blood cultures in neonatal infection screens is justified on clinical grounds, however, their results present particular problems in interpretation. The most common isolate from neonatal blood cultures is coagulase negative staphylococci, although these are rarely considered significant isolates due to their association with skin flora contamination. The presence of contaminant staphylococci in a blood culture is a common factor in prolonging an initial course of prophylactic antibiotics while awaiting confirmation from the laboratory.

Umbilical stump infection (omphalitis)

The umbilical stump is colonised by bacteria at birth and, while the bacterial load may be reduced by cleansing and topical administration of antiseptics, it is a site that is still prone to infection. The administration of antiseptics has also been shown to delay the drying and separation of the cord and, since all bacteria cannot be eradicated from the stump site, this may increase the duration of vulnerability to umbilical stump infection. It is normal to find some redness at the edge of the skin as the cord separates, but any greater sign of infection, such as discharge of pus, requires attention. The main causes of infection are *Staphylococcus aureus*, coliform bacilli and *Beta haemolytic streptococci*. As well as damage to the umbilical site, there is further risk of systemic spread of infection, so this condition should always be given close attention.

The use of umbilical arterial catheters has been documented to correspond to an increased risk of systemic infection in pre-term neonates. Therefore, when these are in place, scrupulous attention must be given to cord care.

Gastro-intestinal infections

Gastroenteritis is now a relatively uncommon occurrence in NNUs in the developed world. The main infectious causes are of viral aetiology, since improved infection control measures and general hygiene have reduced the chance for spread of bacterial gastroenteritis. Occasional outbreaks, due to bacterial pathogens, do still occur, with enteropathogenic *E. coli* and *Salmonella sp.* being implicated. In all cases of gastroenteritis, isolation of the infected infant is required, with careful assessment of fluid balance to prevent dehydration and electrolyte imbalance. Oral rehydration therapy is of limited value in neonates, so intravenous fluids will be required.

Necrotising enterocolitis (NEC) is a condition of uncertain aetiology. Many factors, such as congenital heart defects, exchange transfusions and early enteral feeding, predispose to this condition. The current explanation for its cause is that, rather than being a primary infection caused by specific pathogens, the initial event leading to NEC is an episode of intestinal ischaemia (Coit, 1999). This then allows invasion of the intestinal mucosa with normal, gas-producing bowel flora such as *E. coli* and *Clostridium sp.*, giving rise to the formation of the characteristic gas pockets. (For a more detailed discussion of necrotising enterocolitis, *see* Chapter 8.)

Urinary tract infections

Urinary tract infections (UTI) occur in neonates either as a result of ascending infection or as a secondary infection during bacteraemia. In cases of repeated infection, subsequent follow-up may be required to exclude obstructive abnormalities of the urinary tract, as there is a strong correlation between these and infection. The overall incidence of neonatal UTI ranges from 0.1–1.0% in all babies, with male infants experiencing between three and eight times the infection rate found in female infants (Stork, 1987). In pre-term infants of less than 2500 grams birthweight, UTI rates of 3–10% have been reported (Eliakim et al., 1997).

Diagnosis of neonatal UTI is made difficult due to problems associated with obtaining clean-catch urine specimens for analysis. Both bag urine specimens and free-flowing specimens are suitable, but are prone to contamination. If these produce inconclusive results, a supra-pubic aspirate may be performed. The type of specimen container used is also important, since often only very small volumes of urine can be collected. The standard urine specimen containers contain boric acid powder, which acts as a preservative and prevents subsequent multiplication of bacteria during transit to the laboratory. This allows accurate estimations of the bacterial number at time of sampling to be made. However, if the urine specimen container cannot be filled to the recommended level, the concentration of boric acid can reach bactericidal levels, resulting in a decrease in bacterial count. This can be overcome by using sterile universal containers for small volumes of urine, but, in this case, the specimen must be transported to the laboratory without delay to prevent any bacteria multiplying and giving inaccurate culture results.

NON-BACTERIAL INFECTIONS

Toxoplasma gondii

Toxoplasma gondii is a protozoan parasite whose natural host is members of the cat family, with the domestic cat being the main primary host in Europe. Human infection is as a result of either direct contact with cat faeces or indirect contact with contaminated foods. This may be by ingestion of unwashed vegetables, contaminated with infective sporocysts, or by ingestion of undercooked meat from secondary hosts that have been infected and developed infective tissue cysts.

Severe infection occurs in 10–20% of infected neonates with clinical features of hydrocephalus, retinochoroiditis, cerebral calcification, hepatitis, pneumonia, myocarditis and myositis. Antimicrobial therapy is available for confirmed cases of congenital toxoplasmosis and consists of a combination of anti-parasitic drugs, normally taken for a year.

Rubella

Congenital rubella infection is a rare occurrence in the UK, with only approximately 20 cases being reported annually. However, public awareness is very high, due to vaccination programmes that have been in place since 1970. The best-known clinical manifestations of congenital rubella infection are cataracts and heart defects. Other common manifestations are bone lesions, cryptorchidism, diabetes mellitus, hepatomegaly, splenomegaly, meningoencephalitis, microcephaly, patent ductus arteriosus, pulmonary stenosis and retinopathy.

As well as the actual nursing care delivered to the infected neonate, attention must be given to the fact that these neonates are highly infective and excrete large amounts of the rubella virus. Studies have shown that at 3 months approximately 60% were still actively excreting organisms but, by a year, continued excretion was very rare. The infected neonate should be isolated and cared for by members of staff who have antibodies to rubella. Since occasional cases of reinfection have been documented, it is advisable to exclude any members of staff who are potentially pregnant, even if antibodies to rubella have previously been detected. Advice should also be given to the parents not to expose the infant after discharge home to women who may be pregnant, until the risk of excretion has diminished.

Herpes simplex virus (HSV)

Two types of HSV are major pathogens: HSV-1 causes cold sores, generally around the mouth and nose, and HSV-2 is the major cause of genital herpes (although cross-infection may occur with both HSV-1 and HSV-2). In adults, infection with both HSV-1 and HSV-2 occurs first as a primary infection; the lesion heals and the virus then remains latent in the cells of the central nervous system. The latent virus may then be reactivated to produce lesions at the site of original infection. In contrast to the other infections covered by the TORCH acronym, HSV only rarely causes intra-uterine infection. Infection normally occurs during delivery, since active maternal genital herpes results in the shedding of virus by the mucous membranes of the cervix and vagina.

Perinatally acquired HSV infection presents in three forms:

- localised mucocutaneous infection (20%);
- localised neurological infection (30%); and
- disseminated infection (50%).

When only the mucous membranes are involved, the lesions will appear in 9–11 days and there is only a low chance of long-term sequelae. The more serious neurological infections present later, at 15–17 days, and result in mortality in 20% of untreated cases, with 60% of survivors suffering long-term sequelae. In cases of disseminated HSV infection, the clinical manifestations appear in 9–11 days and include brain, liver and skin involvement, with 80% mortality in untreated cases. With appropriate antiviral treatment (acyclovir for at least 10 days), this mortality is reduced to 20%, with 50% of survivors suffering long-term sequelae.

Neonates with HSV infection should be isolated to prevent spread of infection until antiviral treatment is complete. Since HSV-1 infection in adults is very common, and transmission, under non-mucosal contact situations, is rare, staff with cold sores need not be excluded from work, as long as standard infection control procedures are practised.

Cytomegalovirus (CMV)

CMV is the most common cause of congenital infection, resulting in approximately 120–180 symptomatic cases, annually, in England and Wales. CMV is one of the herpes viruses and, therefore, the neonatal congenital infection can be either as a result of primary maternal infection during pregnancy or reactivation of latent infection, occurring during pregnancy. Almost all of these neonates, who exhibit symptoms at birth, will suffer long-term sequelae.

The clinical manifestations of congenital CMV infection include hepatomegaly, splenomegaly, cerebral calcification, microcephaly, prolonged jaundice, petechiae, thrombocytopenia and pneumonitis. In addition to these symptomatic neonates, an equal or slightly greater number who are infected, yet asymptomatic at birth, can be expected to develop long-term sequelae later in life, of which the main symptom is deafness.

Perinatal infection also occurs, at time of delivery, if active maternal infection is present. Neonates may not be infected at birth, but studies have shown that breast-feeding and close contact with a seropositive mother is a major source of infection in early life. Neonates with CMV infection excrete large amounts of virus and are potentially infective to health-care staff. However, standard infection control procedures have been shown to be effective in preventing transmission to staff and other infants, so isolation is not required.

Respiratory syncytial virus (RSV)

RSV infection in neonates is one of the few exclusively nosocomial viral infections in neonates. There have been no proven cases of intra-uterine infection, with transmission occurring either from aerosol inhalation or contact with infected material in the NNU, or by contact with infected visitors or members of staff, who are often asymptomatic. Infants with suspected or proven RSV infection should be nursed in isolation and any members of staff or visitors with signs of infection (in adults, often only a mild cold) need to be excluded from the unit.

In mild infections, the main symptoms are rhinorrhoea and coughing. In severe infection, bronchiolitis is seen. Neonates with predisposing factors, such as congenital heart defects and bronchopulmonary dysplasia, are more prone to develop these severe infections. Another consequence of RSV infection is viral otitis media, which presents in up to 20% of cases.

Human immunodeficiency virus (HIV)

Congenital infection with HIV can occur as a result of transplacental infection, intranatal infection or neonatal infection through breast-feeding. The highest risk of transmission is to infants at the time of delivery. Antenatal screening programmes have indicated cost-effectiveness (Rivera-Alsina, 2001). If the mother's positive status is known antepartum, antiretroviral medications are given to her to reduce the viral load and the risk to the infant. Plans are made to deliver the infant by elective caesarean section and some units advocate chlorhexidine wash following delivery. Infants of mothers who are HIV-positive are given a 6-week course of antiretroviral therapy and breast-feeding is largely discouraged (Chaudhry, 2001; Shah and McGowan, 2001).

As the general health of women with HIV has improved, there will probably be more HIV-exposed infants born. Under normal circumstances, providing these infants are well, they will be managed on post-natal wards and NNU staff will not come into frequent contact with them. However, pre-term birth or birth complications can occur and disrupt carefully made plans. If extended treatment in the NNU is required, staff must be aware of the increased susceptibility to infection of these infants and provide care accordingly. Immunisation against common childhood infections has been shown to be beneficial and so should be encouraged. As in the case of a hepatitis B infection risk, all specimens sent for pathology examinations should indicate the high-risk status of the specimen.

Hepatitis B virus (HBV)

Congenital HBV infection is predominantly a perinatal infection since intra-uterine infection accounts for fewer than 5% of cases. The main clinical significance of congenital HBV infection are the long-term sequelae of cirrhosis and hepatocellular carcinoma, with acute neonatal hepatitis occurring very rarely. The risk of neonatal transmission is related to the time of maternal infection, as well as the serological markers present at the time of delivery, with infection in the third trimester and presence of HBsAG giving the highest correlation with neonatal infection. Most neonates who are congenitally infected will develop HBsAG antibodies at around 2–3 months of age and will progress to the chronic carrier state.

In an attempt to prevent perinatal infection from HBV-positive mothers, active immunisation with HBV vaccine will be given to the infant, as will passive immunisation with anti-HBV immunoglobulin, according to the infectivity of the maternal infection at delivery. Studies have shown that breast-feeding does not increase the risk of neonatal transmission in HBsAG-positive mothers and should not, therefore, be discouraged.

Measures to reduce the risk of infection to health-care staff must be implemented where neonates are born to HBV-infected mothers. These will depend on local infection control policy and also on the serological status of the mother. In order to warn pathology staff who deal with specimens from these babies, the risk of HBV infection should always be marked clearly on any request forms.

CONCLUSION

The diagnosis, treatment and care of neonates with infection is a complex subject and it has been possible to give no more than an overview here. For more information on cases of infection caused by pathogens that are not detailed here, and for further knowledge, other works may be studied. Drawing on these resources will allow nursing staff to deliver care in a more informed way, not only to the neonate but also to the family, who will need reassurance if their infant is ill due to infection.

REFERENCES

Chaudhry, S. (2001) HIV-positive mothers who breast-feed may die sooner, *British Medical Journal* **322**(7298), 1324

Coit, A.K. (1999) Necrotising enterocolitis, *Journal of Perinatal and Neonatal Nursing* **12**(4), 53–66

DHSS and PS, Scottish ISD(D)5 Collaborative Group (2000) *Trends in Sexually Transmitted Infections in the United Kingdom, 1990 to 1999*, Public Health Laboratory Data, London

Donowitz, L.G. (1989) Nosocomial infection in neonatal intensive care units, *American Journal of Infection Control* **17**(5), 250–7

Eliakim, A., Dolfin, T., Korzets, Z., Wolach, B. and Pomeranz, A. (1997) Urinary tract infection in premature infants: the role of imaging studies and prophylactic therapy, *Journal of Perinatology* **17**(4), 305–8

Fanaroff, A.A., Korones, S.B., Wright, L.L., Verter, J., Poland, R.L., Bauer, C.R., *et al.* (1998) Incidence, presenting features, risk factors and significance of late-onset septicaemia in very low-birthweight infants, The National Institute of Child Health and Human Development Neonatal Research Network, *Pediatric Infectious Disease Journal* **17**(7), 593–8

Holt, D.E., Halket, S., de Louvois, J. and Harvey, D. (2001) Neonatal meningitis in England and Wales: 10 years on, *Archives of Disease in Childhood, Fetal and Neonatal Edition* **84**(2), 85–9

Jones, B.L., Gorman, L.J., Simpson, J. Curran, E.T., McNamee, S., Lucas, C.*et al.* (2000) An outbreak of Serratia marcescens in two neonatal intensive care units, *Journal of Hospital Infection* **46**(4), 314–19

Levine, C.D. (1991) Premature rupture of membranes and sepsis in pre-term neonates, *Nursing Research* **40**(1), 36–41

Mullett, M.D., Cook, E.F. and Gallagher, R. (1998) Nosocomial sepsis in the neonatal intensive care unit, *Journal of Perinatology* **18**(2), 112–15

Rivera-Alsina, M. (2001) HIV screening program in pregnancy deemed cost-effective, *Journal of Reproductive Medicine* **46**, 243–48

Schuchat, A. (1999) Group B streptococcus, *Lancet* **353**(9146), 51–6

Shah, S. and McGowan, J. (2001) Preventing HIV transmission during pregnancy, *Infections in Medicine* **18**(2), 94–105

Slack, M.P., Azzopardi, H.J., Hargreaves, R.M. and Ramsay, M.E. (1998) Enhanced surveillance of invasive *Haemophilus influenzae* disease in England, 1990 to 1996: impact of conjugate vaccines, *Pediatric Infectious Disease Journal* **17**(9 Suppl.) S204–7

Slagle, T.A., Bifano, E.M., Wolf, J.W. and Gross, S.J. (1989) Routine endotracheal cultures for the prediction of neonatal sepsis in ventilated babies, *Archives of Disease in Childhood* **64**(1), 34–8

Spaans, W.A., Knox, A.J., Koya, H.B. and Mantell, C.D. (1990) Risk factors for neonatal infection, *Australian and New Zealand Journal of Obstetrics and Gynaecology* **30**(4), 327–30

Stork, J.E. (1987) Urinary tract infection in children, *Advances in Pediatric Infectious Diseases* **2**, 115–34

15 Neonatal nutrition

Sarah Illingworth

Aims of the chapter

This chapter presents an overview of the nutritional needs of the infant in the neonatal unit. It reviews some of the many difficulties in feeding the small and premature infants, the recommended daily nutritional requirements and promotes a multidisciplinary team approach. The nutritional requirements of premature infants and the various means of nutritional management, including the use of breast milk, breast milk fortifiers and formula milk, and methods of feeding are all discussed.

INTRODUCTION

A wide range of problems may be encountered in the nutritional management of premature infants, yet optimal nutrition is critical in the NNU. Meeting the nutritional needs of the increasing number of very immature infants is important in ensuring their survival after birth, and their subsequent growth and development. An infant of less than 28 weeks gestation will survive for less than a week if no nutrition is provided (Williams, 1991).

Feeding premature infants of varying levels of maturity, size and sickness is challenging to everyone involved in their care. It is essential that each infant's nutritional requirements are assessed individually to ensure that the most appropriate feeding plan is chosen. Close monitoring is then required.

CAUSES OF NUTRITIONAL PROBLEMS ASSOCIATED WITH VERY PREMATURE INFANTS

Low nutritional reserves at birth

The nutrient stores of a premature infant are severely limited. During the last trimester of pregnancy there is a relatively large deposition of nutrients, which these infants miss out on by being born prematurely. A premature infant of 1 kg has energy reserves that allow for survival for only 4 days with no energy intake, and a premature infant of 2 kg has energy reserves that will last for only 12 days (Robertson and Bhatia, 1993). It is partly because of these limited stores that premature infants have increased requirements for many nutrients when compared with larger, term infants.

Physiological immaturity

The nutritional requirements of premature infants are also affected by the fact that many body systems – for example, the gastro-intestinal tract, renal function and skin – are immature. This also affects the infants' ability to tolerate certain nutrients.

During pregnancy one of the placenta's many functions is to act as a modified gastro-intestinal tract. When the infant is born prematurely the gastro-intestinal tract is immature. In general the infant remains unable to feed from the breast or bottle until at least 32–34 weeks gestation. In addition the absence or immaturity of suck, swallow, cough, and gag reflexes increases the risk of aspiration pneumonia (Tudehope and Steer, 1996). Premature infants can also have problems because of underdeveloped smooth muscle and poor sphincter control. Gastro-oesophageal reflux is common. Organised peristalsis normally appears at about 34 weeks gestation. There is an increased incidence of ileus in infants before 34 weeks (Williams, 1991).

The skin is another immature body system that affects the premature infant's nutritional requirements. The skin of a premature infant of less than 28 weeks gestation is thin and poorly keratinised and as a result there is a lot of fluid loss through the skin. These losses mean the premature infant has increased requirements for fluid (Williams, 1991).

High nutrient requirements for growth

Achieving a post-natal growth rate that reinstates the premature infant on their intra-uterine growth curve for weight, length and head circumference is often used as a reasonable estimate of adequate growth until 36–38 post-conceptional weeks (Tsang et al., 1993). Growth velocity is higher at 25 or 30 weeks gestation than at term. The aim of nutritional management of the premature infant is to support this growth rate and allow the infant to adapt to extra-uterine life. The nutritional requirements of these premature infants are greater than at any other time in human life partly because of the need to support this growth rate.

NUTRITIONAL REQUIREMENTS OF THE PREMATURE INFANT

A number of sources discuss the nutritional requirements of premature infants (ESPGAN, 1987; Tsang et al., 1993). For a brief summary of their recommendations, see Table 15.1. For a more in-depth understanding, see the original works.

Water

The guidelines by Tsang and co-workers (1993) and ESPGAN (1987) recommend that enteral-fed premature infants should receive between 150–200 mls/kg/day of water. Some infants will need to be fluid-restricted for a variety of reasons, including patent ductus arteriosus (Robertson and Bhatia, 1993). Volumes of up to 200 mls/kg per day are often necessary to supply sufficient nutrients and cope with the massive insensible water losses that very premature infants have through their immature skin.

Table 15.1 Nutritional needs of the stable premature infant

	Nutrients	Enteral recommendations (kg/day)
Bulk	Energy (kcal)	105–130
	Protein (g)	3.0–3.6[a]
		3.6–3.8[b]
	Carbohydrate (g)	3.8–11.8[a]
		3.8–11.4[b]
	Fat (see text) ratio	4.4–5.7 g/100 kcal
Fat-soluble vitamins	Vitamin A (IU)	700–1500
	Vitamin D (IU)	150–400
	Vitamin E (IU)	6–12
	Vitamin K (IU)	8–10
Water-soluble vitamins	Vitamin C (mg)	18–24
	Thiamin (μg)	180–240
	Riboflavin (μg)	250–360
	Pyridoxine (μg)	150–210
	Niacin (mg)	3.6–4.8
	Folate (μg)	25–50
	Vitamin B_{12} (μg)	0.3
Examples of added elements	Sodium (mg)	46–69
	Chloride (mg)	70–105
	Potassium (mg)	78–120
	Calcium (mg)	120–230
	Phosphurus (mg)	60–140
	Magnesium (mg)	7.9–15
	Iron (mg)	2.0
	Iodine (μg)	16–45
	Zinc (μg)	1.5–2.0[b]
		1.2–1.7[a]
	Selenium (μg)	1.3–3.0

Modified from Tsang et al. (1993)
[a]Infants < 1000 g
[b]Infants > 1000 g

Energy

Tsang *et al.* (1993) recommend 110–120 kcal/kg per day whereas ESPGAN (1987) recommends 130 kcal/kg per day with a minimum of 110 kcal/kg per day and a maximum of 165 kcal/kg per day. Energy is required for resting metabolism, thermoregulation, activity and production of new tissue. A high level of handling of the premature infant will lead to increased energy requirements, as will incomplete absorption of milk and poor temperature regulation.

Protein

The current recommendations by Tsang and colleagues (1993) divide protein intake recommendations into two groups according to birthweight:

<1000 grams   3.6–3.8 g/kg/day
>1000 grams   3.0–3.6 g/kg/day

The aim of providing this amount of protein is to match the intra-uterine protein gain of a normal foetus and match long-term growth and psychomotor development of a term infant of the same post-conceptional age.

It is crucial to get the balance of protein to energy correct. When energy intake is low, protein cannot be fully utilised for tissue synthesis. If the energy intake is sufficient, the same level of protein intake can be used for tissue synthesis, resulting in improved weight gain.

An excessive intake of protein can cause problems, although an increased intake of protein may be needed initially following severe illness. If increased protein intake is indicated there must be careful monitoring of the infant's growth rate and urea and electrolyte levels.

Fat

Fat is important for energy and for fatty acids. Fat is a major source of energy for the premature infant. It provides approximately 50% of dietary energy and is necessary for the transport of fat-soluble vitamins. The guidelines of Tsang and colleagues (1993) recommend 4.4 to 6.0 g/100 kcal, which is the amount usually provided by mature term human milk.

Certain fatty acids, known as the long chain polyunsaturates (LCPs), are important in the development of the brain, the nervous system and the functioning of the eye. The premature infant's ability to make these LCPs from other fatty acids is limited. Decsi and Koletzko (1994) report that premature infants fed a formula without LCPs develop rapid LCP depletion of plasma and tissue lipids. This is associated with reduced visual acuity during the first post-natal months. They conclude that LCP enrichment of formula is desirable for premature infants. Breast-fed premature infants receive LCPs in human milk. An ESPGAN report (1991) recommended that LCPs be added to pre-term formulas in amounts typical of human milk. Tsang and colleagues (1993) recommend that the LCPs' arachidonic acid and docosahexaenoic acid may be considered essential nutrients for infants who weigh less than 1750 grams, who experience difficulty or delay in maintaining full enteral feeding greater than 100 kcal/kg/day. They recommend that the intake of both of these fatty acids for these infants should be 0.25% kcal. These recommendations are theoretical rather than practical with respect to LCP supplementation of formula milk.

Vitamins

Vitamin A: the recommendations for vitamin A intake vary depending on the presence or otherwise of chronic lung disease. The increased requirement in premature infants with chronic lung diseases is recommended because vitamin A is thought to aid recovery.

No lung disease   700–1500 IU/kg/day
Chronic lung disease   1500–2800 IU/kg/day

Vitamins B and C: the recommendations by Tsang and colleagues (1993) for the water-soluble vitamins (the B vitamins and vitamin C) are summarised in Table 15.1 (*see* page 302).
Vitamin D: a deficiency of vitamin D in infancy results in rickets (Neu *et al.*, 1990). Tsang and colleagues (1993) recommend 150–400 IU/kg/day with the aim of providing 400 IU/day, which should be sufficient. They state that intakes need not exceed 800 IU/day in the presence of adequate mineral intake during the first 6 months of life.

Minerals

Calcium, magnesium and phosphorous are essential minerals for tissue structure and function. The metabolism of these minerals is interrelated. Calcium and phosphorus form the major inorganic constituents of bone. During the last trimester of pregnancy there is a huge accretion of calcium and phosphorus. An infant born at term is made up of approximately 30 g of calcium whereas an infant born at 26 weeks gestation is made up of approximately 6 g of calcium (Ziegler *et al.*, 1976). A deficiency particularly of calcium and phosphorus has been identified as a significant aetiological factor in bone disease (with reduced bone mineralisation), common in these premature infants (Bishop *et al.*, 1993).

The recommendations by Tsang and colleagues (1993) are summarised in Table 15.1.

Tsang *et al.* (1993) recommend that the premature infant should receive iron supplementation of 2 mg/kg/day and that this should be started by 2 months of age. This amount of iron is needed because premature infants are born with inadequate iron stores (Williams, 1991).

NUTRITIONAL MANAGEMENT OF THE PREMATURE INFANT

The way nutritional requirements are met will depend on the age, size and health of the infant. The best method of feeding and the most appropriate nutritional source will be decided by staff caring for the premature infant, taking into consideration the parents' preferences with regard to such issues as bottle- or breast-feeding.

When to feed

For relatively large premature infants (those who weigh more than 1500 grams) who are well, there are few contra-indications to enteral feeding within the first 24 hours after birth (Robertson and Bhatia, 1993).

In the case of smaller premature infants there is more debate about when to feed enterally. Berseth (1992) showed that premature infants fed hypocaloric enteral nutrition early showed enhanced maturation of small intestinal motor activity and peptide responses to food. The study also showed that infants who were enterally fed early were able to tolerate full oral nutrition sooner and had shorter hospital stays. Hypocaloric enteral feeds or gut priming or minimal enteral feeding (for example, 0.5ml/hour of enteral feed) can be used as an adjunct to parenteral nutrition in the very premature infant. Neu and colleagues (1990) reviewed the evidence and recommended that, although parenteral nutrition can provide full nutrition for growth of the very premature infant, small priming doses of enteral feeds should begin as soon as possible. This enteral feeding would not be for nutritional purposes but to prevent mucosal atrophy, improve tolerance to subsequent enteral feeds, prevent cholestasis, and induce the secretion of potentially trophic gut hormones.

Total parenteral nutrition is indicated in premature infants whose bowel is being rested because of necrotising enterocolitis or major bowel surgery. Parenteral nutrition is also indicated in very premature infants who are unable to tolerate full enteral feeds initially. Very premature infants and sick, less premature infants will require parenteral nutrition in the early days or weeks (Williams, 1991). The aim of parenteral nutrition is to provide nutrients by vein, without complications (Menon, 1992a).

How to feed

As the premature infant is usually unable to feed by mouth until at least 32–34 weeks gestation, a tube will be required to give or support the infant's enteral nutrition (Shaw and Lawson, 1994). Tube feeding can be accomplished by continuous feeds or by bolus feeds (Neu et al., 1990). Silvestre and colleagues (1996) looked at continuous versus intermittent feeding methods and summarised that premature infants in a stable condition achieved similar growth and had comparable lengths of hospital stay regardless of feeding method. It did appear that continuous feeds were better tolerated in the very premature infant who had feeding problems. Continuous feeds are also better tolerated in the early stages of feeding in the infant with respiratory disease (Williams, 1991).

When giving continuous feeds it is good practice to draw up only 4 hours of milk at a time. Syringes are positioned at an angle as this aids the dispersion of fat.

Nasogastric, nasojejunal or, less commonly, gastrostomy tubes are used to feed infants on the NNU. The gastrostomy tube may be necessary to allow enteral feeding in an infant with a tracheo-oesophageal fistula who is not selected for early repair (Shaw and Lawson, 1994). Tubes may be passed via the oral rather than nasal route; some doctors prefer this, as infants are predominantly nasal breathers (Neu et al., 1990). A survey of regional neonatal intensive care units on feeding policies for the ventilated premature infant showed that intragastric and bolus feeding were used more frequently; only two out of the 32 units gave intrajejunal feeds. When ventilation was no longer required the majority of the units surveyed moved towards bolus and intragastric feeds. Intrajejunal feeds are sometimes given as they may reduce the danger of reflux and milk aspiration in the trachea, although data to confirm this is sparse, and intra-jejunal feeding also has its own risks (Neu *et al.*, 1990).

Increasingly, breast-feeding is promoted in the NNU. Breast-feeding can be problematic at the best of times even with a large, demanding term infant. For the mothers of pre-term infants the difficulties are compounded. Even if it is stable enough to be allowed access to the breast, the infant may be too small and weak to adequately stimulate the flow of the mother's milk. The mother herself may be unwell and the lack of privacy and the experience of a breast pump may not be helpful in establishing lactation. Strategies for enhancing the expression of breast milk include bilateral breast pumping (Groh-Wargo *et al.*, 1995), kangaroo care (Cattaneo *et al.*, 1998) and supporting the mother to express while by her infant's cot-side. Mothers may also be worried about the amount of milk being produced and taken (Hedberg Nyqvist, 2001).

There has been some concern over infant confusion between the nipple and the artificial teat, which may inhibit the latching on and the effective suck on the breast. To address this, some neonatal nurses are advocating the use of soft moulding cups rather than bottles and teats. One study however highlighted reluctance by nurses to introduce cup feeding on to the NNU. Concerns related to parents' abilities and to the risks of pouring the milk into the infant's mouth (Hedberg Nyqvist and Strandell, 1999). Further studies advocate cup feeding, stating that it is cost-effective, allows the infant to be discharged earlier and may promote successful breast-feeding in the pre-term infant (Ritchie, 1998). The neonate is innately tuned in to root, latch, suck and swallow. Further studies are required to support this innovation.

Human milk

Human milk is well tolerated by the premature infant and has a unique composition, providing immunological protection against infection (Tudehope and Steer, 1996). The composition of human milk enhances absorption and utilisation of fat, zinc and iron. In addition, human milk has a low renal solute load (Quan *et al.*, 1994). By providing food for her infant the mother is more involved in the care and emotional bonding is enhanced (De Curtis *et al.*, 1999).

Lucas and Cole (1990) showed a reduction in the incidence of necrotising enterocolitis in premature infants fed human milk compared with similar infants fed formula milk. There is also evidence that premature infants fed their own mother's breast milk had higher IQ scores at 7.5–8 years when compared with those who were not. The exact reasons for these findings are not known (Lucas *et al.*, 1992a).

Breast milk is normally the feed of choice for premature infants, and mothers are encouraged to express milk for their infants until they are able to breast-feed. A survey of all UK regional intensive care units by McClure and colleagues (1996), which looked at feeding policies for ventilated pre-term infants, showed that all units preferred to use expressed maternal milk if available.

Pre-term human milk has a higher concentration of protein, sodium and chloride than term breast milk but there is considerable variation in protein, lactose, fat and energy content between different mothers (Tudehope and Steer, 1996). Nutritionally, human milk may be deficient in some of the nutrients for the growing premature infant (Quan *et al.*, 1994); human milk fortifiers (*see* page 308) increase its nutrient content.

Promoting lactation

The mother's diet and lifestyle can affect the quality and the quantity of breast milk produced. The Department of Health (1991) report on dietary reference values for food energy and nutrients for the UK recommends that lactating women should have increased intakes of energy, protein, and many vitamin and minerals. For most breast-feeding or expressing women, adequate nutrition will be provided by increased quantities of a normal varied diet based on a healthy eating principle (Thomas, 1994). Thomas's general dietary guidelines (1994) for lactating women are summarised below:

- Eat regularly.
- Let your appetite guide how much you eat.
- Eat a varied diet, including food from all the main food groups.
- Do not try and lose weight while you are breast-feeding.
- Drink plenty of fluids.
- Avoid too much alcohol, coffee, and tea.

Women who are expressing should be advised to express regularly to maximise lactation. Occasional breast-feeds, if possible, should be encouraged as these help to maintain milk supply (Royal College of Midwives, 1998). Although it may be unavoidable, mothers should avoid getting too stressed. Lactating women should also be advised not to smoke as smoking reduces the volume of milk produced (Garrow and James, 1996).

Human milk storage

Freshly expressed milk provides the most benefits for the very premature infants but it is not always practical to provide this. Expressed breast milk (EBM) for a mother's own infant can be stored by refrigeration or by freezing. When fresh breast milk is stored in a refrigerator the total bacterial colony count increases with time (Jocson *et al.*, 1997). This research supports the current recommendation of using refrigerated EBM within 24 hours.

When storage is required for longer than 1 day, supplies of breast milk must be frozen; this is usually for a maximum of 3 months. Freezing is accompanied by a loss of some vitamins (Bank *et al.*, 1985). Freezing can also disrupt milk fat globules (Wardell *et al.*, 1981).

When expressed breast milk is being stored it should be clearly labelled with the infant's name, the date and the time expressed. It is good practice to defrost the oldest first and use it in the sequence it was expressed. Breast milk can be given at room temperature but should be used within 4 hours.

Human milk fortification

Nutritionally, human milk may be deficient in many nutrients for the growing premature infant (Quan *et al.*, 1994). This has led to the development of human milk fortifiers, which increase the nutrient content of human milk. The use of fortified breast milk has increased in the UK. A survey of all UK regional intensive care units by McClure *et al.* (1996) looked at feeding policies for ventilated pre-term infants and found that, in 1994, 72% of units sometimes fortified expressed breast milk and that 13% routinely fortify expressed breast milk. In 1987 only 5% of units fortified expressed breast milk. The reason for deciding to fortify was concern about the infants' weight gain when fed only expressed breast milk. Tsang *et al.* (1993) summarised six trials looking at fortification of human milk and found increases in rates of weight, length and head circumference gain in the infants fed fortified milk.

There are concerns, however, that human milk fortifiers may lead to feed intolerance (Metcalf *et al.*, 1994).

A number of different breast milk fortifiers are available in the UK, all of which have a slightly different nutritional composition and come in a powder form:

- Nutriprem Breast Milk Fortifier (Cow & Gate);
- Eoprotin (Milupa);
- SMA Breast Milk Fortifier (SMA).

Low birthweight formula

If breast milk supplies are insufficient or unavailable, it may be decided that the infant should be formula fed. There are several low-birthweight formulas available. In the absence of human milk, low-birthweight formulas are the most appropriate substitute (Tudehope and Steer, 1996). A survey of all UK regional intensive care units by McClure *et al.* (1996), which looked at feeding policies for ventilated pre-term infants, showed that the use of low-birthweight formulas has increased. They concluded that the use of low-birthweight formulas reflects more awareness of their nutritional benefits.

Low-birthweight formulas contain higher levels of protein, energy, fat, vitamins, and minerals than term formulas. These formulas are often used until a premature infant reaches 2 kg or 2.5 kg, or is discharged home from hospital. According to Ehrenkranz and colleagues (1989), low-birthweight formulas have been shown to support weight gain and nutrient retention at rates approximating the third trimester of pregnancy. Table 15.2 shows the composition of four low-birthweight formulas available in the UK.

Follow-on low-birthweight formula

Many premature infants are discharged from NNUs on term formulas, which are suitable for healthy term babies. Follow-on low-birthweight formulas contain higher levels of many nutrients than term formulas. A comparative study (Lucas

Table 15.2 Compositions of low-birthweight formula (compositions taken from manufacturer's information)

Nutrients per 100 mls	Cow & Gate Nutriprem	Farley's Osterprem	Milupa Pre-Aptamil	SMA LBW
Energy (kcal)	80	80	80	82
Protein (g)	2.4	2	2.4	2
Fat (g)	4.4	4.6	4.4	4.4
Calcium (mg)	100	110	100	80
Phosphorus (mg)	50	63	50	42.5
Sodium (mg)	41	42	41	35
Iron (mg)	0.9	0.04	0.9	0.8
Vitamin D (μg)	5	2.4	2.4	1.5

et al., 1992b) looked at the effect on growth and clinical status between infants fed exclusively normal term formula and infants fed exclusively follow-on low-birthweight formula premature. They found increases in linear growth and weight gain in the infants who received the follow-on low-birthweight formula. Bishop and colleagues (1993) suggested that the use of a follow-on low-birthweight formula had a significant positive effect on bone growth and mineralisation.

One major drawback of follow-on low-birthweight formulas is the cost, as they are not available on prescription or in exchange for milk tokens. Table 15.3 shows the composition of the two follow-on low-birthweight formulas that are available in the UK.

Table 15.3 Compositions of follow-on low-birthweight formula (compositions taken from manufacturer's information)

Nutrients per 100 mls	Cow & Gate Nutriprem 2	Farley's Premcare
Energy (kcal)	74	72
Protein (g)	1.8	1.85
Fat (g)	4.1	3.96
Calcium (mg)	90	70
Phosphorus (mg)	45	35
Sodium (mg)	25	22
Iron (mg)	1.1	0.65
Vitamin D (μg)	1.6	1.3

Term formula

Standard infant formulas are designed for full-term infants and do not meet the specific nutritional needs of premature infants on the whole, although term formulas are often fed to larger, more mature pre-term infants. Whey-based formulas are normally used. Table 15.4 shows the composition of four whey-based term formulas available in the UK.

Table 15.4 Compositions of term formula (compositions taken from manufacturer's information)

Nutrients per 100 mls	Cow & Gate Premium	Farley's First Milk	Milupa Aptamil	SMA Gold
Energy (kcal)	67	68	67	67
Protein (g)	1.4	1.45	1.5	1.5
Fat (g)	3.5	3.82	3.6	3.6
Calcium (mg)	54	39	66	46
Phosphorus (mg)	27	27	42	33
Sodium (mg)	19	17	23	16
Iron (mg)	0.5	0.69	0.7	0.8
Vitamin D (μg)	1.4	1.0	1.0	1.1

Specialised infant formula

Specialised formulas may need to be used if a premature infant has malabsorption or has a condition requiring them (for example, in chylothorax, a condition in which the lymphatic drainage channels have been disrupted and lymph drains into the thorax). A recognised complication of cardiac surgery would need a specialised formula such as Monogen (SHS). Specialised formula milks should only be used when needed. It must be remembered that on the whole specialised formula milks are produced to meet the lower nutritional requirements of term infants rather than those of pre-term infants and may therefore need fortifying.

Weaning

Term infants are normally ready to start solids between 4–6 months of age, but the pre-term infant is unlikely to be able to cope with solids at this age. It is difficult to be exact about the stage at which a premature infant will manage solids. Weaning should not begin before 16 weeks of age. If weaning is delayed until the premature infant is 16 weeks corrected age, then the infants are surviving on milk alone for a prolonged period. The Department of Health (1994) report on weaning and the weaning diet suggests that a reasonable compromise may need to be adopted and weaning can be advised when the infant weighs at least 5 kg, has lost the extrusion reflex and is able to eat from a spoon.

The following equation has been suggested for calculating the point at which a premature infant is ready for solids (Shaw and Lawson, 1994):

16 weeks + ½ (prematurity) = weaning date
therefore, for an infant born at 26 weeks gestation the weaning date would be 23 weeks (16 weeks + ½ (14 weeks) = 23 weeks)

In this case, weaning could be introduced at 23 weeks chronological age provided the infant is 5 kg and has lost the extrusion reflex and is able and willing to eat from a spoon.

Suitable first solids should be of a smooth consistency and bland taste, for example, baby rice, pureed soft fruits or pureed non-fibrous vegetables.

GROWTH MONITORING AND GROWTH EXPECTATIONS

Achieving a post-natal growth rate that reinstates the premature infant on their anticipated intra-uterine growth curve for weight, length and head circumference is a reasonable estimate of adequate growth until 36–38 post-conceptional weeks (Tsang et al., 1993). Measurements of weight, length and head circumference are important as, used together, they provide a means of identifying premature infants who are not achieving an adequate growth rate. The most commonly used measures of growth in premature infants are weight and head circumference, but these do have limitations (Griffin et al., 1999). It is important not to use weight alone to measure growth.

Weight

Serial measurements of the infant's weight should be taken. Over a long period of time these measurements are a rough but useful indication of overall nutritional adequacy (Menon, 1992b). It should be remembered that weight is not only affected by nutritional status, but also by changes in the fluid balance of premature infants. Weight measurements also give little information on the compositional nature of growth (Griffin et al., 1999). It is important to take note of the weight of the attachments on the infant and to subtract this weight from the total (Menon, 1992a). Serial measurements of bodyweight should be plotted on an appropriate centile chart. Using a centile chart as a standard, a guide of expected weight gain might be approximately 15–18 g per kg/day, up to 2 kg, then 25–30 g per day thereafter.

Length

Measurement of length is considered to be the best indicator of nutritional adequacy and it most closely relates to lean body mass (Griffin et al., 1999). Crown to heel length is often measured and there are stadiometers that will fit inside an incubator to measure body length. This method of measuring means that the infant will need to be frequently handled, which is often poorly tolerated (Menon, 1992a). Another measurement of linear growth in premature infants is knee–heel length, which may be measured with less disturbance to the infant (Menon, 1992a). It is assumed that this measurement is representative of growth of the whole body, but Griffin and colleagues (1999) found that knee–heel length was a less accurate predictor than crown–heel length and less reproducible. Crown–heel length where possible should be measured serially, plotted on an appropriate centile chart, and used along with weight and head circumference measurements to assess growth.

Head circumference

Growth in head circumference is usually measured weekly and gives a rough indication of brain growth (Menon, 1992a). It should be remembered that head growth is spared during nutritional stress (Griffin *et al.*, 1999).

CONCLUSION

There are many challenging nutritional problems encountered on the NNU which require a multidisciplinary team approach. The neonatal nurse is in an ideal position to work with dieticians, the family and doctors to ensure adequate nutrition, growth and development of the infant.

REFERENCES

Bank, M.R., Kirksey, A., West, K. and Giacoia, G. (1985) Effect of storage time and temperature on folacin and vitamin C levels in term and pre-term human milk, *American Journal of Clinical Nutrition* 41(2), 235–42

Berseth, C.L. (1992) Effect of early feeding on maturation of the pre-term infant's small intestine, *Journal of Pediatrics* 120(6), 947–53

Bishop, N.J., King, F.J. and Lucas, A. (1993) Increased bone mineral content of pre-term infants fed with a nutrient-enriched formula after discharge from hospital, *Archives of Diseases in Childhood* 68(5), 573–8

Cattaneo, A., Davanzo, R. Uxa, F. *et al.* (1998) Recommendations for the implementation of the kangaroo mother care for low-birthweight infants, *Acta Paediatrica* 87, 440–5

De Curtis, M., Candusso, M., Pieltain, C. and Rigo, J. (1999) Effect of fortification on the osmolality of human milk, *Archive of Disease in Childhood Fetal Neonatal Edition* 81(2), 141–3

Department of Health Report on Health and Social Subjects 41 (1991) *Dietary Reference Values for Food Energy and Nutrients for the United Kingdom*, HMSO, London

Department of Health Report on Health and Social Subjects 45 (1994) *Weaning and the Weaning Diet*, HMSO, London

Decsi, T. and Koletzko, B. (1994) Polyunsaturated fatty acids in infant nutrition, *Acta Paedaitrica Suppl* 395, 31–7

Ehrenkranz, R.A., Gettner, P.A. and Nelli, C.M. (1989) Nutrient balance studies in premature infants fed premature formula or fortified preterm human milk, *Journal of Pediatric Gastroenterology and Nutrition* 8(1), 58–67

ESPGAN (1987) Nutrition and feeding of pre-term infants, *Acta Paediatricia Scandinavica* [supplement] 336

ESPGAN (1991) Comment on the content and composition of lipids in infant formulas, *Acta Paediatricia Scandinavica* 80, 887–96

Garrow, J.S. and James, W.P.T. (1996) *Human Nutrition and Dietetics*, Churchill Livingstone, Singapore

Griffin, I.J., Pang, N.M., Perring, J. and Cooke, R. J. (1999) Knee–heel length measurement in healthy preterm infants, *Archive of Disease in Childhood Fetal Neonatal Edition* 81(1), 50–5

Groh-Wargo, S., Toth, A., Mahoney, K. *et al.* (1995) The utility of a bilateral breast pumping system for mothers of premature infants, *Neonatal Network* 14(8), 31–5

Hedberg Nyqvist, K. (2001) The development of pre-term infants' milk intake during breast-feeding: influence of gestational age, *Journal of Neonatal Nursing* 7(2), 48–52

Hedberg Nyqvist, K. and Strandell, E. (1999) A cup feeding protocol for neonates: evaluation of nurses' and parents' use of two cups, *Journal of Neonatal Nursing* 5(2), 31–6

Jocson, M.A.L., Mason, E.O. and Schanler, R.J. (1997) The effects of nutrient fortification and varying storage conditions on host defense properties of human milk, *Pediatrics* 100(2), 240–3

Lucas, A. and Cole, T.J. (1990) Breast milk and necrotising enterocolitis, *Lancet* 336, 1519–23

Lucas, A., Morley, R.M., Cole, T.J., Lister, G. and Leeson-Payne, C. (1992a) Breast milk and subsequent intelligence quotient in children born preterm, *Lancet* 339, 261–4

Lucas, A., Bishop, N.J., King, F.J. and Cole, T.J. (1992b) Randomised trial of nutrition for preterm infants after discharge, *Archives of Disease in Childhood.* 67(3), 324–7

McClure, R.J., Chatrath, M.K. and Newell, S.J. (1996) Changing trends in feeding policies for ventilated preterm infants, *Acta Paediatrica* 85, 1123–5

Menon, G. (1992a) Parenteral nutrition for the neonate, *British Journal of Intensive Care* May/June, 185–92

Menon, G. (1992b) Monitoring nutrition in intensive care neonates, *British Journal of Intensive Care* April, 149–55

Metcalf, R., Dilena, B., Gibson, R., Marshall, P. and Simmer, K. (1994) How appropriate are commercially available human milk fortifiers? *Journal of Paediatrics and Child Health* 30(4), 350–5

Neu, J., Valentine, C. and Meetze, W. (1990) Scientifically based strategies for nutrition of the high-risk low-birthweight infant *European Journal of Pediatrics* 150(1), 2–13

Quan, R., Yang, C., Rubinstein, S., Lewiston, N.J., Stevenson, D.K. and Kerner, J.A. (1994) The effect of nutritional additives on anti-effective factors in human milk, *Clinical Pediatrics* 325–8

Ritchie, J.F. (1998) Immature sucking response in premature babies: cup feeding as a tool in increasing maintenance of breast-feeding, *Journal of Neonatal Nursing* 4(2), 13–17

Robertson, A.F. and Bhatia, J. (1993) Feeding premature infants, *Clinical Pediatrics.* 32(1), 36–44

Royal College of Midwives (1998) *Successful Breast-feeding*, Holywell Press, Oxford

Shaw, V. and Lawson, M. (1994) *Clinical Paediatric Dietetics*, Blackwell, Oxford

Silvestre, M.A., Morbach, C.A., Brans, Y.W. and Shankaran, S. (1996) A prospective randomized trial comparing continuous versus intermittent feeding methods in very low-birthweight neonates, *The Journal of Pediatrics* 128(6), 748–52

Thomas, B. (1994) *Manual of Dietetic Practice*, Blackwell Scientific Publications, Oxford

Tsang, R., Lucas, A., Uauy, R. and Zlotkin, S. (1993) *Nutritional Needs of the Preterm Infant: Scientific Basis and Practical Guidelines*, Williams and Wilkins, Baltimore, MA

Tudehope, D. and Steer, P.A. (1996) Annotation which milk for the preterm infant? *Journal of Paediatrics and Child Health* 32(4), 275–7

Wardell, J.M., Hill, C.M. and D'Souza, S.W. (1981) Effect of pasteurization and of freezing and thawing of human milk on its triglyceride content, *Acta Paediatrica Scandinavia* 70, 467–71

Williams, A.F. (1991) Feeding of very low-birthweight infants, *Postgraduate Update* 326–33

Zeigler, E.E., O'Donnell, A.M., Nelson, S.E. and Komon, S.J. (1976) Body composition of the reference fetus, *Growth* 40(4), 329–41

16 Neonatal pharmacology

Helen Chadwick

Aims of the chapter

This chapter introduces the neonatal nurse to the basics of pharmacology. The methods of drug administration are discussed and the means by which these are absorbed considered. Some factors of drugs metabolism are reviewed and some of the most common drugs administered on the neonatal unit described.

INTRODUCTION

The safe and effective use of medicine in neonates is a complex area. From birth sometimes as early as 23 weeks gestation, to 4 weeks post term, a neonate's ability to handle a medicine will vary considerably due to changes in drug disposition. Medicine disposition refers to the handling of a medicine through absorption, distribution, metabolism and excretion. These processes are affected by gestational age, weight for dates, the concurrent disease state and the condition of the infant. There is an increasing trend to use medicine in this age group and it is paramount that those administering medicines have an understanding of how the infants are likely to respond.

ABSORPTION

This is the passage of a drug from its site of administration, through tissues or cell membranes and into the circulation. With intravenous administration, this does not need to be accounted for, but the intramuscular, percutaneous, oral and rectal routes are all subject to the effects of absorption.

Oral absorption

Drug absorption from the oral route can be affected by a number of factors (Table 16.1), and for this reason is not ideal.

For a medicine to be absorbed from the gastro-intestinal tract, it must be mainly in a lipid-soluble, unionised form. The pH affects drug ionisation and solubility. An acidic (low) pH favours absorption of acidic drugs, and a basic (high) pH favours the absorption of basic drugs. Gastric acid secretion is the main determinant of gastric and duodenal pH; it appears to be variable at birth, and rarely present in neonates of less than 32 weeks gestation. Acid secretion patterns in the neonatal period are generally reduced, and may be related to the presence or absence of enteral feeding (Hyman *et al.*, 1983).

Table 16.1 Factors affecting oral drug absorption

Patient factors	Drug factors
• Gastric emptying	• Pharmaceutical form
• GI tract acidity	• Ability of drug to cross membrane
• Food	• Ionisation at gastric pH
• Disease state	• Molecular weight

The unpredictability of gastric acid secretion and gastric and duodenal pH leads to variability in oral drug absorption. The relatively higher, more alkaline pH may enable basic drugs such as penicillins to be more rapidly and completely absorbed than acidic drugs such as phenobarbitone, when compared with adults.

The rate of gastric emptying may be delayed in newborns and infants up to 6 months of age. Intestinal motility is also affected by cardiovascular, metabolic and neurological disease. Bowel surgery will reduce motility and increase acid secretion and also reduce the surface area available for absorption. As most drugs are absorbed in the small intestine, this will slow the rate of absorption, delay the onset of effect and lower the peak concentration of drug in the plasma. For drugs degraded by stomach acid, such as penicillin, reduced gastric emptying will result in a higher proportion of the drug breaking down and less being absorbed.

Many factors affect gastric acid secretion, gastro-intestinal motility and drug absorption. Biliary function, when reduced, will lower the absorption of lipid-soluble drugs and vitamins. The presence of bacterial flora in the gastro-intestinal tract differs in neonates and this affects drug absorption. Some bacteria are able to metabolise drugs. Reduced peristaltic activity may result in the drug being in contact with the site of absorption for a longer period of time, and increase absorption.

Although oral administration can be a safe and effective route for drug delivery, the unpredictable and erratic absorption of drugs must be taken into consideration. This is important when consistent, predictable plasma concentrations or complete absorption are required.

Rectal absorption

Rectal administration is useful if the oral and intravenous routes are unavailable. Absorption by this route is also affected by factors such as pH. The pH of the rectal area is slightly alkaline. The drugs most suitable for rectal administration are those that are mainly unionised at this pH and sufficiently lipid-soluble to cross cell membranes. Drugs are formulated for rectal administration in solution and as a solid suppository. Absorption is more rapid from solutions than from suppositories, as there is a delay while the suppository dissolves. Accurate dosing can be difficult in the neonate as suppositories are usually formulated in adult doses.

Intramuscular absorption

Absorption following intramuscular (IM) administration depends on how well the drug disperses after injection and on the blood supply to the local area. Drugs need to be lipid-soluble to cross the muscle tissue into the blood, and stable at muscle pH.

Blood supply is often compromised in infants with poor peripheral blood flow, as with respiratory distress syndrome, hypotension or cardiac failure. 'Drug pooling' can occur when perfusion is poor. When there is an improvement in blood flow, the drug can be rapidly absorbed and this may result in toxicity or adverse effects.

The major limiting factor on the use of the intramuscular route is the small muscle mass of premature infants and neonates. This, together with the resultant variable absorption, means this route of administration is usually avoided except where intravenous access is not possible. The IM route is routinely used with vitamin K, which is more reliably absorbed in this way than when given by mouth.

Topical absorption

In neonates, especially premature infants, the epidermis is thin and immature, and acts as a poor barrier to the absorption of agents applied to the skin. The ratio of skin surface area to body weight is much greater than that of an adult and can result in relatively greater amounts of a topically applied drug being absorbed. Any trauma (burns or inflammation) will increase drug absorption into the bloodstream (Tyrala and Hillman, 1977). Toxic effects of topical hydrocortisone, hexachlorophene and phenol have been reported, and extreme caution should be used when applying any topical agent to neonatal skin. Consideration should be given to the toxic effects if absorption occurs. Topical absorption could prove to be an effective route of administration in the future, but further research is required.

Due to the variability in drug absorption in the neonate, it is usual to use the intravenous route of administration. The oral, rectal and intramuscular routes are usually reserved for those infants who are not seriously ill and who are haemodynamically stable.

DISTRIBUTION

Distribution is the spread of the drug once it has entered the body. It is affected by a number of factors:

- route of administration;
- body composition;
- plasma protein binding;
- tissue binding;
- vascular perfusion.

The route of administration is also important in drug distribution. A drug administered orally will pass through the liver before entering the systemic circulation (first pass metabolism). If extensive metabolism occurs, very little drug may be left for systemic action. Intravenous administration results in the drug entering straight into the bloodstream and direct distribution to the heart and lungs. This can result in a risk of anatomical damage (DoH, 2001) and an increased risk of toxicity.

Volume of distribution

This is the theoretical volume in which a drug distributes. If a drug is water-soluble (for example, gentamicin), it will stay in the water content of the body. Any fat-soluble drugs will distribute into the fat. As a result, when the volume of these components changes, the concentration of the drug in the bloodstream is altered.

Total body water is increased in the neonate due to a large extracellular fluid load and a small amount of fat (see Figure 16.1). This effect is more exaggerated the more premature the neonate. It results in lower plasma levels of water-soluble drugs, which stay mainly in the extracellular fluid when administered in an equal dose based on mg/kg of body weight compared with adults or older children; in other words, they are more dilute. Drugs affected include the aminoglycosides (gentamicin, tobramycin), penicillins, and non-depolarising neuromuscular blockers (pancuronium, vecuronium). If an infant has oedema, the effect will be more pronounced and drug level interpretation will be even more difficult.

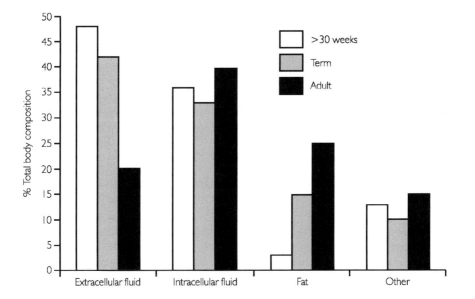

Figure 16.1 Neonatal body composition as a percentage of total body weight

With a fat-soluble drug, less of the drug is distributed into the fat, resulting in higher plasma concentrations. Some of the drug will bind to plasma proteins such as albumin. As only free drug can bind to its target site, less is available for systemic action. Neonates have reduced levels of these proteins so more of the drug is free and available for action, possibly resulting in an exaggerated pharmacological or toxic response. This may account for the lower therapeutic level of theophylline required in neonates (6–12 mg/l) when compared with adults (10–20 mg/l).

Agents such as other drugs or body compounds can displace drugs bound to plasma proteins from their binding sites. Bilirubin is one such agent. Increased production and delayed excretion of bilirubin, which occurs in the first few days of life, can lead to higher free drug levels. Therapeutic drug monitoring is not always helpful in predicting this toxicity as most assay methods measure total drug and not free drug.

The converse is also true, and drugs can displace bilirubin from its plasma protein binding sites. This may lead to higher levels of free bilirubin and result in central nervous system toxicity (Kernicterus).

Drugs that bind to plasma proteins depend on the structure of the drug. Plasma protein binding effects only become clinically significant if a drug is highly protein-bound (for example, phenytoin).

Tissue binding and uptake of drugs is also altered in neonates compared with adults. The increased penetration of many drugs into the central nervous system (morphine, fentanyl, diazepam) may be explained by an immature blood–brain barrier, and results in greater CNS concentrations at low doses or plasma levels.

The concentration of drug available for pharmacological action is influenced by a number of factors and these can result in a larger dose being required than for an adult on a mg/kg basis. However, despite lower plasma levels, the concentration at the site of action may be greater, leading to enhanced pharmacological action. Doses of drugs used in neonates must be carefully chosen and preferably based on controlled studies and pharmacokinetic information. Extrapolation from paediatric or adult doses is unsatisfactory.

METABOLISM

Many drugs undergo metabolism before excretion from the body. Many organs and tissues, including the lungs, gastro-intestinal tract, kidneys and blood, are capable of metabolising drugs. However, the liver is the major organ responsible for drug metabolism. Some drugs, such as gentamicin, are not metabolised and are excreted unchanged by the renal system.

At birth the hepatic enzymes responsible for metabolism are not fully functional, or may act differently from the way they act later in life. This can result in drugs such as theophylline, morphine and diazepam remaining in the body for long periods of time.

Neonates may also have different enzyme action, which may metabolise drugs in a different way. This may result in the production of pharmacologically toxic or active metabolites, or they may be just as effective as in the adult system. With paracetamol, for example, little difference is seen between the metabolism of the neonate and the adult.

Following birth, liver function and enzyme systems mature at varying rates. Blood flow and liver size are relatively greater in infants than in adults and, as liver enzymes mature, a period of increased drug metabolism, compared with adults, can occur. A number of disease states (RDS, hypoxaemia, septicaemia) can alter liver function, resulting in rapid changes during the neonatal period. In general, drug metabolism by the liver is decreased in the neonate, and this effect is even more marked in the premature infant. Careful monitoring of drug plasma levels and therapeutic response is required.

ELIMINATION

Most drugs and metabolites rely on the kidneys for excretion. Renal function develops late in gestation, at about 34 weeks, and so it is markedly reduced in the pre-term neonate. Following birth, renal function develops at a rate dependent on gestation, post-conceptional age and concurrent disease state. Cardiovascular disease and hypoxia can delay this development. Due to the reduced renal function, drug excretion can be poor in the neonate and, although it improves gradually, drug dosages remain variable.

Drugs can also affect renal function, as a number of commonly used drugs on the NNU are nephrotoxic (aminoglycosides), or can reduce renal blood flow, (indomethacin). Other drugs may increase renal blood flow (dopamine) and improve renal elimination.

For those drugs (aminoglycosides, penicillins, pancuronium, frusemide) excreted mainly unchanged by the kidneys, or having active metabolites, renal function needs to be monitored carefully to prevent toxicity and ensure adequate therapeutic effect.

THERAPEUTIC DRUG MONITORING

Therapeutic drug monitoring (TDM) is the measurement of drug levels in a body fluid, usually serum, to determine whether the drug is within certain concentration limits known to be safe and effective. The level needs to be high enough to be therapeutic but low enough to prevent toxicity.

TDM is more important in neonates than in any other group of the population. The incidence of adverse drug reactions is much greater in neonates than in infants, children or adults. Often, adverse drug reactions are unexpected or difficult to attribute to a specific drug therapy. Careful monitoring may improve recognition of these.

Drugs requiring close monitoring are generally those with a small difference between an effective level and a toxic level, that is, a narrow therapeutic range.

Drugs that require serum level monitoring include:

- aminoglycosides;
- theophylline;
- phenytoin;
- digoxin.

Due to the variations in drug distribution, metabolism and elimination, therapeutic concentrations of drugs may differ between adults and neonates. Plasma levels need to be considered in conjunction with the clinical state of the infant and the therapeutic response seen. For example, anti-epileptic drug levels may be slightly low but the infant may be seizure-free.

A number of factors can affect the serum levels obtained from the laboratory. This may lead to inappropriate adjustments in dosage, increasing the risk of toxicity or ineffective dosing. The most important factor is the time of sampling in relation to the dose. A peak level must be taken long enough after the dose is given to allow the drug to be fully distributed throughout the body, while trough levels should be taken immediately before the next dose. Sampling times vary between drugs and are generally standardised based on adult experience and studies.

The time of the dose and time of sampling should always be recorded to allow serum level interpretation.

Drug administration

Intravenous administration

The intravenous route is the main route of drug administration to neonates and presents a number of problems.

Drug delivery via a syringe pump is the method of choice when precise rates of drug delivery are required (or large volumes used), as it allows complete control over the time and rate of administration. With the antegrade infusion method, the drug is injected in the direction of flow via a 'Y' site attached to a primary infusion fluid. This can result in large variations in predicted drug delivery times at the low infusion rates commonly used in neonates.

The characteristics of the syringe pump or infusion pump may be important. Fluctuations in blood pressure during a dopamine infusion to a premature neonate have been reported (Schulse *et al.*, 1983). Low-pressure infusion pumps have reduced these problems, but careful consideration is still required.

The intraluminal diameter of intravenous tubing is important in determining the characteristics of drug infusions. Tubing with a smaller intraluminal diameter causes an increase in the speed of flow of the infusion fluid (DoH, 2001). This reduces the time required for drug delivery, reduces the flush volume and prevents delays in drug delivery.

The material from which the intravenous tubing is made should also be considered. Some drugs, such as insulin, paraldehyde and glyceryl trinitrate, are absorbed on to certain plastics, causing variations in drug delivery. Leeching of substances from various disposable intravenous administration products is also a problem with paraldehyde infusions. Specialist advice from the pharmacy department should be sought to determine the infusion tubing available for administration of these products. Generally, polyethylene-lined administration sets are recommended.

The use of bacterial and particulate in-line filtration devices is now common. Intravenous solutions contain varying quantities of particulate matter, which may produce phlebitis or even pulmonary granulomas. Certain drugs (such as insulin) may bind to such filters, while others (such as liposomal amphotericin) may not pass through. Again, specialist pharmacy advice should be sought.

Inadequate mixing of drug additions to intravenous infusion bags or between the drug solution and the primary infusion fluid can result in inaccurate and dangerous administration of large drug doses. Squeezing of intravenous infusion bags is not an effective method of mixing additives. The bag should be inverted several times to ensure even dispersal of the drug. This is particularly important when potassium is added to large-volume intravenous bags. Suitable dilutions of drug solutions should be used to prevent differences in specific gravity resulting in the drug settling out or floating in the primary infusion fluid. This is a particular problem when low infusion rates are used and can be reduced by using narrow-bore tubing.

Many drugs are administered by 'IV push'. This term is ambiguous and should be discouraged. All drugs administered to neonates should be given a minimum of 5 minutes to allow adequate mixing with blood and removal from the injection site. This avoids large localised concentrations of drug solution, which can cause phlebitis or toxicity. Specific problems can occur, due to high local drug concentrations; these may include seizures, cardiac arrhythmias and hypotension. Adult administration rates should not be applied to neonates, as the dilutional effects of the systemic circulation following drug administration are vastly different.

The use of small dosage volumes, which are often encountered in the neonatal intensive care unit, can cause difficulty. Often, formulations of a suitable strength to enable precise and easy dosage measurement, are not commercially available. The inadvertent administration of the dead-space volume if a syringe is flushed, can lead to drug toxicity when concentrated drug solutions are used.

Incompatibility between intravenous drugs is important when two or more drugs are mixed in the same line. Careful consideration is equally important, whether mixing with a primary infusion fluid or another drug solution via a 'Y' site connection. Mixing of drug solutions is to be discouraged, although, with an infant in a critical state, and a limited number of access ports, there is often little choice.

Incompatibility can be either physical or chemical. Physical incompatibility is the most obvious and results in formation of precipitate or a cloudy solution. Chemical incompatibility is less obvious, but results in drug inactivation or even conversion to toxic substances. Pharmacy advice should be sought before attempting to administer drugs together or with an infusion fluid with which compatibility is unknown.

Some drugs are also sensitive to light and can be affected by phototherapy, especially when low infusion rates are used.

Local policies and procedures for intravenous drug use, covering reconstitution, dilution and administration, are essential for safe and effective drug delivery to neonates.

Oral administration

The administration of oral medication is not without complications. The risk of aspiration should be considered, even in the presence of a nasogastric tube. This is particularly important whenever an oral preparation has a particularly high or low pH. When using a nasogastric tube to administer drugs, an inadequate flush volume may not clear the tubing following drug administration. This may result in a proportion of the dose remaining in the tubing.

Incompatibility can also occur with oral dosage forms. The administration of some drugs (such as phenytoin) in the presence of enteral feeds can reduce absorption (Bauer, 1982).

The use of hypertonic oral medications may also be associated with the development of necrotising enterocolitis (White and Harkavy, 1982; Atakent et al., 1984).

Advice as to when to administer some of the less commonly used drugs in relation to feeds should be sought from the hospital pharmacist.

DRUG FORMULATION

The majority of commercially available drug products are formulated for use in adults with little consideration to their potential use in neonates. Many dosage forms are presented in strengths or concentrations that require accurate measurement of small dosage volumes. Appropriate techniques should be used to avoid errors in such measurements, taking into account the dead space of syringe hubs and needles.

The concentration of drug solutions is important in avoiding pain and phlebitis at the injection site, or adverse effects on the gastro-intestinal tract. These complications can be avoided by simple dilution to specified concentrations before administration and may also prolong the patency of an intravenous line or reduce the risk of necrotising enterocolitis.

The use of certain intravenous preparations orally may overcome some problems, as injections are often formulated without preservatives to minimise irritation at the site of injection. However, this should only be undertaken after pharmaceutical advice has been sought and safety confirmed.

Many drug preparations contain other ingredients, as well as the active constituent. These may be preservatives, formulation stabilisers, impurities or even flavourings, and have been associated with adverse effects, including intraventricular haemorrhage, metabolic acidosis, cardiac arrhythmias, seizures, and hypersensitivity reactions (American Academy of Paediatrics, 1985). It is important to investigate and assess the constituents of a drug formulation before administration to neonates. Advice can be obtained from pharmacists or drug manufacturers.

MEDICINES COMMONLY USED ON THE NNU

This section has been written to give an overview of some of the more commonly used drugs on the NNU. It is not intended to be a pharmacopoeia and current guidelines should be observed when prescribing.

Reflux

Table 16.2 Drugs and medicines used in cases of reflux

Medicine	Use	Adverse effects	Interactions
Domperidone	Traditionally an antiemetic, more recently used in gastro-oesophageal reflux; has a pro-kinetic effect on the upper gut	Has some central action, so may cause acute dystonic reactions	Effects may be antagonised by anti-muscarinics and opioid analgesics
Gaviscon Infant[R]	Reacts with stomach acid, producing a raft on top of the stomach contents; acts as a mechanical barrier to reflux	High sodium content; may cause hypernatraemia	None reported
Ranitidine	Inhibits gastric acid secretion; used in severe reflux where oesophagitis has occurred	Hypersensitivity reactions including urticaria, fever, bronchospasm, hypotension and anaphylactic shock; may occur after a single dose; liver function tests can be altered transiently	None reported

Infection

Antibiotic use varies across the country depending upon local resistance patterns. Table 16.3 lists some of the commonly used antibiotics.

Table 16.3 Use of antibiotics in cases of infection

Medicine	Use	Adverse effects	Interactions	TDM
Aciclovir	An antiviral agent used to treat herpes simplex and varicella-zoster viral infections	Severe inflammatory reactions have been reported at the site of injection; can impair renal function	There is an increased risk of renal damage when used concurrently with other nephrotoxic drugs	None
Amoxicillin	An aminopenicillin, similar to ampicillin; a broad-spectrum antibiotic active against a wide range of organisms, including listeria	GI upset, rash	None relevant	None
Amphotericin B	Anti-fungal agent used to treat systemic fungal infection; a valuable but toxic medicine; a small test dose is usually given before each course to exclude anaphylactic reaction	Nephrotoxicity; the conventional formulation will give rise to some degree of renal impairment in >85% of patients; anaemia common; hypokalaemia, flushing, generalised pain, convulsions, leucopenia and anaphylaxis may occur; infusion-related effects include fever, vomiting and rigors; the liposomal formulation has fewer renal and infusion-related side-effects and can be used where nephrotoxicity develops	Other nephrotoxic drugs; hypokalaemia may cause digoxin toxicity; corticosteroids may enhance potassium depletion	Close monitoring of renal function
Benzylpenicillin	A penicillin antibiotic; often used in combination with gentamicin as first-line prophylaxis	Allergic reactions	None relevant	None

Continued

Table 16.3 Continued

Medicine	Use	Adverse effects	Interactions	TDM
Cefotaxime	Broad spectrum cephalosporin antibiotic; often used in neonatal meningitis; should not be used alone if infection with listeria is suspected	Usually transient and mild; those reported include candidiasis, rash, fever, transient increase in liver function tests and diarrhoea	High doses used in combination with aminoglycosides or diuretics may impair renal function	None
Flucloxacillin	Antibiotic of choice for penicillinase-resistant staphylococci	GI upset, rash, hepatitis and cholestatic jaundice (may occur several weeks after stopping treatment)	None relevant	None
Fluconazole	Anti-fungal agent often used in the management of systemic *Candida albicans* infection	GI upset, rashes; mild and transient increases in liver enzymes	Increased plasma levels of midazolam, theophylline, phenytoin	None
Gentamicin	Aminoglycoside antibiotic, used to treat Gram-negative bacterial infection; does not penetrate the CSF very well	Nephrotoxicity and ototoxicity if recommended blood levels are exceeded	Increased risk of ototoxicity and nephrotoxicity with cephalosporins, vancomycin, frusemide and amphotericin	Take levels around third dose; trough level immediately before the third dose and peak level 1 hour post dose; aim for a trough of > 1.5 mg/l and a peak of 5–8 mg/l
Metronidazole	Used in the treatment of anaerobic bacterial infection, a range of protozoal infections, after gastro-intestinal surgery and in the management of necrotising enterocolitis	GI upset is the most common; CNS effects such as drowsiness have been reported; skin rashes and urticaria	Concurrent barbiturate use can reduce the plasma levels of metronidazole	None
Trimethoprim	Often used to treat and prevent urinary tract infection	Most frequent are rash, pruritis and GI upset; more serious skin reactions have occurred; possible haematological abnormalities	May increase levels of phenytoin and digoxin	None

Continued

Table 16.3   Continued

Medicine	Use	Adverse effects	Interactions	TDM
Vancomycin	A glycopeptide, active against most Gram-positive bacteria; often used to treat systemic staphylococcal infection from infected central lines	Ototoxicity and nephrotoxicity have been reported, usually when used in combination with gentamicin; if given too rapidly, can cause histamine release resulting in pruritis and erythema – the red-man syndrome	Care when used with other potentially nephrotoxic drugs, e.g. aminoglycosides and amphotericin	Take levels around third dose; trough level immediately before the third dose and peak level 1 hour after the end of the infusion; aim for a trough of 5–10 mg/l and peak of 20–40 mg/l

Respiratory system

Dexamethasone

Dexamethasone is a potent glucocortocoid steroid. It accelerates surfactant production in the pre-term foetal lung, reducing respiratory death in this group of neonates. In pre-term infants with bronchopulmonary dysplasia (BPD), dexamethasone can reduce the amount of time that an infant requires ventilation or remains in oxygen after extubation. However, dexamethasone is not without adverse effect. It is associated with an increased risk of infection and, in those on diuretics, nephrocalcinosis; rises in blood glucose and blood pressure, and an increased risk of gastro-intestinal haemorrhage and retinopathy of prematurity (ROP). When used for over 10 days, it causes adrenal suppression for 2–4 weeks. Use of dexamethasone should be reserved for infants who remain ventilator-dependent and doses and duration of treatment should be kept as low as possible.

Surfactants

Surfactant deficiency was first recognised as the cause of the respiratory distress seen in pre-term infants in the first 2–3 days of life in 1959. The introduction of surfactant treatment in the 1980s has been associated with significantly improved survival in pre-term neonates who have neonatal respiratory distress syndrome. The effect of combined antenatal steroids and post-natal surfactant is more effective than either of these treatments alone.

Surfactants can be divided into two main groups: natural (produced from extracts of animal lung) and synthetic. Both groups are effective in the treatment and prevention of respiratory distress syndrome. However, comparative trials demonstrate greater early improvement in the requirement for ventilator support, less risk of pneumothorax, and fewer deaths associated with natural surfactant extract treatment. Natural surfactant may be associated with an increase in intraventricular haemorrhage, although the more serious haemorrhages (Grades 3 and 4) are not increased. Despite these concerns, natural surfactant extracts would seem to be the more desirable choice when compared with currently available synthetic surfactants.

Surfactant is administered via the endotracheal route and for this reason is only given where an infant is already ventilated. It is usual to give surfactant to those infants born at less than 32 weeks gestational age as soon as it is clear that they are oxygen-dependent. Some units give it prophylactically to all intubated infants born at less than 30 weeks.

Natural surfactants can cause a rapid decrease in ventilator requirements and infants receiving these medicines require careful monitoring and adjustment of ventilator settings.

Caffeine

In an infant with recurrent episodes of apnoea, the methylxanthines (theophylline and caffeine) are thought to stimulate breathing efforts, and have been used in clinical practice since the 1970s. The mechanism of their action is not certain, although possibilities include increased chemoreceptor responsiveness, enhanced respiratory muscle performance and generalised central nervous system excitation.

While there are no long-term data on effectiveness and safety of caffeine, it appears to have similar short-term effects on apnoea/bradycardia to theophylline. However, caffeine has potential therapeutic advantages over theophylline due to its higher therapeutic ratio, more reliable enteral absorption and longer half-life, which allows once-daily dosing. For these reasons it is the recommended preparation for the treatment of apnoea.

Patent ductus arteriosus (PDA)

Indomethacin, an inhibitor of prostaglandin synthesis, is now recognised as being useful in the management of symptomatic PDA. Maintenance of the duct is prostaglandin-dependent. Inhibition of the prostaglandin formation by indomethacin results in closure of the PDA in 80% of cases.

Indomethacin should not be used where the infant has serious coagulation disorders or has necrotising enterocolitis.

REFERENCES

American Academy of Paediatrics on Drugs (1985) Interactive ingredients in pharmaceutical products, *Paediatrics* 76, 635–43
Atakent, Y., Ferrara, A., Bhogal, M. *et al.* (1984) The adverse effects of high oral osmolar mixtures in neonates, *Clinical Paediatrics* 23, 487–91
Bauer, L.A. (1982) Interference of oral henytoin absorption by continuous nasogastric feedings, *Neurology*, 32 (5), 570–2

Department of Health [DoH] (2001) Review of the deaths of four babies due to cardiac tamponade associated with the presence of a central venous catheter, Department of Health, London

Hyman, P.E., Feldman, E.J., Ament, M.E., Byrne, W.J. and Euler, A.R. (1983) Effect of external feeding on the maintenance of gastric acid secretory function, *Gastroenterology* **84**, 341–5

Schulse, K.F., Graff, M., Schimmel, M.S., *et al.* (1983) Physiologic oscillations produced by an infusion pump, *Journal of Paediatrics* **103**, 796–8

Tyrala, E.E. and Hillman, L.S. (1977) Clinical pharmacology of hexachlorophene in newborn infants, *Journal of Paediatrics* **91**, 481–6

White, K.C. and Harkavy, K.L. (1982) Hypertonic formula resulting from added oral medications, *American Journal of Diseases of Childhood* **136**(10), 931–3

FURTHER READING

Ainsworth, S.B., Beresford, M.W., Milligan, D.W.A., Shaw, N.J., Matthews, J.N.S., Fenton, A.C. *et al.* (2000) Pumactant and poractant alfa for treatment of respiratory distress syndrome in neonates born at 25–29 weeks gestation: a randomised trial, *Lancet*; **355**, 1387–92

Halliday, H.L., Ehrenkranz, R.A. (2001) Delayed (>3 weeks) post-natal corticosteroids for chronic lung disease in pre-term infants (Cochrane Review). In: *The Cochrane Library*, 3, Update Software, Oxford

The Northern Neonatal Network (2000) *Neonatal Formulary 3*, BMJ Books, London

Royal College of Paediatrics and Child Health (1999) *Medicines for Children*, RCPCH, London

Steer, P.A., Henderson-Smart, D.J. (2001) Caffeine versus theophylline for apnoea in pre-term infants (Cochrane Review). In: *The Cochrane Library*, 3, Update Software, Oxford

17 HOME DISCHARGE

Doreen Crawford and Liz Sampson

Aims of the chapter

This chapter focuses on the nursing management of infants discharged home with additional, sometimes extraordinary, needs. Consideration is given of the period of transition and the support offered to the families at home. The chapter uses infants with chronic lung disease that remain oxygen-dependent as examples of ongoing care. They may require continuous oxygen therapy and management and tend to be the infants most often affected by prolonged hospitalisation.

INTRODUCTION

Most surviving pre-term infants will have been discharged home by the time they reach term. There are, however, a small but increasing number of infants with continuing problems who, without special planning and consideration, would remain in hospital for a prolonged period. These infants were sometimes referred to as 'geriatric neonates' and their care tended to fall between the neonatal units and the children's hospitals. Evidence now indicates that early discharge is good for infants and good for families. In addition, the policy saves resources, releases cots and makes the most use of highly skilled staff (Hallam *et al.*, 1996).

Infants with ongoing chronic problems tend to fall into the following groups (although some infants may have problems that overlap):

- neurological problems;
- feeding problems;
- congenital or acquired abnormalities needing surgical intervention perhaps resulting in stoma or urinary diversions;
- complications of ventilation such as tracheostomy or bronchopulmonary dysplasia (BPD) or chronic lung disease (CLD).

CHRONIC LUNG DISEASE AND BRONCHOPULMONARY DYSPLASIA

BPD is described as a chronic pulmonary condition of infants who have experienced respiratory failure. They remain oxygen-dependent for at least 28 days and have associated clinical and radiological findings. It is recognised to be a complication of barotrauma from mechanical ventilation and oxygen toxicity following respiratory distress, although there is evidence that the predisposing factors are changing with extensive use of surfactant (Bancalari and del Moral,

2001). Other infants will develop chronic lung disease as a result of recurrent aspiration, patent ductus arteriosus, acute or chronic infections and apnoea of prematurity (Rojas *et al.*, 1995; Bancalari, 2001). They may also have been ventilated, usually for a shorter period. They remain oxygen-dependent and have associated radiological findings of severe hyperinflation alternating with areas of increased density.

There are theoretical differences between the two conditions of CLD and BPD, but for all practical purposes the two terms have largely merged. 'CLD' may be used more widely to include BPD as it covers the whole spectrum. The management and treatment remain much the same.

These infants can be very demanding and irritable as they mature and will often stretch their carers to their limits. An understanding of the condition and the reasons why breathing is such hard work can be of great benefit when coping with the stress of caring for them. As always, a nursing priority is to provide a safe environment and high standards of care to allow for optimum growth and development.

Impact of the environment

Mature infants with CLD are easily stressed. Prolonged hospitalisation creates insecurity, which, added to the lack of individual attention, results in irritable and demanding behaviour. This can lead to hypoxia, which inhibits growth and contributes to a continuing cycle of events (see Figure 17.1).

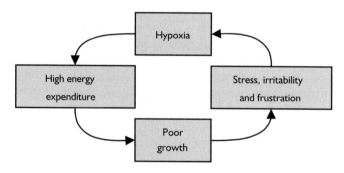

Figure 17.1   Hypoxia cycle

To provide an optimal environment for growth and, therefore, for recovery, it is necessary to avoid stress and hypoxia, as well as providing a satisfactory nutritional intake. This is not always easy to achieve in hospital. The ultimate answer to avoid these complications is early discharge home.

Pathophysiology of chronic lung disease

As a result of their chronic lung disease, these infants consume excessive amounts of energy because of their increased effort to breathe. To understand why, each area of the respiratory tract can be considered in relation to the symptoms that the infant suffers.

Small airways

There is dysplasia of respiratory epithelium and excessive mucus production, which leads to narrowing of the airways. This causes an increased resistance to airflow, increasing the work of breathing.

Alveoli

There are areas of severe hyperinflation, alternating with areas of increased density, due to collapse or fibrosis. This causes poor lung compliance with the high intrathoracic pressures needed to expand the lungs, which increases the work of breathing. The emphysematous areas receive excessive amounts of ventilation but are poorly perfused. The increased work of breathing causes over-ventilation and, therefore, carbon dioxide retention. The areas of collapse are inefficient units of ventilation and gas exchange resulting in hypoxaemia. To compensate, the respiratory rate increases, making breathing more difficult.

Pulmonary vascular bed

Alveolar hypoxia causes the vascular bed to constrict and the pulmonary artery pressures to increase, which can lead to pulmonary hypertension and right heart failure. This is mainly reversible but persistent hypoxaemia leads to persistent pulmonary hypertension and to irreversible disease (cor pulmonale). It is this which, in the past, has led to the significant mortality of these infants.

Adequate oxygenation is essential to the survival of these infants. Even a mild degree of chronic hypoxaemia can have general effects. These may include sleep disturbances and poor growth, as well as the effects that can be associated with acute apnoeic episodes and respiratory infections.

The ultimate cure for chronic lung disease is the natural growth and maturation of normal lung tissue, which will occur with increasing age and weight gain. Many infants have a long struggle to achieve this, with many hurdles to get over during the first few years, and it is during this period that a high standard of nursing care, and individual love and care from the family, are critical.

Management of BPD/CLD

Most hospitals now run some form of neonatal community services, allowing infants with chronic lung disease to be discharged home, to be cared for by their families. Close monitoring support and supervision is provided by a team of people who are familiar with pre-term lung disease and the requirements of oxygen therapy, until the infant no longer needs oxygen and its growth and development are satisfactory. This form of care management ensures minimum risk to the infant and minimal anxiety to the family. These infants remain extremely vulnerable but being at home is the best place for them.

By the time infants with chronic lung disease graduate to the special care nursery, although still small, they may be quite mature. It is usually at this point that the parents will start to feel frustration. Following the rollercoaster ride of the neonatal period, through intensive and high-dependency care, the parents' expectations may have risen about the possibility of taking a healthy infant home. They may have seen other equally sick infants, of similar age, get better and be discharged or transferred. In comparison, their infant's progress may seem to have come to a standstill.

Parents need a very positive approach with respect to their infant's condition. They need to understand what CLD is, why their infant has it and how it will be managed, including the possibility of discharge while still on oxygen therapy. Oxygen should not be seen as a barrier to discharge but as a part of the ongoing treatment. Providing this is discussed fully with the parents, they can look forward to discharge like any other parent. A degree of apprehension can be seen as normal and probably applies to all parents taking a new infant home from hospital or a neonatal unit.

PLANNING NURSING CARE

Infants with CLD can present with minimal symptoms and few ongoing problems, or may have multiple problems associated with their condition. Planning for their care is based on individual assessment, to identify and meet their specific needs. A multidisciplinary team meeting will develop an individual management plan. The parents will have been included in the consideration of their infant's care throughout the stay in hospital and will also be invited to planning meetings. Parents appreciate information and this can be a contributory factor to the satisfaction they feel towards the health care that their infant has received (Mancini and While, 2001).

Forward planning is essential, not only to relieve anxiety and to ensure trouble-free discharge, but also because of resource issues. At present, home oxygen is funded by the GP although the support is provided by the NHS Trusts. Other consumables are provided by a combination of prescription and hospital issue. The parents must be clear as to who is responsible for supplying what and have the appropriate contact names and numbers. There should also be some attempt to identify potential problems and contingency plans should be drawn up. Potential problems can generally be subdivided into the following categories:

- breathing;
- nutrition, feeding and growth;
- development;
- infant care issues;
- family coping and stress.

It is important to remember that the level of nursing care and supervision needs to be reduced, gradually, as the infant and parents are prepared for discharge. A satisfactory transition period is vital; one of the hardest things for parents to do is to believe that their infant is safe in their care with less intensive monitoring (Turrill, 1999). Parents can become very dependent on equipment and staff and may find it difficult to make their own decisions about their infant, with direct professional advice (Redman, 1993). To avoid this, parents must be involved with planning and carrying out as much of their infant's care as possible, although this will be determined by their home commitments, particularly when there are siblings to consider. It is important to get the transitional phase right to equip the parents to cope with life at home. Some mothers have felt isolated following discharge and unequipped for the challenges of caring for these infants at home (Manns, 2000). The ideal following discharge is a balance between support and professional intrusion in family life.

Oxygen

The infant's needs
The main problem for these infants is their inability to maintain adequate oxygenation without additional inspired oxygen. They need a continuous concentration of inspired oxygen to maintain a stable and consistent oxygen saturation.

Once extubated, or weaned from CPAP, an infant with chronic lung disease will be transferred to incubator, headbox or nasal prong oxygen in order to provide the specific concentration required to maintain adequate saturations. Several attempts will have been made to wean the infant off oxygen. Once it is clear that this is not going to be possible, for home discharge to be considered the infant would have to be tolerating nasal prong oxygen and to have remained stable on this form of management. Particular attention would be paid to any changes in SaO_2 during activities, especially when sleeping, feeding, playing or crying, and during procedures. Any changes in levels may indicate an unstable oxygen requirement.

Administration of oxygen
There are different types of nasal cannula available and all have their advantages and disadvantages; they are generally well tolerated. The double nasal cannula, which comes in several sizes, is placed in the nostrils and secured to the cheeks by tape. They can sometimes be difficult to secure in very small infants, as the prongs tend to slip out. As the infant matures they can actually be kept in position without any tape. The main concern with this method is that an active infant can remove them and, as they can be worn as a necklace or spectacles, close supervision is required to maintain the infant's safety as well as oxygenation. The lumens of these cannulae are very fine and can get blocked up easily, particularly during colds. During periods of illness, such as upper respiratory tract infection (URTI), a higher flow tends to be necessary because of the nasal discharge.

A single catheter, either size 5 or 6 FG, is inserted via one nostril into the nasopharynx. The distance that this is inserted is determined by measuring the distance from the tip of the nose to the eyebrow (in the very small infant) or from ear to nostril (for the larger infant). The catheter can then be secured to one cheek and tucked into the clothing at the back to prevent pulling or kinking of the catheter. This method is generally tolerated well, although some infants may have increased nasal secretions for the first few days, particularly if the catheter is not inserted far enough. It is not so easily removed and, during cold, the nasal discharge is largely bypassed.

Oxygen can be provided by a concentrator or by cylinders and a number of low flow oxygen meters are available to regulate the flow. These allow for delivery of oxygen from 1.0 l/min down to 10 cl/min but probably the most useful and widely used is the 100–500 cl/min type. Humidity is useful for some infants and can also be included in the circuit.

Most paediatricians like to keep the oxygen saturation above 90% at all times but it is not always appreciated how even mild hypoxia can cause pulmonary hypertension. Some infants are far more sensitive than others. The only way to identify an infant's response to oxygen, and increased SaO_2, is by echocardiogram to measure pulmonary artery pressures. If this facility is not available, it is probably preferable to maintain SaO_2 at 94–97%, at all times, to minimise the risk of irreversible pulmonary hypertension and, at the same time, allow for better growth. Most infants are by this time past the risk of retinopathy.

Monitoring

Once an infant has been established on nasal oxygen therapy, and his or her condition and oxygen requirements have been stable for some days, the necessity of continuous monitoring should be considered. While in hospital, most infants are monitored as a back-up to professional observation, to help nurses care for the infant safely. Monitors are a source of anxiety for parents and frequently create a degree of dependency. It is not unusual to see parents staring at the monitor rather than at their infant. When planning a discharge, intermittent monitoring is preferable, to give the parents a chance to familiarise themselves with looking at and assessing their infant's breathing pattern and general well-being without relying on the monitor. An apnoea monitor is probably the only monitor needed continuously at this time.

There will always be the exception as some infants may be less stable and require variable oxygen concentrations, depending on their level of activity. These infants would probably go home initially with continuous monitoring facilities.

The frequency with which an infant with CLD oxygen saturation level should be monitored will vary between units and depends on their clinical stability. For example, fairly random intermittent monitoring for a couple of half-hour periods would give a fairly comprehensive overview of how the infant is coping. Ideally, the infant would be assessed through a sleep, while being handled, and during and after feeding. The SaO_2 probe should be securely attached and there should be good pulse volume and no movement artefact. Overnight recording of saturations should be performed if there has been an increase in oxygen requirements as these infants are sometimes at risk during sleep of intermittent sleep hypoxia (Zinman *et al.*, 1992).

Most oximeters have a memory facility to enable the downloading of 8 hours of recording on to a personal computer or a two-channel printer. These are especially useful for the older infant with a more regular sleep pattern, enabling accurate monitoring of trends as quiet and REM sleep states are easily identified.

Feeding and growth

Growth failure is a significant problem for many infants with chronic lung disease. Growth is essential for repair and development of lung tissue as well as for general development and feeding. Nutrition is a major issue and central to the success of care at home. Trying to achieve adequate growth can be extremely difficult and frustrating, both for the infant and for carers, and requires good nutritional intake and oxygenation.

One of the main factors for poor growth is the increased energy expenditure for breathing. Studies have shown a 25% increase in energy expenditure for such infants, compared with those without lung disease (Yeh *et al.*, 1989). Other factors related to growth failure may be chronic hypoxia, poor nutritional intake, gastro-oesophageal reflux, vomiting, emotional stress and deprivation.

Increased oxygen may be needed to compensate for the increased respiratory effort and hard work required to feed, and may make feeding easier to cope with. Hypoxia during feeding can increase the risk of aspiration, respiratory distress, apnoea and bradycardia.

Nutrition

Many infants with CLD or BPD may have their fluid intake restricted to avoid fluid overload and heart failure. Whether restricted or not, a high calorie intake will be necessary to compensate for their high-energy expenditure.

Low-birthweight formulas will provide a high calorie and mineral intake and it may be necessary to continue these formulas after discharge, particularly if the infant is on a fluid-restricted diet or has an inadequate nutritional intake due to poor feeding. Some infants may need additional calorie supplements as well.

For many infants with CLD, it may be thought that breast milk and breast-feeding alone will not provide adequate nutrition. The infant may be prescribed a combination of low-birthweight milk or other additives to be mixed with the breast milk. Alternatively, a modification of the feeding regime could be made to ensure a mix of high-calorie bottle feeds as well as a continuation of the enjoyment of breast-feeding. There are many positive benefits of breast-feeding, apart from calorie intake, and more research is required to inform practice. It can be very difficult for a mother who has always been told that 'breast is best', to be advised that her infant also needs formula milk and other concoctions. This needs sensitive handling by medical and nursing staff.

Follow-on milk formulas for pre-term infants have now been developed (*see* Table 15.3) as the next step in nutrition, once low-birthweight milk is discontinued. This milk continues to provide additional energy, protein and minerals to allow for catch-up growth to continue.

For the older infant with more severe BPD, early weaning needs to be considered as a means of increasing energy intake without an increase in fluid intake. This tends to be well received and enjoyed by the infant, and can make a significant difference to growth. Close liaison and follow-up with a paediatric dietician is essential to advise on the optimal nutritional requirements needed to promote growth, while in hospital, during discharge planning, and continuing at home.

Feeding problems

Some of these infants will be poor, disorganised feeders. They may continue to have feeding problems, long after the usual age for sucking and swallowing co-ordination has been reached. Most will be taking some feeds orally by the time of discharge, although they can still be struggling to achieve an adequate intake.

These feeding problems may be attributed to prolonged ventilation and oral endotracheal intubation, which have resulted in hypersensitive and deformed palates. Some infants may simply be too tired by the effort to breathe, suck and swallow. Other infants may not feed well because of residual neurological damage. For nursing management, the following points should be considered when planning a feeding programme:

- optimal oxygenation to avoid increased respiratory distress;
- a quiet environment, with minimal distractions for the infant and his feeder;
- feeding by a limited number of nurses (with experience of feeding these types of infants), along with the parents, to allow a consistent and regular feeding habit to develop;
- a clear feeding plan, to provide the necessary encouragement and support for sucking and swallowing co-ordination. This would take into account the individual preference for the appropriate teat, flow and the temperature of the milk. Some infants, who may have poor oral muscle tone and poor oral reflexes, require support of the lower jaw and gentle stimulation to encourage sucking. Their tongue and jaw movements may be less controlled and they may have poor cheek stability and inadequate lip seal;
- the parents, with support, are the right people to feed their infant and this helps to develop a relationship and pattern, prior to discharge. Often, the infant's feeding improves after discharge because of the consistency in handling and the developing relationship with the parents.

The paediatric speech therapist may also play an important role during the early management of the sick neonate, particularly for those infants who have delayed oral feeding and for assessing oral-motor function. They may advise on alternative feeding regimes and oral stimulation, and are often a good source of different feeding teats and bottles to try.

Management of the disorganised feeder is a subject covered by Vandenberg (1990); this text is important reading for neonatal nurses.

Some infants may require continued nasogastric tube feeding for a prolonged period. This need not be a barrier to discharge, provided there is adequate support in the community. Tube feeding is probably more demanding at home than oxygen therapy. The worst scenario is that the feeding situation can leave the parents feeling inadequate about the infant's continued inability to feed. The parents are by far the best people to get oral feeding established so it is important for their confidence and faith in themselves to remain high. Under normal circumstances, feeding an infant is a source of mutual joy and satisfaction. For these infants and their parents it can become a source of frustration and many problems.

Gastro-oesophageal reflux and vomiting

Pre-term infants have a higher incidence of gastro-oesophageal reflux (see Chapter 8). Repeated vomiting and regurgitating with small aspirations will further damage the delicate lung tissue. Infants who reflux milk may have intermittent episodes of desaturations or apnoea and bradycardia. A 24-hour pH study or a barium swallow will be needed to confirm this. If this proves to be positive, treatment can be started. This includes thickening of feeds, giving antacids such as Gaviscon, and careful positioning. The infant needs to be nursed tilted and prone, either supported in a cot or in a reflux chair. This is generally enough to improve the problem. If reflux persists, domperidone may be effective.

If reflux is not positively identified, there are many other factors that may contribute to excessive vomiting. Diuretics are emetic and can aggravate the situation. Often these infants find it difficult to bring up wind and then vomit when they eventually manage to burp. Excessive coughing can cause an infant to vomit, and this can, in time, develop into a behavioural problem, when the infant learns that vomiting brings attention. Excessive vomiting can be frustrating and distressing for parents, particularly after discharge and it needs early management to minimise the problem whenever possible.

Development

Many very low-birthweight infants will have moderate to major delay in development because of their prematurity and need for neonatal intensive care. This likelihood increases with the sicker and smaller infants. Infants with added complications such as BPD remain even more vulnerable and the developmental delay is not always apparent at the time of discharge.

In the nursery it is important that nurses are able to recognise the factors that produce stress and the effect that it may have on the infant. Care should be planned to minimise stress and provide an optimal environment for long-term developmental outcome. Factors such as noise, bright lights, pain, and inappropriate and excessive handling can all be reduced by adopting sensitive attitudes to care, and by careful planning of care. Massage is another method recognised for its advantage in reducing stress. Chapters 4 and 12 discuss ways to reduce stress and enhance development on the NNU.

Teaching parents to understand what causes stress, and how to reduce it, is an important part of the nurse's role.

Skin-to-skin contact

Skin-to-skin contact ('kangaroo care') between mother and infant can be a very effective method of reducing stress, promoting good relationships, enhancing development, improving milk production and can result in improved oxygenation. The infant is placed naked, except for a nappy, between their mother's breasts in an upright position. Held like this, the mother, more naturally, talks or sings and gently strokes the head. Breathing becomes more relaxed as the SaO_2 rises and they become very calm and content. It also has a very positive effect for the mother, in boosting her confidence in handling the infant. This model of care will have been promoted throughout the infant's stay in hospital and the parents should be encouraged to put time aside for the continuation of the practice after discharge.

Motor delay

At home, it may become apparent to the parents that their infant has a degree of motor delay. It is inevitable that their child will be compared unfavourably with friends' full-term infants, whose progress will appear to be so much faster. It is important that the parents understand, before discharge, that developmental delay is possible and has to be seen in context. It may be significant, not only because of the infant's prematurity and poor health after birth, but also because of the time spent in hospital. The majority will catch up but it may take 2 or 3 years, or even longer.

A full physiotherapy assessment may be helpful to identify any significant problems, so that advice can be given to parents on positioning and exercises to perform. The infant may also be involved with a play therapist. These strategies can provide the infant with every opportunity to catch up with their development, without forming bad habits. Parents will need support and encouragement if their infant has significant delay. Regular developmental assessments will be done either by the hospital or community child development team.

Infant care issues

These infants can be less than tolerant of handling and care routines. In addition, they can be clammy, sweaty little individuals who would benefit greatly from frequent baths and changes of clothes, providing they are well. The care that can be provided at home is more flexible than the care that tends to be available in a hospital and the bath can be timed to coincide with the infant's 'good spells'. Forward planning, to organise all that is needed for the bath and change beforehand, will reduce the amount of time the infant has to hang around. The parents may plan their day so that there are always two people around during this time of day, to provide a spare pair of hands if required.

Positioning

Department of Health recommendations regarding Sudden Infant Death (2000) include the advice to lay infants on their backs. Parents will be very anxious about what position is safe and right for their child (Crawford, 2000), particularly as some infants with CLD may breathe and oxygenate better when nursed prone and tilted at an angle. Prior to discharge the infant needs to be monitored supine and prone to see if there is a significant change in SaO_2, and the issues need to be discussed between neonatal staff and the parents.

Input from the physiotherapist is useful at this stage as many of these infants have adopted poor posture. Their respiratory effort, particularly if they are hypoxic, may have encouraged them to arch their backs and extend their necks, to make the work of breathing easier.

Medication

Some infants may only be on vitamins and iron by the time they are discharged. Others may be on a selection of drugs including diuretic therapy, anti-reflux therapy, mineral supplements, calorie supplements, bronchodilators and steroid inhaled therapy. The number of drugs can be overwhelming for the parents, who must be given the opportunity and time to familiarise themselves with administering them, particularly because of the minute doses involved, and also to understand the importance and action of each drug.

Family coping and stress

The importance of the parents' role in caring for their infant cannot be overemphasised. Families with an infant with CLD may have multiple problems to overcome prior to taking their infant home and will need individually tailored support and advice.

When first approached about taking the infant home on oxygen, most parents will feel extremely anxious about their ability to cope and about the effect that it may have on their family life. They may ask questions about the safety of oxygen in the home and about the risks to the infant. Parental confidence will increase as they spend more time with their infant. They will come to understand their infant's personality more, and be able to anticipate any problems and identify any needs. With increased confidence they may make useful changes to the plan of care, which should be respected by the nursing team.

The mother's time with the infant may be limited, because of other children, or because the family live a long way from the hospital, particularly if there are financial implications of travel. The earlier the concept of home oxygen therapy is discussed with the parents – at least as a possibility – the more easily they will be able to accept it. They need to accept that their infant is not 'normal' and that their expectations may have to change. An understanding of CLD or BPD will enable them to accept the problem and allow them to plan and look forward to the infant's discharge.

Some parents may need the opportunity to talk about their feelings and to express their anxieties and fears. A psychologist, as an independent member of the team, can play an important role during this period. A social worker may also be involved, particularly if there are financial or housing problems, which make it difficult to take a small, vulnerable infant home. Benefits are available to some families. Parents may find it helpful to speak to a family who have already taken an infant home on oxygen, or contact the BPD support group or the Nippers Group.

The involvement of so many people can lead to conflicting advice and, more than anything else, these parents need consistency. The named nurse/primary nurse, or person who is identified to prepare the family for discharge, needs to build up a good relationship of trust and communication.

DISCHARGE PREPARATION AND PLANNING MANAGEMENT AT HOME

An increasing number of very low-birthweight infants are surviving, but many remain oxygen-dependent because of CLD. It is increasingly popular and cost-effective to send these infants home (Hallam *et al.*, 1996). To ensure that they are safe and happy, and there are no major problems and trauma to the family, close supervision and management in the community are essential.

Before the infant is sent home on oxygen, there needs to be an identification of the teams who will provide follow-up care, support and supervision. The following options are currently available:

- A hospital-based neonatal community nurse may be available, whose responsibility is to follow up all of the pre-term infants being discharged, or a combined unit/community post, which may only follow up infants with ongoing problems.
- Paediatric community teams, with at least one member having neonatal experience, may become responsible for the infant with ongoing problems.
- Discharge into the responsibility of the GP and the health visitor is not uncommon but less frequent these days. Major problems may develop because of the lack of experience and understanding of CLD. The infant will require frequent visits back to the hospital for day or overnight monitoring and assessment.

Close liaison between the hospital paediatrician managing the infant and the community team is vital, and there should be some input from the NNU prior to discharge, to allow a problem-free transitional period from hospital to home.

Allowing a neonatal nurse to make an occasional visit when the unit is quiet does not provide a reliable and supportive community service to the family. This may be detrimental to all concerned, as some families become very dependent on unit staff.

The Royal College of Physicians (1992) gives very clear recommendations on how oxygen-dependent infants and children should be followed up (and by whom), and guidelines in respect of equipment, monitoring and education and liaison.

CRITERIA FOR DISCHARGE

- The infant is feeding, preferably by bottle or breast (supplementary NGT feeding will be considered).
- The infant is gaining weight.
- Nasal oxygen therapy is well tolerated.
- There are preferably two adults in the home, or a single parent who is well supported.
- Home conditions are adequate, with a telephone installed.
- The infant has no other medical complications.
- There is good support from the GP and health visitor.

Once the team has made a decision with the parents to send the infant home, a target date should be set. This gives the parents time to organise their home life and the hospital time to set up and implement a teaching programme for the parents.

The teaching programme includes:

- changing and securing the nasal catheter or prongs;
- use of oxygen equipment;
- resuscitation;
- assessment of breathing;
- clinical signs of hypoxia;
- administration of medications;
- maintaining a safe environment.

The use of oxygen in the home, and the safety factors regarding storage and changing cylinders, need to be discussed. Concentrators are the safer option, as there is no need to store a large supply of cylinders. Parents need to understand the risks with smoking and naked flames and should adopt a non-smoking policy in the home.

Full resuscitation in the event of collapse should be taught (Crawford and Marro, 1993). The correct use of an apnoea monitor is also explained and practised. Considerable time should be spent teaching the parents how to assess their infant's normal breathing pattern and how this may change if the infant were unwell, or if there was accidental disconnection of the oxygen supply. Parents may need to experience the way their infant looks and behaves when hypoxic.

Parents need to understand the risks of respiratory viruses, particularly during the first year. It is important to stress the need to avoid contact with small children with coughs and colds, and crowded environments, such as super-markets, schools, GP surgeries and 'well baby' clinics. This could be very difficult if there are siblings in the family but it is still important for parents to be aware of the risks. Home visits by the GP or health visitor may have to be arranged.

Prior to discharge, parents are asked to be resident in the unit for at least 24 hours, and to care for their infant in their own room, away from the unit. This gives them the opportunity to take full responsibility, while support is still close at hand. It also gives them an insight into their infant's needs and demands over a 24-hour period and an indication of how their lives are going to change. Alternatively, the parents could be offered the opportunity to take the infant out on escorted visits home for the morning or for the day on a couple of occasions, to get used to having the infant at home and to see whether any problems arise.

EQUIPMENT AND LIAISON

Advance planning allows time for the necessary arrangement and preparation of equipment and time for liaison with all those who are going to be concerned with the infant's management.

There are currently two options available for supplying oxygen in the community (both are prescribed by the GP):

- Oxygen cylinders with a standard bullnose head are supplied and delivered by the local chemist. A system for delivering a low flow (less than a litre) needs to be supplied by the hospital. For infants on a very low flow of oxygen (less than 100 cl), with the likelihood of stopping oxygen in a relatively short time, cylinders may be the most appropriate method of supply.
- For infants on long-term therapy, with higher requirements, an oxygen concentrator is the preferred choice of supply. This is an electrical machine, which plugs into the domestic electricity supply and takes in ambient air, separates oxygen from nitrogen and other gases and supplies oxygen-enriched gas to the infant, reaching a concentration of 96%. This is also available on prescription and is supplied by companies with contracts to regional health authorities. A low-flow meter needs to be ordered (as an extra item) when arranging for the fitting of a concentrator.

Cylinders can be arranged within a few days but it may take up to a week to have a concentrator supplied and fitted in the home. The best method needs to be discussed with the GP and parents, and the equipment must be organised in advance. A portable oxygen system is an essential equipment for the family, but is not available on the drug tariff and has to be supplied by the hospital. Holidays will need to be planned well in advance.

The source of the disposable items for these infants depends very much on different health authorities and on who is providing the community care. The infant's suitcase is usually well packed with at least a month's supply of disposables, but it must be clear where further supplies will come from.

A discharge summary is completed, with copies made available for the parents, GP and health visitor. Immunisations for these children are recommended and will have been kept up to date. Arrangements for follow up appointments are made according to local policy, commonly in a month's time.

Parents find the day of discharge a time of mixed emotions; it is a day they have anticipated (but never believed would happen) for a long time. There is excitement, mingled with apprehension and it is definitely not a good day to give any more information. Everything should be made ready 24 hours before, in order to make the day as smooth and trouble-free as possible. It is useful for the parents to have an information booklet, including all the information and teaching that has taken place, a checklist for equipment and a discharge care plan, with medications.

Good communication and liaison between the hospital and the community health team is essential for ongoing management. Infants on diuretics will require frequent urea and electrolyte level tests, which may be performed at home. Any infants who remain on oral or inhaled steroids will need to have periodic measurement of blood pressure. These investigations may be performed by the community nurse or by the GP.

An on-call service is available for most parents. Surprisingly, very few parents use it for urgent problems but it does give an extra sense of security, particularly in the first few weeks, while they are trying to gain confidence in the equipment and experience in care. Alternatively, the parents may have open access to the paediatric ward at their local hospital.

CONTINUING MANAGEMENT

The need to monitor the infant's SaO_2 applies at home, just as it does in hospital. While the infant is still small it is not difficult to monitor, through a sleep and feeding cycle. However, as infants get older and more active, monitoring can become more of a problem. During the day they will be far more stable and consistent with their saturations, and short monitoring periods are sufficient. Infants should be monitored overnight every few weeks, or if there is a change, up or down, with oxygen requirements, or if they are unwell. This is something that parents manage very well and, as the infants get older and have a more settled sleep pattern, the information recorded is very accurate.

Feeding can be a frustrating experience at home. Most infants improve when discharged but occasionally an infant may slow down and fail to complete feeds. This is especially common if they have a cold, with increased mucus and a cough. Antibiotics are often prescribed prophylactically depending on the GP.

Bronchodilator therapy is usually prescribed at the first sign of a wheeze, and this can make a significant improvement. Oxygen flow may be increased a little to ensure good oxygenation; these infants are very vulnerable (to episodes of hypoxia) when unwell because of increased respiratory effort and sensitive airways. Most hospitals have an open-door policy, and the infants can be admitted directly to the paediatric ward if necessary.

WEANING FROM OXYGEN

The point at which to reduce oxygen depends very much on the individual infant's stability. Full monitoring during weaning is crucial, so as not to compromise the infant. Once infants are maintaining saturations above 96%, in minimal oxygen, they will be monitored for a short period in air. If the SaO_2 does not drop below 94%, parents will be advised to disconnect the oxygen for an hour or two each day, while the infant is awake. Over a 2-week period, if saturations remain good, this period off oxygen will be increased, until the infant is off oxygen all day while awake. The infant will still need to be monitored, in air, during daytime sleeps. If they continue to maintain above 94%, oxygen will be stopped all day, awake and asleep.

It is important, at this point, to identify which infants have lower SaO_2 when asleep (Sekar and Duke, 1991). Before stopping oxygen at night, an overnight recording, in air, will be done, along with an echocardiogram, before a final decision is made. Infants with severe lung disease can have a significant fall in saturations when asleep, despite having a SaO_2 above 94%, in air, when awake, and will still require oxygen overnight. A very small number may still be on oxygen past 2 years of age and these children will continue to need visiting and support, but probably only on a fortnightly or monthly basis.

The infant will continue to be monitored for the first month after stopping oxygen and a repeat overnight recording will be done before discontinuing visits. The infant can then be handed over to the care of the health visitor.

CONCLUSION

Caring for these infants at home can be hard work for the parents and will put many demands on the family environment and relationships. It works well, provided that the parents are properly prepared before discharge and receive the support they need at home. Parents are the best people to care for their infants but they are expected to learn a significant amount in a short period. Success depends on good communication and trust during the preparation for discharge. If this is not present, difficulties will arise and parents may end up bitterly regretting the experience. This could have a harmful effect on their own relationship and on their relationship with their child, and result in diminished faith in the health services.

Changes in the National Health Service have emphasised the importance of community care and this is seen as the way forward. There will be more infants with additional and extraordinary needs going home. The nurses have a responsibility to ensure a safe and happy discharge, with appropriate management. Care in the community should enable these infants to grow and develop happily and safely.

REFERENCES

Bancalari, E. (2001) Changes in the pathogenesis and prevention of chronic lung disease of prematurity, *American Journal of Perinatology* **18**(1), 1–9

Bancalari, E. and del Moral, T. (2001) Bronchopulmonary dysplasia and surfactant, *Biology Neonate* **80**(5), 7–13

Crawford, D. (2000) Are we further forward or just re-mixing the message? *Paediatric Nurse* 12(8), 20–22

Crawford, D. and Marro, G. (1993) As easy as ABC, *Paediatric Nurse* 5(3), 12–13

Department of Health [DoH] (2000) *Reduce the Risk of Cot Death*, HMSO, London

Hallam, C., Rudbeck, B. and Bradley, M. (1996) Resource use and costs of caring for oxygen-dependent children; comparison of hospital and home care, *Journal of Neonatal Nurses* 2(2), 23–25

Mancini, A. and While, A. (2001) Discharge planning from a neonatal unit: an exploratory study of parents' views, *Journal of Neonatal Nursing* 7(2), 59–62

Manns, S. (2000) Life after SCBU: long-term effects on mothers at home with a child with bronchopulmonary dysplasia and on home oxygen, *Journal of Neonatal Nursing* 6(6), 193–6

Redman, C. (1993) Putting the family back in control, *Child Health* 1(3), 112–16

Rojas, M., Gonzar, A., Bancalari, E. *et al.* (1995) Changing trends in the epidemiology and pathogenesis of neonatal chronic lung disease, *Journal of Pediatrics* 126(4), 605–10

Royal College of Physicians (Chairperson M. Silverman) (1992) *Domiciliary Oxygen Therapy for Children: A Report of a Working Group of the Committee of Thoracic Medicine*, RCP, London

Sekar, K. and Duke, J. (1991) Sleep apnoea and hypoxaemia in recently weaned premature infants with and without BPD, *Paediatric Pulmonology* 10, 112–16

Turrill, S. (1999) Interpreting family-centred care within neonatal nursing, *Paediatric Nursing* 11(4), 22–24

Vandenburg, K. (1990) Nippling management of the sick neonate in the ITU; the disorganised feeder, *Neonatal Network* 9(1), 9–15

Yeh, T., McClenan, D., Ajayi, O. *et al.* (1989) Energy expenditure in the CLD infant, *Pediatrics* 114, 448–51

Zinman, R. *et al.* (1992) Oxygen saturations during sleep in patients with bronchopulmonary dysplasia, *Biology Neonate* 61, 69–75

APPENDIX I: USING THE EDINBURGH POST-NATAL DEPRESSION SCALE

The Edinburgh Post Natal Depression Scale (EPNDS) was designed to detect early signs of PND and to set out the procedures that should be followed on detection in order to safeguard the family. It was recommended that the screening be carried out by a member of the primary health care team, normally the health visitor, at about the time of the 6-week post-natal check. It consists of a number of questions (*see below*), which are then scored. High scores indicate the need for further assessment, help and support. The management on which to form the framework of care for a woman with PND will be based on the integrated expertise from the community, maternity and psychiatric services.

Unfortunately, the mother of a very sick infant in the NNU may not be at home receiving the care and support of the family health visitor and may be at greater risk of depression. The neonatal nurse needs to be familiar with the early signs of depression and, where possible, should facilitate access to a health visitor so that these women do not 'fall through the net'.

(The Edinburgh tool is replicated by kind permission of the CRAG.)

THE EDINBURGH POST-NATAL DEPRESSION SCALE (EPNDS)

The mother should complete the EPNDS at 6–8 weeks after the birth, around the time of the post-natal visit. She should complete it on her own, whether she is at home or at the clinic. The scale is simple to use. The 10 questions are as follows:

1 **I have been able to laugh and see the funny side of things:**
   a   As much as I always could
   b   Not quite so much now
   c   Definitely not so much now
   d   Not at all

2 **I have looked forward with enjoyment to things:**
   a   As much as I ever did
   b   Rather less than I used to
   c   Definitely less than I used to
   d   Hardly at all

3 **I have blamed myself unnecessarily when things went wrong:**
   a   Yes, most of the time
   b   Yes, some of the time
   c   Not very often
   d   No, never

4 **I have been anxious or worried for no good reason:**
   a   No, not at all
   b   Hardly ever
   c   Yes, sometimes
   d   Yes, very often

5 **I have felt scared or panicky for no very good reason:**
   a   Yes, quite a lot
   b   Yes, sometimes
   c   No, not much
   d   No, not at all

6 **Things have been getting on top of me:**
   a   Yes, most of the time. I haven't been able to cope at all
   b   Yes, sometimes I haven't been coping as well as usual
   c   No, most of the time I have coped quite well
   d   No, I have been coping as well as ever

7 **I have been so unhappy that I have had difficulty sleeping:**
   a   Yes, most of the time
   b   Yes, sometimes
   c   Not very often
   d   No, not at all

8 **I have felt sad and miserable:**
   a   Yes, most of the time
   b   Yes, quite often
   c   Not very often
   d   No, not at all

9 **I have been so unhappy that I have been crying:**
   a   Yes, most of the time
   b   Yes, quite often
   c   Only occasionally
   d   No, never

10 **The thought of harming myself has occurred to me:**
   a   Yes, quite often
   b   Sometimes
   c   Hardly ever
   d   Never

Mothers are asked to indicate which answers come closest to 'How you have felt in the past 7 days, not just how you feel today.'

Mothers who score above a threshold of 12/13 are likely to be suffering from a depressive illness of varying severity; nevertheless, the EPDS score should not override clinical judgement.

Appendix II: Methods of assessment of gestational age

Dubowitz and Dubowitz

The Dubowitz and Dubowitz (1970) method of assessing gestational age (Figure II.1) involves the scoring of neurological and external criteria within the first 5 days of birth. The total score is read against a graph (Figure II.2) to give a post-birth estimation of gestational age.

Some notes on techniques of assessment of neurological criteria

Posture

Observed with infant quiet and in supine position. Score 0: arms and legs extended; 1: beginning of flexion of hips and knees, arms extended; 2: stronger flexion of legs, arms extended; 3: arms slightly flexed, legs flexed and abducted; 4: full flexion of arms and legs.

Square window

The hand is flexed on the forearm between the thumb and index finger of the examiner. Enough pressure is applied to get as full a flexion as possible, and the angle between the hypothena eminence and the ventral aspect of the forearm is measured and graded according to diagram. (Care is taken not to rotate the infant's wrist while doing this manoeuvre.)

Ankle dorsiflexion

The foot is dorsiflexed on to the anterior aspect of the leg, with the examiner's thumb on the sole of the foot and other fingers behind the leg. Enough pressure is applied to get as full flexion as possible, and the angle between the dorsum of the foot and the anterior aspect of the leg is measured.

Arm recoil

With the infant in the supine position the forearms are first flexed for 5 seconds, then fully extended by pulling on the hands, and then released. The sign is fully positive if the arms return briskly to full flexion (Score 2). If the arms return to incomplete flexion or the response is sluggish it is graded as Score 1. If they remain extended or are only followed by random movements the score is 0.

Leg recoil

With the infant supine, the hips and knees are fully flexed for 5 seconds, then extended by traction on the feet, and released. A maximal response is one of full flexion of the hips and knees (Score 2). A partial flexion scores 1, and minimal or no movement scores 0.

Popliteal angle

With the infant supine and his pelvis flat on the examining couch, the thigh is held in the knee–chest position by the examiner's left index finger and thumb supporting the knee. The leg is then extended by gentle pressure from the examiner's right index finger behind the ankle and the popliteal angle is measured.

Heel-to-ear manoeuvre

With the baby supine, the baby's foot is drawn as near to the head as it will go without being forcing. The distance between the foot and the head is observed, as well as the degree of extension at the knee, and both are graded according to the diagram. The knee is left free and may draw down alongside the abdomen.

Scarf sign

With the baby supine, the examiner takes the infant's hand and tries to put it around the neck and as far posteriorly as possible around the opposite shoulder. The manoeuvre is assisted by lifting the elbow across the body. The examiner observes how far the elbow will go across and grades according to illustrations. Score 0: elbow reaches opposite axillary line; 1: elbow between midline and opposite axillary line; 2: elbow reaches midline; 3: elbow will not reach midline.

Head lag

With the baby lying supine, the hands (or the arms if a very small infant) are grasped and the infant is pulled slowly towards the sitting position. The position of the head in relation to the trunk is observed and graded accordingly. In a small infant the head may initially be supported by one hand. Score 0: complete lag; 1: partial head control; 2: able to maintain head in line with body; 3: brings head anterior to body.

Ventral suspension

The infant is suspended in the prone position, with the examiner's hand under the infant's chest (one hand in a small infant, two in a large infant). The degree of extension of the back and the amount of flexion of the arms and legs are observed. The relation of the head to the trunk is also noted. All observations are graded according to the diagrams.

If scores differ on the two sides, take the mean.

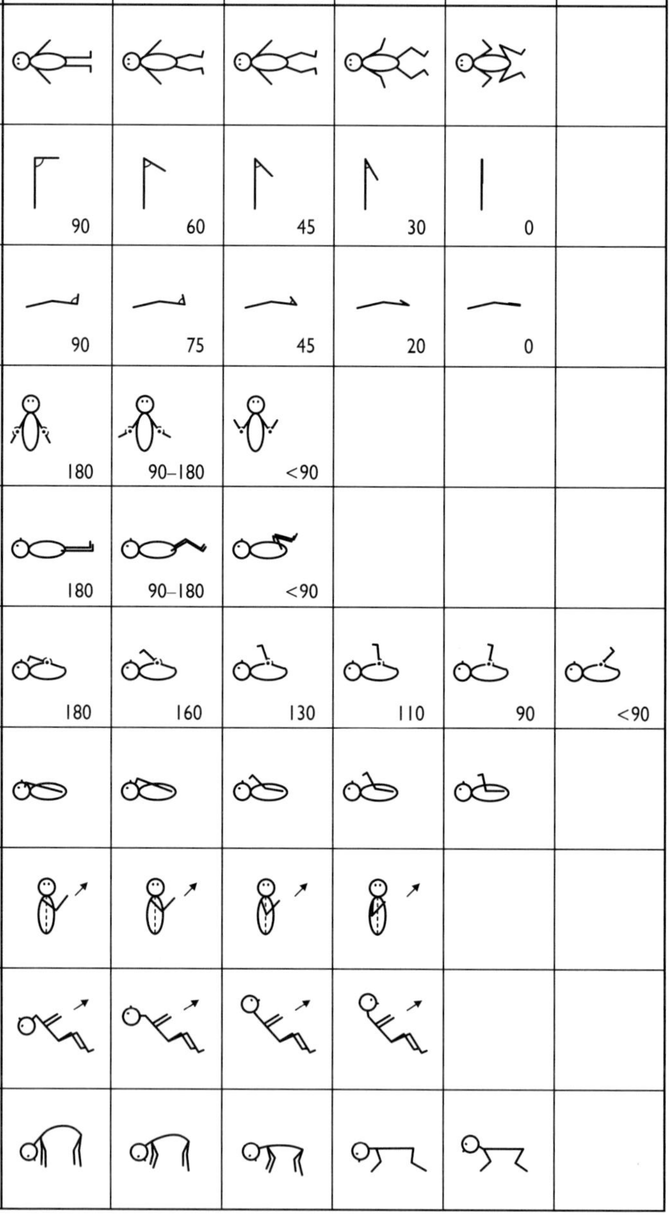

Neuroligical sign	Score					
	0	1	2	3	4	5
Posture						
Square window	90	60	45	30	0	
Ankle dorsiflexion	90	75	45	20	0	
Arm recoil	180	90–180	<90			
Leg recoil	180	90–180	<90			
Popliteal angle	180	160	130	110	90	<90
Heel to ear						
Scarf sign						
Head lag						
Ventral suspension						

Figure II.1 *Assessment of gestational age*

Reproduced from Dubowitz L.M.S, Dubowitz, V. and Goldberg, C. (1970) Clinical assessment of gestational age in the newborn infant, The Journal of Pediatrics July 77(1), 1–10, by kind permission of the authors and Journal of Pediatrics.

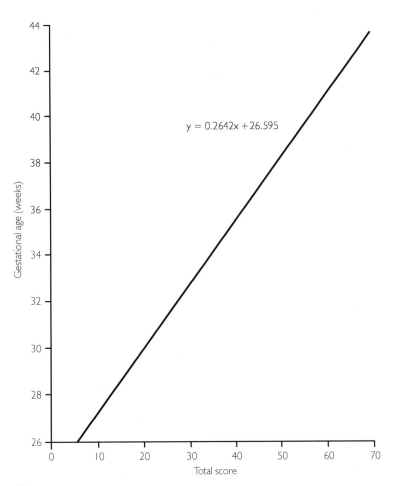

Figure II.2 *Post-birth estimation of gestational age (Dubowitz and Dubowitz, 1970)*

APPENDIX III: NORMAL VALUES

Table III.1   Neonatal electrolyte and urea ranges

	Pre-term	**Neonatal**
Sodium (Na) mmol/l	130–140	130–145
Potassium (K) mmol/l	4.5–7.0	4.0–6.0
Chloride (Cl) mmol/l	90–115	92–110
Calcium (Ca) mmol/l	1.9–2.8	2.0–2.9
Phosphate (PO_4) mmol/l	1.1–2.6	1.8–3.0
Magnesium (Mg) mmol/l	0.62–1.27	0.7–1.15
Glucose mmol/l	2.0–5.5	2.5–5.5
Creatinine μmol/l	50–120	55–150
Urea mmol/l	1.5–6.7	2.0–5.2

Table III.2   Blood gas values

	Pre-term	**Neonatal**
pH	7.3–7.4	
$PaCO_2$	4.6–6.0	kPa (35–45 mm Hg)
PaO_2	7.3–12	kPa (55–90 mm Hg)
Bicarbonate	18–25	μmol/l
Base excess	−2–2	μmol/l

APPENDIX IV: ABBREVIATIONS AND GLOSSARY OF KEY TERMS

ABO	Blood groups
ANNP	Advanced Neonatal Nurse Practitioner – a neonatal nurse who has undergone additional educational and skills training and practices an extended role
APIB	Assessment of Pre-term Infant Behaviour
APGAR	A scoring system used at birth to determine health status of the newborn infant
CAT scan	Computerised axial tomography – a non-invasive investigation, which gives details of altered anatomy or disease
CMV	Cytomegalovirus – a contagious and infectious virus, which can damage the infant
CNEP	Continuous negative pressure – a mode of support designed to encase the body in a sub-atmospheric pressure to facilitate more effective self-ventilation
CNS	Central nervous system – the brain and spinal cord
CO$_2$	Carbon dioxide
CPAP	Continuous positive airway pressure – a constant pressure designed to maintain the airways open
CPB	Cardio-pulmonary bypass – an intra-operative procedure, which maintains the circulation and can facilitate a bloodless cardiac field for the surgeon to work on
CSF	Cerebro-spinal fluid – the fluid that bathes the brain and spinal cord
CVVH	Continuous veno/venous haemofiltration – a method of eliminating toxins from the blood via a circuit
DSVNI	Distress Scale for Ventilated Newborn Infants
ECG	Electrocardiograph – tracings taken that monitor the electrical activity of the heart
ECMO	Extracorporeal membrane oxygenation – a means of oxygenating the infant. Blood is taken from the body and flows through a specialist circuit
ELBW	Extremely Low Birth Weight (below 1.000 gms)
ET	Endo-tracheal tube – artificial tube maintaining patency of the trachea
G$_6$PD	Glucose 6 phosphate dehydrogenase – an inherited condition affecting the infant's metabolism
GFR	Glomerular filtration rate
GI	Gastro-intestinal – the anatomical structures relating to the digestive system
HFV	High-frequency ventilation – a mode of ventilation designed to deliver breaths at a higher than physiological rate

IMV	Intermittent mandatory ventilation/volume – a mode of ventilation designed to deliver measured pressures or set volumes of gas
IBCS	Infant Body Coding System
IPPV	Intermittent Positive Pressure Ventilation – a mode of ventilation designed to rhythmically deliver inflation pressures to ventilate the lungs
IUGR	Intra-uterine growth retardation
IM	Intramuscular – directly into the muscle
IV	Intravenous – directly into the vein
LBW	Low Birth Weight (below 2.500 gms)
NBAS	Neonatal Behaviour Assessment Scale
NBW	Normal Birth Weight (2.500 gms or more)
Neonatal	The first 28 days of life
Newborn	The brief period following separation from the mother before 24 hours old
NFCS	Neonatal Facial Coding System
NNU	Neonatal unit – a speciaist unit caring for the sick infant
O_2	Oxygen
PD	Peritoneal dialysis – a method of eliminating toxins using the peritoneal membrane
PEEP	Positive end expiratory pressure – sustained residual pressure maintained at the end of a ventilated breath
Perinatal	The first 7 days of life
pH	Potential hydrogen – the amount of acidity/base in a substance
PIP	Positive inspiratory pressure – maximum pressure delivered through a ventilator circuit
PIPP	Premature Infant Pain Profile
PO_2	Partial pressure oxygen – pressure exerted by oxygen gas molecules
Post-term	Infants born in excess of 42 weeks gestation
Post-operative	Nursing actions that take place following surgery
Premature	Immature development of the infant
Pre-operative	Nursing activities and actions required before the infant has surgery
Pre-term	Infants born before 37 weeks completed gestation
PROM	Prolonged rupture of membranes – when the infant's amniotic sac is leaking or ruptured and is not followed by the infant's birth within 24 hours
Rh	Rhesus antibodies on the red blood cell
SaO_2	Saturations of oxygen – the amount of oxygen present in the blood circulation
SG	Specific gravity – a measure of solutes suspended in fluid medium

SGA	Small gestational age
TcPO$_2$	Transcutaneous oxygen
TDWL	Transdermal water loss – fluid loss through the infant's skin
Term	Infants born between 37 and 42 completed weeks of gestation
TORCH	Toxoplasmosis others (e.g. syphilis) rubella cytomegalovirus, Herpes simplex/hepatitis/HIV
TPN	Transparenteral nutrition – feeding an infant directly into the circulation
UAC	Umbilical venous catheter – a catheter passed into the umbilical vein, to access the circulation
Utero-placental	The interface between the uterus and the placenta
UVC	Umbilical venous catheter – a catheter passed into the umbilical vein, to access the circulation
VLBW	Very Low Birth Weight (below 1.500 gms)

INDEX

Abdominal
  distension 95, 151, 162, 164
  measurement 153
  tenderness 95
Abdominal wall defect 156
Abortion 23, 45
Abuse 23, 35, 43
  alcohol 43, 45, 52
  domestic 43
  drugs 43
  NAI 53
  neglect 45
  prevention 43, 339, 344
  sexual 44, 52
Accountability 10, 15, 17
Acid alcohol fast bacilli 291
Acid base balance 208
Acidosis 112, 119, 142, 206, 207, 216, 220,
  232
  metabolic 84, 151, 155
Acrocyanosis 175
Activated clotting time 193
Acute pain 37, 247, 250
Acute tubular necrosis 210
Acyclovir 296
Adenosine 198
Adolescent mother 36, 43, 46, 52
Adrenaline 91, 197
Adrenogenital syndrome 212
Advanced Neonatal Nurse Practitioner 7, 273
Advocacy 14, 26, 32, 36, 40, 245
Aerobic respiration 142
Affected limb,withdrawal of 249
AGA, see Gestational age, appropriate size for
Airborne transfer 283
Airway resistance 97, 124, 331
Albumin 90, 210, 219, 318
Alder Hey Children's Hospital 16
Aldosterone 206
Alfentanyl 262
Alkalosis 143, 215
Allitt Report 35
Altitude complications 283
Alveolar cells 118, 331
Aminoglycoside 213, 217, 317
Amniotic fluid and sampling 94, 105, 111, 119
Amphotericin 213, 321
Anaemia 98, 105, 153, 190, 214
Analgesia 37, 152, 157, 160, 165, 192, 245
Anastomosis 154, 162
Anencephaly 227, 235, 239
Angiography 190

Anomalous venous drainage 189
Antalgic position 251
Antenatal care 23, 214
Antenatal scan 148, 156, 159, 161, 200
Antepartum haemorrhage 111
Anti D 111
Antibacterial agent 158
Antibiotic 192
  administration 287
  broad spectrum 152, 157, 165, 237
  prophylactic 151, 159, 162, 185, 190, 287
Anticoagulation 193
Anticonvulsant therapy 238
Antidiuretic hormone 88, 93, 232
Anuria 214
Aortic coarctation 184, 189
Aortic valve stenosis 185
Aortic valvotomy 185
APGAR system 73, 75, 209, 231
Apnoea 73, 95, 151, 166, 247, 327
  monitor 334
  terminal 232
Appendectomy 165
Arnold-Chiari malformation 236
Arrhythmia 110, 191, 207, 232, 321
Arterial calcification 212
Arterial catheter 134, 294
Arterial line 127, 134, 154, 182
Ascites 114
Aseptic technique 152, 158
Asphyxia 90, 93, 98, 150, 231, 233
  birth 136, 212, 231
  effects of 232
  neonatal 73
Aspirate
  bile stained 153
  gastric 163
  intermittent 156
Aspiration pneumonia 121
Assessment
  eyes 82
  fluid balance 88
  genitalia 82
  gestational age 81
  serum electrolytes 87
  tools 83
Assessment of Pre-term Infant Behaviour 256
Asystole 194
Atelectasis 98, 119, 136, 331
Atresia 94, 156, 160
Atrial septal defect (ASD) 185
Atropine 197

Attention deficits 59
Attention span 246
Auto Immune Deficiency Syndrome (AIDS) 291
Autonomy 5, 18, 24, 39, 40

Bacteraemia, symptomatic 210
Bacteria, proliferation 151
Bacterial flora 315
Ballard 83
Balloon septotomy 190
Barotrauma 129, 329
Bartters syndrome 215
Beckwith Wiedmann Syndrome 159
Beneficence 18, 21, 24
Benzodiazepine 233
Beta haemolytic streptococci 289, 294
Bicarbonate 78, 219
   buffering system 142, 208
   dialysis 220
   ions 142, 208
Bile salts 94
Biliary atresia 114
Biliary cirrhosis 114
Biliary function 315
Bilirubin 105, 318
Bilirubinometry, transcutaneous 106
Birth trauma 247
Birthweight
   extremely low 79
   low 79
   normal 79
   very low 79, 92
Bladder
   distended 209
   manual expression 140, 236
   palpation of 209
   percussion of 209
Blalock-Hanlon procedure 188
Blood
   coagulation 92
   contaminated culture 294
   count 289
   cross-matching 154
   culture 107, 238, 288, 293
   donor 109
   gas 110, 129, 142, 289
   glucose 89, 128, 153, 159, 191, 218
   group 107
   replacement 110
   specimens 153
   tests 107
   transfusion 150, 154, 206
Blood-brain barrier 105
Blood glucose 89
Blood pressure 110, 153, 157, 183
   fluctuation 230, 231

four limb 183
   measurement of 182
Blood vessels, rupture of 230
Body movement 249
Bombesin 95
Bonding 63
Bone mineralisation 92, 93
Boric acid container 287, 295
Bowel
   deflated 138, 156
   dilated 151
   evacuate 140
   exposed 156
   hernia 138, 158
   inactive 140, 151
   ischaemic 156, 165
   loops 151
   obstruction 151
   perforation 156
   problems 236
   resection 155
   surgery 154, 315
   thickened 151
Bradycardia 95, 132, 153, 166, 181, 250
Brain abscess 190
Brain injury 232
Brain stem 227
Breast-feeding 63, 108, 304
   advantages 306
   anxieties 114, 306
   hepatitis B 298
   HIV 297
   pumps 306
Breast milk 286, 306
   composition 95, 307
   expressed 151, 177, 306
   fortifier 307
   good practice 307
   immunoglobins 286
   infection risk 307
   protective factors 95
   storage 307
   unfortified 93
Breast milk jaundice 113
Breast pumps 126
Breast tissue 82
British Heart Foundation 176
British Hypertensive Society 215
Bronchial mucosa 132
Bronchiolitis 297
Bronchodilator 339
Bronchodysplasia 211
Bronchopulmonary dysplasia 129, 205, 297, 326, 329
Bronze Infant Syndrome 108
Brow contraction 248
Brown fat 83

Bulging fontanelle 237
Burden of treatment 20, 135, 204, 332

Caesarean section 72, 129, 286
Caffeine 166, 198, 327
Calciferol 93, 304
Calcitonin 92
Calcium 207, 304
  burns 208
  metabolism 92, 207
  regulation 92, 207
  resonium enema 207
Calcium carbonate 208, 217
Calcium chloride 208
Calcium gluconate 207
Calorie intake 86, 302, 335
Cancer 247
Candida albicans 290
Capillary return 95, 158
Captopril 215
Carbonic acid 142, 208
Cardiac catheterisation 175, 179
Cardiac decompensation 212
Cardiac enzymes 178
Cardiac failure 176, 232, 316
Cardiac lesions during transfer 282
Cardio-pulmonary bypass 185, 187, 193
Cardiorator 180
Cardiovascular disease 319
Cardioversion 182
Cataract 295
Catecholamine 97, 212
Catheter
  blocked 221
  peritoneal 218
  suction 163
  Tenckhoff 218
  umbilical 150, 152
  urinary 140, 153
Centile chart 311
Central line 91
  tip specimen 287
Central nervous system 206, 296, 318
Central venous pressure 158
Cerebral blood flow 231, 250
Cerebral calcification 295
Cerebral cortex 228, 245
Cerebral hemispheres 228
Cerebral infarction 212
Cerebral oedema 220, 232, 238
Cerebral oxygenation 132
Cerebral palsy 59, 239
Cerebral vascular accident 190
Cerebrospinal fluid 228, 230, 238, 293
Chemical peritonitis 156
Chest drain 141, 163, 196
Chest physiotherapy 133, 250

Child protection 47, 53, 54, 130
Chlamydia trachomatis 288, 292
Chlamydial conjunctivitis 293
Chlamydial pneumonia 293
Choanal atresia 76, 122
Cholangiogram 107
Chorionic villus sampling (CVS) 111
Chromosomal abnormality 80, 81, 159
Chronic liver failure 114
Chronic lung disease 119, 122, 304, 329
Chronic pain 247, 251
Chvostek's sign 208
Chylothorax 195, 310
Circadian rhythm 258
Circulation, poor 151, 158
Circumcision 250, 261
Cirrhosis 114, 298
Civil law 15
Clinical audits 33
Clinical governance 33
Clonazepam 233
Clostridium 294
Coagulase negative staph 292
Coarctation 211, 216
Code of Professional Conduct (UKCC) 13,
  21, 27
Cognitive skills 60
Cold stress 84, 90
Colic 247
Coliform bacilli 289, 294
Collagen 99
Colostomy 155, 165
Colostrum 95, 135, 286
Communication skills 63
Communication with parents 277
Community care 106, 342, 344
Computerised axial tomography 239
Confidential information 42
Congenital heart defect 172, 174, 294, 297
Congenital heart disease 171, 174
Congenital infection 81, 213, 297
Congenital nephrotic syndrome 215
Congenital pneumonia 121
Congenital syphilis 292
Congenital toxoplasmosis 295
Congestive cardiac failure 175, 189
Conjoined twins 24, 40
Conjugated bilirubin 105
Conjunctivitis 290, 293
Consent 38, 190
  informed 190
  legal 39
  obtaining 154
  parental 38
  proxy 39
  refused 40
  surgical 157

Consequentialist theory 18
Constipation 140
Continuous arteriovenous haemofiltration 218
Continuous positive airway pressure 122, 123, 153
Continuous veno/venous haemofiltration 218
Convulsions 185, 233, 282
Coombs test 107
Coping ability 239
Coping skills 15
Cor pulmonale 331
Corneal abrasion 108
Cortical necrosis 232
Cortical-medullary necrosis 213
Counselling, genetic 159
Counselling of parents 156, 192
Creatinine 209, 210, 219
Credible voice 15
Crigler-Najjar Syndrome 112
Cry, types of 247, 250
Cryptorchidism 296
Cultural factors 67
Curare 139
Cushing's disease 212
Cyanosis 161, 175, 188
Cystic fibrosis 114
Cystic kidney disease 205
Cystic lesions 114, 228
Cytomegalovirus 107, 112, 215, 296, 297

Deafness 297
Dehydration 93, 206, 212, 220, 294
Development 81
  brain 227, 303
  critical period 226
  gastro-intestinal 94, 148, 158, 164
  lung 97, 117, 121, 331
  muscle and fat 81
  psychomotor 303
  skin 99
Developmental
  milestones 58, 238
  needs 58
  problems 59, 238, 337
  process 58
  progress 60, 62
Dexamethasone 326
Diabetes mellitus 296
Diabetic mothers 89
Dialysis 204, 216, 233
Diamorphine 130, 152, 262
Diaphragmatic fatigue 120
Diaphragmatic hernia 97, 122, 164
  antenatal diagnosis 141
  Bochdalek type 137
  congenital 137
  Morgagni type 137

surgical repair 140
transfer 282
Diaphragmatic paralysis 195
Diarrhoea 108, 206
Diazepam 233, 318
Dietary supplementation 215
Digestive enzymes 94
Digoxin 177, 185, 198, 320
Discharge
  early 106
  preparation 34
Discrimination 35, 36
Distress Scale for Ventilated Newborn Infants 256
Diuresis 86, 93
Diuretic 112, 207
Dobutamine 199
Documentation 51, 253, 267
  specimen 288
Domperidone 167, 337
Dopamine 140, 198, 232, 319, 320
Doppler 81
Down's syndrome 171, 238
Drash syndrome 215
Drug
  absorption 314
  administration 320, 322
  adverse reaction 319
  delivery via syringe pump 320
  distribution 316
  elimination and excretion 319
  fat soluble 317
  incompatibility 321
  light sensitive 322
  localised concentration 321
  metabolism 315, 318
  nephrotoxic 319
  plasma level 319
  pooling 316
  water soluble 317
  withdrawal 45
Drug-induced respiratory depression 122
Dubowitz 83
Ductus arteriosus 72
Ductus venosus 172
Duodenal atresia 94
Duodenal obstruction 165
Dysplasia 213
Dysplastic kidney disorder 214
Dyspnoea 221

E. coli 286, 289, 293
Ear infection 131
Ears 82
Echocardiogram 162, 212, 334
Eclamptic fit 72
Elastin fibres 99

Electro-cardiograph 175, 179
Electrolyte balance 152, 154, 164, 204, 294
Embolus formation 134
Embryogenesis
　cardiovascular 171
　central nervous system 227, 229
　gastro-intestinal 94, 149
　pulmonary 96, 117
　renal 204
　skeletal-muscular 81
Embryological development 148
Emergency Protection Order 51
EMLA cream 262
Emotional care 65
Emotional sweating 250
Emphysema 119, 331
ENB 405 33
Encephalocele 235
End of life 14
Endocarditis 185, 189
Endocrine system, changes in 250
Endotracheal intubation 107, 129, 181, 230,
　248, 287, 336
Enteral
　drugs 151
　feeding 123, 135, 152, 217
Enterococcus faecalis 289
Enterohepatic circulation 105
Epidural 262
Erythroblastosis foetalis 111
Erythrocytes 90
Erythromycin 292
Essential minerals 304
Essential nutrients 303
Ethical dilemmas 16, 135, 222, 234
Ethical grid 18
Ethical issues 6, 13, 238
Ethics 13
　decision-making 17
　implications for practice 15
　of research 15
　principles 18
European Convention on Human Rights 33
Euthanasia 23, 34
Evidence-based practice 8, 14, 23, 38, 76, 132
Excessive light/noise 66
Exchange transfusion 107, 294
Excitatory amino acids 234
Exomphalos 156
Expiratory coughs 247
Exploitation. 35
Extra-corporeal membrane oxygenation 3,
　125, 193
Extreme pain 247, 251
Extreme prematurity 59
Extremely low birthweight 59, 79
Eye contact 62

Eyes 82
Eye-squeeze 248

Fabricated illness by proxy 44
Facial expression 62, 248
Facial palsy 212
Faecal streptococci 289
Failure to thrive 45, 184, 214, 215
Fallot's tetralogy 175, 187, 189
Family-centred care 7, 26, 32, 41, 58, 60, 67,
　136, 138, 177, 192, 236
Feeding
　additives 166, 335
　bolus 166, 305
　breast milk 306
　by mouth 305
　by tube 123, 167, 305, 337
　cardiac infant 177
　complications 95, 231
　continuous 166, 305
　cup 306
　difficulties 130, 336
　early 150
　effort 335
　enteral 94, 301, 304
　formula 308
　gastrostomy 305
　growth-restricted 96
　gut priming 95
　in TOF 161
　introduction 94
　low birthweight formula 308
　oral 335
　parenteral 95, 151, 152, 154, 157, 159,
　　160, 165, 305
　policy 96, 306
　regrade 153, 165
　safety 305
　specialist formula 308
　term formula milk 93
　thickeners 166
　transpyloric 166
Fentanyl 262, 318
Fibrin 221
Filtration device 321
Finite resources 15
First smile 63
Fistula 161, 162
Floppy infant 238
Flucloxacillin 292
Fluid
　balance 88, 109, 128, 152, 154, 158, 191,
　　216, 301
　challenge 209, 216
　depletion 216
　intra/extracellular 86, 318
　loss 156, 159

overload 152, 206, 216, 218, 219, 232
  peritoneal 219
  restriction 216
  retention 210, 214
  shift 87
  status 212, 216
Flying squad (*see* transfer) 139
Foetal
  activity 81
  breathing 96, 97, 120
  circulation 72, 172
  distress 72
  gas exchange 121, 172
  haemoglobin 121, 143
  heart sounds 81
  hypoxia 94, 119, 121, 172
  lungs 96, 117, 118, 172
  pain 37, 245
  Rh disease 98
  rights 37
  ultrasound 209
  welfare 51
Foetal alcohol syndrome 45, 234
Folic acid 217, 235
Fontanelle, bulging 237
Foramen ovale 72, 172, 174
Formula milk 151, 300, 335
Frusemide 93, 199, 232, 319
Fungal peritonitis 221
Futile treatment 21, 23, 135, 189

G-6PD 107, 111, 112
Galactosaemia 107, 112
Gas exchange 118, 176, 270
  impaired 136
  physiology 124
Gastric acid 166, 314, 315
Gastric aspiration 107, 153
Gastroenteritis 286, 294
Gastro-intestinal abnormality 150, 329
Gastro-intestinal haemorrhage 326
Gastro-intestinal motility 167, 315
Gastro-oesophageal reflux 165, 301, 339
Gastroschisis 155, 281
Gastrostomy 162, 305
Genetic counselling 238
Genetic engineering 222
Genital herpes 296
Genitalia 82
Gentamicin 152, 287, 317
Geriatric neonate 329
Gestational age 23, 96, 205
  appropriate size for 79
  assessment of 79, 81
  small for 79
Gilbert's syndrome 112
Glaucoma 247

Glenn procedure 188
Glomerular filtration rate 205
Glomerulonephritis 211, 289
Glomerulus 205, 208
Glucagon 89
Glucocortocoid steroid 326
Glucogenesis 90
Gluconate 208
Gluconeogenesis 90
Glucose and insulin infusion 207
Glucose concentration 220
Glucose dialysate 221
Glucuronic acid 105
Glucuronidase 105
Glucuronyl transferase 105
Glyceryl trinitrate 320
Glycogen 84, 89
Glycosuria 92
Gonococcus 290
Gonorrhoea 290
Goodness or rightness 19
Gram negative infection 286
Gram stain 288
Griffiths Report 38
Growth
  intra-uterine 300, 311
  measurment of 311
  post-natal 311
  restriction 80, 90
Gustave-Roussy Child Pain Scale 256
Gut priming 95, 135, 305

Haem oxygenase inhibition 108
Haematuria 210, 213
Haemolysin 289
Haemolysis 105, 206
Haemophilus influenzae 291
Haemopoiesis 105
Haemorrhage 213
  cerebellar 229, 230
  intracranial 229, 234
  intraventricular 228
  periventricular 229
  subarachnoid 229
  subdural 229, 230
Hair 83
Handling, excessive 59, 63, 232
Head circumference 81
Headbox 122, 127, 333
Health budget 15
Health Economics Group 239
Health policy, weaning 310
Hearing 62
  impairment/loss 66, 106
Heart surgery 245
Heparin 219
Heparinised saline 134, 153

Hepatic enzyme 318
Hepatitis 107, 114, 295, 298
Hepatocellular carcinoma 298
Hepatomegaly 176, 296
Hernia 221
Herpes 107, 112
Herpes simplex virus (HSV) 296
Hexachlorophene 316
Holistic care 37
Home discharge 58, 62, 306, 308
Homeostasis 83, 89, 142, 204
Human albumin 140, 232, 281
Human immunodeficiency virus 45, 215, 297
Human Rights Act 32
Humidity
   during transfer 276
   in the incubator 123, 217
   requirement 86, 132, 157, 334
   risks of 292
Hunger 246
Hyaline membrane disease (*see also* RDS) 329
Hydrocephalus 234, 235, 236, 295
Hydrocortisone, topical 316
Hydrogen ion concentration 142, 208
Hydronephrosis 210, 211
Hydrops foetalis 292
Hygiene regulations 237
Hyperaldosteronism 215
Hyperbilirubinaemia 106
Hypercalcaemia 93, 94, 208
Hyperglycaemia 87, 91, 92, 153, 221
Hyperinflation 132, 330
Hyperkalaemia 110, 206, 210, 219
Hypernatraemia 206, 215
Hyperoxia 178, 230
Hyperoxygenation 132
Hyperparathyroidism 93, 208
Hypertension 134, 206, 211, 214, 216, 218
Hyperventilation 132, 139, 250
Hypervolaemia 206
Hypoalbuminaemia 207, 215, 220
Hypoaldosteronism 206, 212
Hypocalcaemia 81, 92, 110, 208, 234
Hypochloraemia 215
Hypoglycaemia 81, 84, 89, 135, 153, 159, 234
Hypokalaemia 135, 207, 215, 221
Hyponatraemia 87, 88, 135, 206, 210, 234
Hypoparathyroidism 207, 208
Hypoperfusion 212
Hypopituitarism 114
Hypoplasia 137, 205, 211, 213
Hypoplastic abnormal aorta 211
Hypoplastic heart 175, 189
Hypoplastic lungs 122, 139
Hypotension 140, 150, 158, 232, 316, 321
Hypothalamus 83, 227

Hypothermia 81, 119, 194
   induced 193
   selective 232
Hypothyroidism 93, 114, 215
Hypotonia 83, 93, 238
Hypovolaemia 164, 205, 216
Hypoxaemia 319, 331
Hypoxia 72, 84, 94, 97, 150, 188, 226, 230, 231, 233, 319, 334
Hypoxic ischaemic encephalopathy 233

Iatrogenic renal disorders 222
Ileostomy 88, 155
Ileus 206
Immune system 286
Immunity
   complement 96
   lymphocytes 96
   lysomes 96
   macrophages 96
Immunoglobulin 96, 237, 286, 298
Inappropriate stimulation 58
Incubator 85, 123, 135, 152
   transport 275
Indomethacin 186, 199, 215, 217, 231, 319, 327
Infant Body Coding System 249, 256, 354
Infant massage 65
Infection 234, 285
   ascending 237
   control 62, 67, 285, 297
   desending 131
   Gram-negative 286
   immunity against 286, 342
   in humidity 292
   intra-uterine 237
   necrotising enterocolitis 151
   nosocomial 285
   perinatal 292, 297
   prevention 156, 178, 237
   risk 157, 285
   screen 107, 285
   signs of 92, 152
   urinary tract 210, 295
Infusion bag 321
Inotropes 165, 270
Insensible loss 82, 87, 159, 302
Inspissated bile 114
Insulin 90, 320, 321
Intensive care, cost of 24
Inter-atrial septal defect 188
Intercostal drain 141
Intermittent mandatory volume 122
Intermittent positive pressure ventilation 122, 196
Interstitial oedema 87
Intestinal ischaemia 294

Intolerable life   23
Intra-uterine growth retardation   72, 292
Intra-uterine transfusion   111
Intracerebral fluid distribution   206
Intracranial haemorrhage   212, 234
Intracranial pressure   132, 236, 250
Intractable pain   262
Intramural gas   151
Intrapleural tension   141
Intra-uterine growth restriction   80
Intravascular coagulation   213
Intravenous dextrose   206
Intravenous feeding   135
Intravenous tubing   320
Intraventricular haemorrhage   181, 228, 327
Intubation
   cold   76, 130
   disadvantages   130
   emergency   76, 138
   nasal   130
   oral   76, 130
   prior to transfer   270
   rapid sequence induction   130
   risk   162
Invasive procedures   19, 285
IQ, lower   81
Iron   286, 304
Ischaemia   213, 228, 232, 234
IUGR   see Intra-uterine growth restriction
IV push   321

Jaundice   104, 297
   breast milk   113
   early   106
   greenish   106
   haemolytic   111
   hepatocellular   111
   obstructive   111, 114
   persistent   210
   profound   106
   prolonged   106
   reoccuring   106

Kangaroo care   65, 306, 338
Karyotyping   159
Kernicterus   105, 234, 318
Kidney function   87, 217
Korotkoff sound   216
Kramer's rule   104

Lactase   94
Lactation   126, 307
Lactoferrin   96, 286
Lactose   94
Ladds bands   165
Laerdal face masks   133
Lancefield groups   289

Language delay   59
Language skills   63
Lanugo   82
Laparotomy   154, 165
Latching on   96, 306
Latex agglutination test   293
LBW   See Birthweight, low
Learning difficulties   59
Left ventricular failure   176
Lethargy   215
Life-and-death decisions   17
Ligamentous arteriosus   174
Ligamentum teres   174
Lignocaine   199, 220, 262
Limbs, abnormal positions of   251
Lipolysis   89
Liposomal amphotericin   321
Listeria monocytogenes   290
Litigation   6, 22, 231, 272, 278
Liver, foetal   105
Long chain polyunsaturates   303
Low birthweight   46, 204, 205
Low birthweight formula   308, 335
Low flow oxygen meter   334
Lumbar puncture   107, 230, 237, 293
Lung development   98, 117, 331
Lymphocytes   96

Macropapular rash   292
Macrophages   96
Magnesium   92, 304
Magnesium sulphate   136
Magnetic resonance scan   239
Malabsorption   310
Malrotation   164
Management
   of NEC   152
   of post-operative bleeding   195
   of reflux   163, 166
   of Repogle tube   162
   of shock   164
   of transfer   282
   of workload   138
Mannitol   232
Massage   337
Maternal diabetes   129, 150
Maternal hypertension   98
Maternal smoking   80
Maternal substance abuse   80, 81
Maternal toxaemia   98
Measurement of head circumference   81, 238
Mechanical lancets   261
Meconium   113
   aspiration   72, 121
   inhalation   136
   passing   151

plugs 136
  staining 136
Medulla oblongata 227
Meningeal irritation 234
Meninges 234, 237
Meningitis 234, 237, 247, 289, 293
Meningococci 286
Meningoencephalitis 296
Menstrual period, last 81
Mental health problems 44, 45
Mesenteric ischaemia, see also NEC 94
Metabolic acidosis 84, 209, 219
Metabolic disturbance 234
Metabolic rate 87
Metabolism 304
  anaerobic 84
  disorders 89
Methicillin-resistant *staphylococcus* 292
Methylxanthine 327
Microbiology request form 288
Microcephaly 296
Micturating cystography 210
Milestones, delayed 238
Milk aspiration 306
Minimal handling 152, 160, 182, 259
Model
  decision-making 40
  ethical 18
  gentle human touch 64
  management 5
  organisational 5
  play 61
Monitors, disadvantages 127
Moral philosophy 16
Moro reflex 249
Morphine 197, 262, 318
Motor co-ordination 59.
Multi-agency working 31, 34, 47, 50, 51, 53
Multicultural society 3, 16, 36, 67
Multicystic dysplasia 210
Multicystic dysplastic kidney disease 214
Multidisciplinary team 3, 50, 54, 67, 130,
    133, 148, 236, 238, 273, 285, 300, 312
  medical 17, 78
  nursery nurse 34, 139
  paramedical staff 17
  Social Services 34, 340
Multiple birth 72
Multiple pregnancy 23, 80
Muscle relaxant 130, 139, 140, 162
Muscle tone 63
Muscular dystrophy 238
Music, therapeutic power of 259
Mycobacterium tuberculosis 291
Myelomeningocele 227, 236
Myocarditis 295
Myositis 295

Narcotic analgesia 262
Narcotic, withdrawal 234
Nasogastric
  aspirate 95, 151, 159
  feeding 63, 123, 128, 305, 337
  tube 152, 166, 177
Nasojejunal feeding 167, 305
Nasolabial furrow 248
Necrosis 134, 232
Necrotic bowel 154
Necrotising enterocolitis 94, 110, 135, 150,
    160, 205, 233, 247, 289, 294, 305, 306,
    322, 327
  transfer 282
Neglect 35, 45
Neisseria gonorrhoeae 287, 290
Neonatal Behavioural Assessment Scale 256,
    354
Neonatal Facial Coding System 248, 256, 354
Neonatal Infant Pain Score (NIPS) 253
Neonatal protection 31, 33, 50
Neonatal services 25
Nephrectomy 215
Nephrocalcinosis 213, 326
Nephrostomy 211
Nephrotic syndrome 206, 213
Nephrotoxic drugs 213
Neural tube 235
Neurogenic bladder 213
Neurological assessment 195
Neurological development 245
Neurological injury 90
Neuromuscular blockers 317
Neuropathology 228, 239
Neurotoxins 234
NHS policy 4, 7, 21, 27, 31, 43
  Working Together to Safeguard Children 47
Nipple confusion 306
Nitric oxide 3, 125, 136, 137, 195, 267, 276
Nitrogen washout 175, 178
Non-maleficence 18, 19, 21, 24
Nosocomial infection 285
Nurse education 8, 34, 273
Nurse induction 35
Nurse prescribing 8
Nurse recruitment 10, 35
Nurse retention 10
Nurse stereotypes 10
Nurse supervision 35
Nursery nurse 8, 34, 139
Nursing contracts 8
Nursing rights 27
Nursing specialist 7, 33, 132
Nutrition programme (*see also* Nutritional
    requirement) 217
Nutritional
  deficiency 304

reserves 300
support 215
Nutritional management 301
Nutritional requirement 301
  energy 302
  fat 303
  minerals 304
  pre-term 304
  protien 302
  vitamins 303
  water 301
Nutritional reserves 135
Nystatin drops 290

Observation
  during transfer 276
  neurological 238
  respiratory 127
Obstructive lesions 183
Obstructive nephropathy 217
Obstructive uropathy 211˙
Oedema 87, 99, 210, 215, 219, 317
  cerebral 220
  prevention of 177
  pulmonary 215
Oesophageal atresia 161, 281
Oesophageal peristalsis 94
Oligohydraminos 209
Oliguria 209, 213, 219
Omentum 220, 221
Omphalitis 292, 294
Omphocele 158
Ophthalmia neonatorum 290
Opisthotonos 237
Optimum development 60
Oral candidiasis 290
Oral stimulation 63
Organ donation 16, 194, 200, 239
Organ retention 16
Oricular acupuncture 262
Oropharyngeal suction 140
Oropharynx 140
Orthodontic problems 130, 336
Orthopnoea, prevention of 177
Osmotic forces 87, 218, 219
Osteomyelitis 292
Overhead heater 127, 206, 217
Oxygen 76, 122, 335
  analyzer 122
  concentration 122
  concentrator 341, 342
  dependency 329, 339
  home therapy 329, 331
  humidity 123, 334
  in the home 341
  low flow meter 334
  portable system 342

requirements 95, 121
safety 143
saturation 66, 143, 216, 250, 334
toxicity 143, 329
weaning off 343
Oxytocin 113

Pacemaker 194
Pain (see also Chapter 12) 22
  assessment tools 37, 256
  avoidance 322
  control 37
  cry 247
  expression 248
  intractable 262
  management 37, 263
  pathway 245
  protocol 263
  responses to 251
Painful stimulus, response to 248
Pancreatic lipase 94
Pancuronium 317, 319
Paracetamol 262, 319
Paraldehyde 233, 320
Paralysed infant 140
Parathyroid hormone 92
Parent information 41, 135, 154, 190
Parental
  adjustment 149
  anxiety 154, 192
  considerations during transfer 272
  orientation 192
  responsibility 51
  skills 45
  support 138, 157, 164, 190, 192
Parenteral nutrition 135, 152, 305
Parenting 61
Patent ductus arteriosus 150, 172, 174, 186,
    189, 205, 296, 327, 330
Pathogens, opportunistic 131
Patient's advocate 245
Peaked T waves 207
Penicillin 292, 315, 317
Perceptual abilities 63
Perforation 151
Perinatal asphyxia 88, 98, 129, 209, 212
Peritoneal dialysis 218
Peritonitis 221
Periventricular leucomalacia 228, 234
Periventricular/intraventricular haemorrhage
    229
Persistent truncus arteriosus 188
Petechiae 297
Phenobarbitone 108, 233, 315
Phenol 316
Phenytoin 233, 318, 320, 322
Philosophies of play 59

Phlebitis 321
Phosphate 93, 207, 208, 210
Phosphorous 93, 304
Photophobia 293
Photosensitivity 109
Phototherapy 87, 107, 108, 206
  disadvantages 109
  home 106
Physical skills 60
Physiological expression 247
Physiological stress responses 64
Physiology
  pain 37
  respiratory 119, 120
Physiotherapist 133, 236, 339
Physiotherapy
  assessment 133
  chest 133, 196
  limb 140, 236
  postural drainage 133
  process 133
  techniques 133
Pierre Robin syndrome 76
Placenta previa 80
Placental infarction 80
Placental insufficiency 98
Plasma catecholamines 250
Plasma loss 158
Plasma protein 318
Plasma protein fraction 140
Plasma, raised urea 219
Play
  care plan 59, 62
  needs 58, 67
  opportunities 59
  philosophy 59
  programme 62
  provision 67
  safety 67
  session 62
  specialist 67
Pleural cavity 141
Pneumococci 286
Pneumonia 126, 161, 292, 295
Pneumonitis 297
Pneumothorax 119, 129, 136, 139, 196, 211, 283
Polycystic kidney disease 214
Polycythaemia 81, 90, 150
Polyhydramnios 161
Polypharmacy 234
Polyuria 92, 93
Poor immune response 285
Portal vein hypertension 114
Positioning 65, 152, 178
  frog 64
  in respiratory distress 127

lordotic 143
Posterior urethral valve 211, 213
Post-natal depression 44
Post-natal growth 311
Potassium 88, 214, 219, 321
  conservation 206
  exchange agent 207
  removal of 220
  supplement 206, 207
Potassium chloride 221
Potter syndrome 214
Pregnancy-induced hypertension 80
Premature Infant Pain Profile (PIPP) 253
Preserving life 19
Primary nursing 138
Professional issues 5, 9, 13, 47
Prognostic indicators 23
Prolongation of suffering 20
Prolonged rupture of membranes 286, 289
Proprioception 59
Prostaglandin 175, 185, 188, 200, 282
Protamine 195
Protection of Children Act (1999). 35
Protective attachment 64
Protein in CSF 293
Proteinuria 213, 215
Pseudohermaphroditism 215
Pseudomonas aeruginosa 291, 293
Psychomotor development 303
Pulmonary
  perfusion 98
  vasoconstriction 84
Pulmonary air leaks 129
Pulmonary arterial hypertension 186
Pulmonary arterial pressure 334
Pulmonary arterioles 72
Pulmonary granuloma 321
Pulmonary hypertension 122, 139, 334
Pulmonary hypoplasia 97, 137
Pulmonary oedema 98, 176
Pulmonary stenosis 183, 296
Pulmonary ventilation 124, 231
Pulse oximetery 127, 143, 175, 276, 334
Pyelonephritis 211, 213
Pyogenic streptococci 289
Pyrexia, rebound 194
Pyridoxine 217

Quality Adjusted Life Years 25
Quality of life 19
Quiet time 65, 259
Quiet wakefulness 246

Radiant heater 74, 110, 135, 155
Range finding 261
Rapid eye movement sleep 246
Rashkind procedure 188

Reduced R wave 207
Reflective practice 9
Reflexology 262
Reflux 165, 306
Reflux nephropathy 211
Reflux (*see also* GOR) 64, 162, 301
Regression 246
Renal
  abnormality 211
  agenesis 205, 214
  bicarbonate loss 208
  disease 209
  dysplasia 211
  impairment 158, 204, 216, 232
  insufficiency 207
  obstruction 204, 212
  scarring 212
  structure impaired 211
  ultrasound 212
Renal arterial stenosis 211
Renal arterial thrombosis 211
Renal development 319
Renal disease
  inherited 214
  intrinsic 211
Renal failure 212
  acute 206
  chronic 206, 215
  end-stage 218
  progressive 215
Renal tract anomaly 214
Renal tubular dysfunction 214
Renal vein thrombosis 210
Replogle tube 161, 281
Research 15
  clinical 38
  consent 39
  need for 8
  study aims 39
  undertaking 38
Resources
  allocation of 4, 24
  cost-effective 129
  finite 13, 27
  play 67
Respiration, laboured 117
Respiratory
  assessment 117
  support 122, 329
Respiratory alkalosis 139
Respiratory depression, drug-induced 122
Respiratory distress 126, 128
Respiratory distress syndrome 88, 128, 186,
  213, 230, 316, 319, 326
Respiratory failure 75, 120, 129, 329
Respiratory function compromised (*see also*
  Chapter 7) 96, 153

Respiratory infection 131, 289
Respiratory muscle failure 117
Respiratory syncytial virus 297
Respiratory therapist 132
Respite facilities 24
Rest 65
Resuscitation 71, 112, 118, 135, 232
  abandon 21, 78, 232
  diaphragmatic hernia 138
  during transfer 272
Retinal damage 108, 143, 296, 326, 334
Retinochoroiditis 295
Rhesus disease 72, 109, 111
Rhinorrhoea 297
Rickets 93
Right ventricular failure 176
Rights issues 20, 31
Rights of the Child 59
Risk assessment 6
Rubella 107, 112, 295

Salbutamol 207
Saline instillation 132
Salmonella 294
Scarlet fever 289
Second trimester 94
Secondary anaemia 105
Sedation 108, 129, 139, 190
Seizure 233
Self-calming strategy 64
Self-determination 19, 24
Sensory deprivation 63
Separation 58
Sepsis 92
Septicaemia 216, 238, 293, 319
Serous fluid 221
Serratia marcescens 289
Serum electrolytes (*see also* Chapter 10) 87
SGA *see* Gestational age, small for
Shape cards 61
Shared Governance 5, 6, 10
Shock 138, 164, 176, 193
Short gasping inhalations 247
Shrill penetrating cry 247
Sibling 61, 66
Sickle cell anaemia 107, 111
Sight 61
Silastic patch/pouch 157, 158, 160
Skin 301
  biology 99
  care 82, 99, 155
  characteristics 82, 99
  damage 100
  drying 82
  functions 99
  infection 289
  integrity of 261

post-term 82
pre-term 81
problems 99
term 82
Sleep
  pattern 65, 335
  prolonged 96
  states 66, 246
Small for gestational age 81
Social interaction 63
Social Services 34
Social skills 60
Sodium 87, 152, 155, 206
Sodium bicarbonate 78, 207, 217
Sole creases 82
Somatostatin 95
Soother, use of 123
Sound spectography 247
Sound stimuli 63
Specialist formula 310
Specimen
  container 287, 295
  documentation 288
  storage 288
  taking 287
Speech development 63
Speech therapist 131, 336
Spherocytosis 111
Sphygmomanometer 215
Spina bifida 235
Spinal cord 227, 228
Spinal muscular atrophy 238
Splenomegaly 296
Staphylococci 293
Staphylococcus albus 292
Staphylococcus aureus 221, 292, 294
Staphylococcus epidermidis 221, 292
States of consciousness 246
Stenosis 134, 156, 160, 183, 189
Stercobilin 114
Stercobilinogen 105
Steroids, antenatal 119
Stimulation
  at birth 97
  hyper-responsive 232
Stoma 154
Stool
  blood-stained 95, 151
  mucousy 164
Stratum corneum 81, 99
Streptococcus 286, 289
Stress 91
  cold 83, 84
  effects of 153
  family 43
  levels 138
  parental 38

perinatal 150
reaction 237
reduction 65
Subarachnoid haemorrhage 230
Subarachnoid space 228
Subdural haematoma 230
Sucking
  mechanics 301, 306
  mechanism 63, 149
  non-nutritive 96
  reflex 162
  response 63
Suction 75, 131
  advantages 131
  continuous 162
  disadvantages 131
  during transfer 281
  need for 176
  oropharyngeal 140
  pressures 131
  risk of IVH 230
  risks of 163
  size of catheter 131
  strength 132
  trans-anastomosis 163
Support systems 46
Suppository 151
Supra-pubic aspirate 295
Supra-pubic catheter 211
Supra-ventricular tachycardia (SVT) 182
Surfactant 74, 118, 129
  accellerated production 326
  artificial 129
  deficiency 98, 129, 326
  production 97, 118
  treatment 129, 326
Surgery, heart 184, 245
Surgical emergency 139, 165, 188
Syphilis 107, 112, 215, 292

Tachycardia 181, 286
  bounding 176
  supra-ventricular (SVT) 182
Tachypnoea 87, 117, 216
TDWL *See* Transdermal water loss
Temperature 83
  core 177
  fluctuation 237
  gap 95, 152, 177, 216
  interpretation of data 177
  peripheral 177, 194
  poor control 84, 127
  regulation 83
Teratogenic 80
Terminal apnoea 231
Tetany 208
Tetralogy of Fallot 175, 187, 189

Thalassaemia 111, 112
The Children Act 1989 21, 59
Theophylline 318, 320, 327
Therapeutic drug monitoring 318, 319
Therapeutic touch 262
Thermoneutral environment 177
Thermoregulation 64, 83, 127, 135, 156,
    191, 236, 250, 302
  brown fat 83
  conduction 84
  convection 84
  during transfer 281
  evaporation 84
  heat shields 135
  humidity 135
  insulation 135
  management of 157
  poor 151
  radiation 84
  unstable 164
Thoracotomy 162, 196, 197
Thrombocytopenia 214, 297
Thrombosis 110, 213
  renal vein 213
Thrombus formation 134, 191
Thrush 290
Thyrotoxicosis 212
Thyroxine 114, 217
Tissue expansion 236
Tobramycin 317
Tolazoline 125, 139
Tongue, taut/cupped 248
TORCH 80, 107, 296
Total parenteral nutrition (TPN) 135, 152,
    195
Touching 64
Toxoplasma gondii 295
Toxoplasmosis 107, 112, 215
Toys 62
Tracheal necrosis 134
Tracheomalacia 122
Tracheo-oesophageal fistula 122, 160, 305
Tracheostomy 130, 131
Trans-anastomstic tube 163
Transdermal water loss 86
Transfer 126, 139, 148, 156
  by air 282
  diaphragmatic hernia 139
  equipment design 274
  hazards during 266
  incubator 192
  in utero 266
  of specimens 288
  policies 273
  preparation for 271
  the process 267
  security of equipment 269

  sick infant 136
  skills of staff 266
  specially trained nurse 7, 273
  stabilisation prior to 269
  team 269
  ventilator 276
Transient tachypnoea of the newborn 120,
    122, 126
Transitional care 34
Transitions at birth 97, 117, 120, 172, 173
Transplantation
  of the heart 189, 194
  of the kidney 215
Transposition of the great arteries (TGA)
    187
Treponema pallidum 292
Tricuspid atresia 188
Trimester, first 204
Trisomy 13 159
Trisomy 18 159
Trisomy 21 159
Tuberculosis 291
Tubular necrosis 232

UKCC 15, 25, 26, 27, 33, 51
Ultrasound scan 81, 148, 179, 205, 216, 230,
    239
Umbilical
  arterial line 129, 150
  catheter 292, 294
  infection 289, 294
  stump infection 289, 294
Unconjugated bilirubin 105, 108
United Nations Convention on the Rights of the
    Child (1989). 21, 32, 47
Upper respiratory tract infection (URTI) 333
Uraemia 220
Ureteric reflux 211
Ureterocele 213
Urethral diverticulum 213
Urethral obstruction 209
Urethral stricture 213
Urinary obstruction 210
Urinary tract dilation 210
Urinary tract infection 210, 289, 294
Urine
  analysis 152
  failure to pass 205
  low output 205
  output 153, 158, 192, 197
  production 87
  retention 236
  specific gravity 177, 197
  specimen 153, 287
  stasis 140, 236
Urokinase 222
Utero-placental insufficiency 81

Vaccination
    programme   291, 295
VACTERL association   161
Value of life   19
Varices   114
Vasoconstriction   83, 84
Vasodilator   125, 194
Vasospasm   134
Vecuronium   317
Venous catheterisation   213
Ventilation   37, 153
    complications   285, 329
    developments   122, 126
    during transfer   270
    high frequency   124
    liquid   126
    long-term   130, 326
    mechanical   129
    need for   153, 154, 231
    negative pressure   125
    nitric oxide   124
    positive pressure   119, 124
    post-operative   165, 194
    pressure control   124
    volume control   124
    weaning   123
    withdrawal of   238
Ventilator
    fighting   124
    synchronisation   124, 130
    transport   276
    trigger   124
    weaning   124
Ventricles   228
    dilated   236
Ventricular overload   176
Ventricular septal defect   185, 188
Ventricular tap   239
Veracity   19
Vernix   82
Vesicoureteral reflux   210
Vesocostomy   211
Viability   14, 118
Virtue ethics   18
Vision   61

Visitation policy   42, 51
Vitamin D   92, 208, 217, 304
Vitamin E   231
Vitamin K   302, 316
Vitamin supplementation   93
Vitamins A, B and C   303
VLBW   See Birthweight, very low
Vocalisation   247
Volvulus   164
Vomit   215
    behaviour   230
    bile stained   95, 151, 164
    milky   95

Water loss, insensible   84
Waterston shunt   187, 188
Weaning   310, 336
Weighing nappies   217
Weight gain   167, 176, 311, 331
Weight loss   86
Werdnig-Hoffman disease   238
White noise   63
Wilm's tumour   215
Withholding/withdrawing treatment   20, 22,
    135
Wolf Parkinson White syndrome   182
Wound care   158, 160, 165, 236
Wound infection   160

Xanthochromia   230
Xenotransplantation   222
X-ray   8, 143
    abdomen   151, 152, 157
    air bronchograms   128
    arterial line   134
    barium   163
    cardiac   179
    chest   126, 157, 162
    chest drain   141
    double bubble   164
    enema   164
    ground glass   128
    neck   161

Zeihl Nilson stain   291